Recent Advances in Magnetic Resonance Imaging in Neuroimaging

nova science publishers
www.novapublishers.com
New York

Neuroscience Research Progress

More information about this series can be found at

Medical Procedures, Testing and Technology

More information about this series can be found at

Maajid Mohi Ud Din Malik
Purnachandra Kawdu Lamghare
Rajesh S. Kuber
Editors

Recent Advances in Magnetic Resonance Imaging in Neuroimaging

nova
science publishers
www.novapublishers.com
New York

DOI: https://doi.org/10.52305/SCEQ6675

Library of Congress Cataloging-in-Publication Data

ISBN: 979-8-90134-244-2 (Hardcover)
ISBN: 979-8-90134-311-1 (eBook)

Published by Nova Science Publishers, Inc. † New York

Contents

Preface

Neurological disorders continue to represent one of the most significant challenges in modern medicine, affecting millions of individuals worldwide and placing substantial burdens on healthcare systems, families, and societies. As our understanding of brain structure and function has evolved from basic anatomical observations to sophisticated insights into neural networks and molecular mechanisms, the role of advanced imaging technologies in neurological diagnosis and research has expanded dramatically, positioning magnetic resonance imaging as an indispensable tool for comprehensive, non-invasive brain assessment. This transformation in neuroimaging capabilities has necessitated a corresponding evolution in how we educate and prepare radiologists, neurologists, neuroscientists, and allied health professionals to harness the full potential of these technologies in addressing the complex spectrum of neurological conditions.

The inspiration for "Recent Advances in Magnetic Resonance Imaging in Neuroimaging" arose from our collective recognition that, while MRI technology has become increasingly sophisticated, a critical gap remained in comprehensive educational resources that could bridge the divide between theoretical physics and clinical application. Traditional approaches to neuroimaging education often compartmentalise technical principles, acquisition protocols, and clinical interpretation, failing to provide learners with the integrated, multidisciplinary perspective that modern neuroimaging practice demands. We recognised the urgent need for a resource that would not only present the fundamental principles of MRI physics but also guide readers through the practical application of advanced techniques, while acknowledging the complex interplay of biological, technical, and clinical factors that influence diagnostic accuracy and research outcomes.

This book represents our commitment to providing radiology students, practising radiologists, neurologists, neuroscientists, imaging technologists, and other healthcare professionals with a comprehensive, evidence-based resource that spans the entire continuum of modern MRI neuroimaging. From the foundational chapters that explore the evolution of magnetic resonance imaging and the fundamental physics underlying signal generation, to advanced discussions of emerging technologies such as ultra-high field imaging, artificial intelligence applications, and novel contrast mechanisms, we have endeavoured to create a resource that is both academically rigorous and clinically relevant. The content systematically progresses from basic concepts to specialised applications, ensuring that readers develop both the theoretical foundation and the practical expertise necessary to implement and interpret advanced neuroimaging studies effectively.

What distinguishes this work from other texts in the field is our deliberate emphasis on integrating multiple imaging modalities and analytical approaches within a cohesive clinical framework. Rather than presenting structural imaging, functional MRI, diffusion imaging, and spectroscopy as isolated techniques, we have integrated these approaches to reflect the reality of modern neuroimaging practice, where optimal diagnostic and research outcomes require the skilful integration of multiple sequences tailored to specific clinical questions and neurological conditions. The inclusion of chapters dedicated to particular disease states—from acute stroke and neurodegenerative disorders to brain tumours and psychiatric conditions—reflects our conviction that practical neuroimaging must be understood within the context of the pathophysiological processes it seeks to illuminate.

Our approach to diverse patient populations and clinical scenarios, including pediatric neuroimaging and emergency protocols, acknowledges that MRI cannot be approached with a one-size-fits-all mentality. Similarly, our exploration of advanced quantitative imaging biomarkers and multimodal integration recognises that neurological assessment increasingly requires sophisticated analytical frameworks that extend beyond traditional qualitative image interpretation. The integration of clinical applications and research findings throughout the text bridges the gap between theoretical knowledge and real-world diagnostic decision-making, helping readers develop the critical thinking skills essential to effective neuroimaging practice.

The inclusion of artificial intelligence and machine learning applications reflects our recognition that neuroimaging is undergoing a profound transformation, with computational approaches continually expanding our analytical capabilities and diagnostic accuracy. By exploring these innovations alongside established techniques, we aim to prepare readers not only for current practice but also for the future of neuroimaging in an era of personalised medicine and precision diagnostics. Our discussion of compressed sensing and accelerated imaging addresses the practical challenges of reducing scan times while maintaining diagnostic quality—a critical consideration in both clinical efficiency and patient comfort.

The chapters on emerging technologies—including chemical exchange saturation transfer imaging, molecular MRI, hyperpolarised imaging, and portable low-field systems—demonstrate our commitment to looking beyond current practice toward the future landscape of neuroimaging. These discussions are particularly relevant as the field moves toward greater accessibility, point-of-care applications, and novel contrast mechanisms that may fundamentally reshape how we visualise and understand brain pathology.

As editors, we bring together expertise from academic radiology, imaging technology, and clinical neuroscience, united by our shared commitment to advancing the science and practice of MRI neuroimaging. We have assembled contributions from leading experts across multiple institutions within the Dr. D. Y. Patil Vidyapeeth family, creating a resource that honours both the technical sophistication of modern MRI and the clinical complexities of neurological diagnosis, while remaining accessible to learners at various stages of expertise. We hope this book will serve not only as an educational tool but also as a catalyst for continued innovation and improvement in how we approach neuroimaging, ultimately contributing to greater diagnostic accuracy, deeper research insights, and better patient outcomes for those with neurological disorders.

We extend our gratitude to all the contributing authors who have dedicated their time and expertise to make this comprehensive volume possible. Their commitment to excellence in neuroimaging education and their willingness to share their knowledge and experience have been invaluable in creating a resource that we believe will serve the neuroimaging community for years to come.

Dr. Maajid Mohi Ud Din Malik
Dr. Purnachandra Kawdu Lamghare
Dr. Rajesh S. Kuber

Acknowledgments

We want to express our heartfelt gratitude to all those who have contributed to the creation and publication of "*Recent Advances in Magnetic Resonance Imaging in Neuroimaging*." First and foremost, we would like to thank the distinguished contributors to this book, including experts in radiology, imaging technology, neuroscience, and allied health sciences from across the Dr. D. Y. Patil Vidyapeeth institutions, who have generously shared their knowledge, expertise, and valuable insights. Their contributions have played a crucial role in making this book a comprehensive and authoritative resource in advanced MRI neuroimaging.

We extend our sincere appreciation to our publisher for their support and belief in this project. Their dedication to disseminating cutting-edge research and facilitating knowledge sharing in medical imaging has been instrumental in bringing this book to fruition.

We would also like to acknowledge the reviewers who provided valuable feedback and constructive criticism during the review process. Their expertise and attention to detail have contributed significantly to the quality, accuracy, and clinical relevance of the content.

Our profound gratitude goes to the leadership and administration of Dr. D. Y. Patil Vidyapeeth, Pune, for fostering an environment of academic excellence and supporting scholarly endeavours. Their commitment to advancing medical education and research has made this collaborative effort possible.

We are deeply thankful to our colleagues at the Department of Radio-Diagnosis, Dr. D. Y. Patil Medical College, Hospital and Research Centre, and the Department of Radiology and Imaging Technology, Dr. D. Y. Patil School of Allied Health Sciences, for their encouragement, professional support, and valuable discussions that have enriched the content of this book.

We extend our appreciation to the radiographers, technologists, and clinical staff whose daily work in acquiring high-quality neuroimaging studies provides the foundation for the advanced techniques and applications discussed throughout this book. Their technical excellence and dedication to patient care continue to inspire our academic pursuits.

We are thankful to our families and loved ones for their unwavering support, understanding, and encouragement throughout the writing and editing of this book. Their patience, spent on countless hours of literature review, manuscript preparation, and editorial work, and their belief in the importance of our work, have been a constant source of motivation.

We acknowledge the patients who have participated in research studies that have advanced our understanding of neuroimaging techniques and their clinical applications. Their contributions to medical science continue to benefit countless others facing neurological challenges.

Lastly, we would like to express our most profound appreciation to the readers of "Recent Advances in Magnetic Resonance Imaging in Neuroimaging"—whether you are students embarking on your journey in medical imaging, practising clinicians seeking to enhance your diagnostic capabilities, researchers exploring new frontiers in neuroscience, or educators preparing the next generation of imaging professionals. It is our sincere hope that this book proves to be an enlightening and informative resource, inspiring further research, innovation, and advancements in MRI technology and its applications in the understanding and diagnosis of neurological disorders.

Dr. Maajid Mohi Ud Din Malik
Dr. Purnachandra Kawdu Lamghare
Dr. Rajesh S Kuber
Editors

Chapter 1

An Introduction to Modern Neuroimaging

Rajesh S. Kuber[1,*]
and Maajid Mohi Ud Din Malik[2,†]
[1]Department of Radio-Diagnosis, Dr. D. Y. Patil Medical College, Hospital and Research Centre, Dr. D. Y. Patil Vidyapeeth (Deemed to be University)- Sant Tukaram Nagar, Pimpri, Pune, India
[2]Radiology and Imaging Technology, Dr. D. Y. Patil School of Allied Health Sciences, Dr. D. Y. Patil Vidyapeeth (Deemed to be University), Sant Tukaram Nagar, Pimpri, Pune, India

Abstract

Magnetic resonance imaging (MRI) has revolutionised our understanding of brain structure and function over the past four decades. This chapter provides a comprehensive overview of the evolution of MRI technology in neuroscience, from its inception in the 1970s to the sophisticated multimodal imaging approaches available today. We trace the development of key innovations, including high-field systems, functional MRI, diffusion imaging, and spectroscopy techniques. The current state of neuroimaging technology encompasses ultra-high field scanners, artificial intelligence-driven analysis, and real-time imaging capabilities that enable unprecedented insights into brain connectivity, metabolism, and disease processes. Clinical applications encompass the diagnosis and monitoring of neurological disorders, surgical planning, and treatment evaluation. In contrast, research applications continue to expand our understanding of cognitive processes, consciousness, and brain-behaviour relationships. This chapter examines emerging trends, including portable MRI systems, ultra-fast imaging sequences, and integration with other neuroimaging modalities, highlighting the transformative potential of these advances for healthcare delivery and neuroscience research.

Keywords: magnetic resonance imaging, neuroimaging, brain imaging, functional MRI, diffusion imaging, SDG 3 - good health and well-being

* Corresponding Author's Email: rajesh.kuber@dpu.edu.in
† Corresponding Author's Email: maajid.malik@dpu.edu.in

In: Recent Advances in Magnetic Resonance Imaging in Neuroimaging
Editors: Maajid Mohi Ud Din Malik, Purnachandra Kawdu Lamghare and R. S. Kuber
ISBN: 979-8-90134-244-2

Introduction

The advent of magnetic resonance imaging has marked one of the most significant milestones in the history of medical science and neuroscience research. Since its introduction into clinical practice in the early 1980s, MRI has revolutionised our ability to visualise the living human brain with unprecedented clarity and detail, fundamentally changing how we diagnose, treat, and understand neurological disorders. Unlike earlier neuroimaging modalities that relied on ionising radiation or invasive procedures, MRI provides exquisite soft-tissue contrast non-invasively, making it uniquely suited for repeated examinations and longitudinal studies of brain structure and function.

The transformation of MRI from a basic physics phenomenon to a comprehensive neuroimaging platform represents a remarkable convergence of physics, engineering, computer science, and medicine. What began as simple anatomical imaging has evolved into a sophisticated toolkit that encompasses functional imaging, diffusion tractography, spectroscopy, perfusion assessment, and quantitative tissue characterisation. Each technological advance has opened new windows into brain organisation and function, enabling investigations that were previously confined to the realm of science fiction. Today's neuroimaging capabilities will allow us to observe the brain in action, map the connections between billions of neurons, detect molecular changes underlying diseases, and visualise tissue properties with millimetre precision.

This chapter provides a comprehensive overview of the current state and future directions of MRI in neuroimaging. We begin by tracing the historical evolution of MRI technology, highlighting key innovations that have shaped the field. We then examine the current landscape of neuroimaging technology, exploring the diverse platforms and techniques available to researchers and clinicians. The clinical and research applications section illustrates the broad impact of MRI across neurology, psychiatry, and neuroscience. Finally, we look toward the future, considering emerging technologies and paradigm shifts that will define the next era of neuroimaging innovation.

1.1. Evolution of Magnetic Resonance Imaging in Neuroscience

The journey of magnetic resonance imaging in neuroscience represents one of the most remarkable technological achievements in modern medicine. The fundamental principles of nuclear magnetic resonance were first described by Felix Bloch and Edward Purcell in 1946, for which they received the Nobel Prize in Physics in 1952 (Bloch, 1946). However, it would take nearly three decades before these principles were successfully applied to medical imaging. The transformation from a spectroscopic technique used primarily in chemistry to a powerful medical imaging modality required numerous technological innovations and conceptual breakthroughs that fundamentally changed our ability to visualise the living human brain.

The first significant step toward medical imaging came in 1971 when Raymond Damadian demonstrated that nuclear magnetic resonance could distinguish between normal and cancerous tissue based on their different relaxation times (Damadian, 1971). This discovery suggested that MRI could provide tissue contrast based on biochemical properties, opening unprecedented possibilities for medical diagnosis. Building on this foundation, Paul Lauterbur introduced the concept of spatial encoding using magnetic field gradients in 1973, creating the first MRI images and establishing the fundamental approach still used today (Lauterbur, 1973). His pioneering work demonstrated that applying gradient magnetic fields could localise the origin of MR signals and reconstruct two-dimensional images. This breakthrough would earn him the Nobel Prize in Physiology or Medicine in 2003.

Peter Mansfield further advanced the field by developing mathematical techniques for rapid image acquisition and introducing the concept of echo-planar imaging (EPI) in 1977, a development that would later become crucial for functional MRI (Mansfield, 1977). Mansfield's contributions to rapid imaging techniques were so significant that he shared the 2003 Nobel Prize in Physiology or Medicine with Lauterbur. The first whole-body MRI scanner was developed in the late 1970s, and by 1980, the first clinical brain images were being produced. These early images, although relatively crude by today's standards, represented a revolutionary advance over existing neuroimaging techniques, such as computed tomography (CT), offering superior soft-tissue contrast without ionising radiation.

The 1980s witnessed rapid technological advancement and clinical adoption of MRI. The development of stronger magnetic fields improved gradient systems, and sophisticated pulse sequences dramatically enhanced image quality and acquisition speed. The introduction of surface coils and phased-array technology improved the signal-to-noise ratio, enabling higher-resolution imaging of brain structures. Researchers began to explore the relationship between MRI signal characteristics and tissue properties, leading to the development of quantitative imaging approaches that could measure T1 and T2 relaxation times, providing valuable insights into tissue microstructure and pathology. Clinical applications expanded rapidly during this period, with MRI becoming the gold standard for detecting brain tumours, multiple sclerosis plaques, and stroke in its acute and chronic phases.

The discovery of blood oxygen level-dependent (BOLD) contrast by Seiji Ogawa in 1990 marked the beginning of functional MRI. It opened an entirely new dimension in neuroscience research (Ogawa et al., 1990). This finding demonstrated that changes in blood oxygenation associated with neural activity could be detected using MRI, enabling non-invasive mapping of brain function. The first functional MRI studies of human brain activity were published in 1991 and 1992, showing activation in primary visual and motor cortices during simple tasks (Belliveau et al., 1991). This breakthrough transformed neuroscience by providing a tool for studying the living, functioning human brain with spatial resolution far superior to that of other non-invasive methods available at the time. Table 1.1 shows key milestones in MRI.

The 1990s and early 2000s witnessed the emergence of diffusion MRI techniques, beginning with diffusion-weighted imaging and evolving into diffusion tensor imaging (DTI), which enabled the visualisation of white matter tracts in the brain (Basser et al., 1994). This technology provided unprecedented insights into brain connectivity and structural organisation, revealing the complex network architecture that underlies brain function. DTI became invaluable for studying neurodevelopment, ageing, and white matter diseases, while also enabling the virtual dissection of fibre tracts for surgical planning. The combination of structural, functional, and diffusion MRI created a comprehensive toolkit for investigating brain structure-function relationships across health and disease.

Table 1.1. Key Milestones in MRI Development for Neuroimaging

Year	Milestone	Contributors	Impact
1946	Nuclear magnetic resonance was discovered	Bloch & Purcell	Established physical principles
1971	NMR differentiation of tissue types	Damadian	Demonstrated medical potential
1973	Introduction of spatial encoding	Lauterbur	Enabled image formation
1977	Echo-planar imaging developed	Mansfield	Enabled rapid imaging
1980	First clinical brain MRI images	Various groups	Clinical implementation began
1990	BOLD contrast discovered	Ogawa et al.	Founded functional MRI
1991	First human fMRI studies	Belliveau et al.	Enabled brain function mapping
2003	7 Tesla human brain imaging	Various groups	The ultra-high field era began
2010	Connectome mapping projects	NIH, EU consortia	Network neuroscience advanced
2020	AI-enhanced reconstruction	Multiple groups	Accelerated imaging revolution

The drive toward higher magnetic field strengths has been a consistent theme throughout the evolution of MRI. While early clinical systems operated at 0.5 to 1.5 Tesla, the development of 3 Tesla systems in the late 1990s provided significant improvements in signal-to-noise ratio and image quality (Vaughan et al., 2001). The subsequent development of 7 Tesla and higher field systems for human imaging further pushed the boundaries, offering unprecedented spatial resolution and sensitivity to subtle tissue contrasts. These ultra-high-field systems have enabled the visualisation of brain structures and functional organisation at mesoscopic scales, revealing details of cortical layers, subcortical nuclei, and vascular architecture that were previously inaccessible in living humans.

Advanced spectroscopic techniques evolved alongside imaging methods, enabling non-invasive measurement of brain metabolites and neurochemistry. Magnetic resonance spectroscopy (MRS) matured from single-voxel acquisitions to sophisticated multi-voxel and spectroscopic imaging techniques, providing spatial maps of metabolite distributions. The development of editing sequences enabled the detection of low-concentration metabolites, such as GABA and glutamate, key neurotransmitters involved in the excitatory-inhibitory balance. These neurochemical imaging capabilities complemented structural and functional MRI, providing a more complete picture of brain physiology and pathology.

The past decade has witnessed the integration of artificial intelligence and machine learning into MRI acquisition and analysis, representing perhaps the most transformative development since the advent of functional magnetic resonance imaging (MRI). Deep learning algorithms have revolutionised image reconstruction, enabling significant reductions in scan time while maintaining or even improving image quality. AI-driven analysis tools can automatically segment brain structures, detect abnormalities, and extract quantitative biomarkers with unprecedented speed and consistency. These developments are democratising advanced MRI techniques, making sophisticated analyses accessible to clinicians and researchers without specialised training.

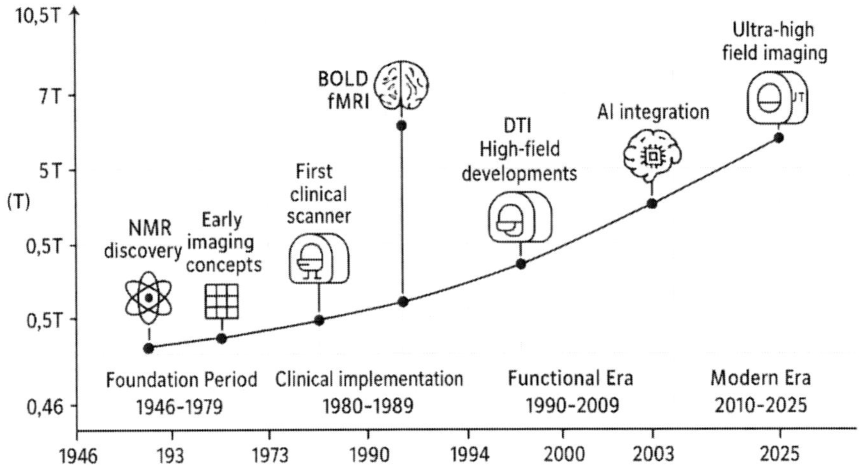

Figure 1. Timeline of major developments in MRI neuroimaging technology.

Figure 1 shows A comprehensive timeline from 1946 to 2025 displaying major milestones in MRI development. The timeline is divided into four eras: Foundation Period (1946-1979) showing NMR discovery and early imaging concepts; Clinical Implementation (1980-1989) showing the first clinical scanners and widespread adoption; Functional Era (1990-2009) showing BOLD fMRI, DTI, and high-field developments; and Modern Era (2010-2025) showing connectomics, AI integration, and ultra-high field imaging. Each milestone is marked with icons representing key technologies, and connecting lines show the relationships between developments. The vertical axis shows the progression of magnetic field strength from 0.5T to 10.5T, while the horizontal axis represents time.

1.2. Current State of Neuroimaging Technology

Contemporary neuroimaging technology represents the culmination of decades of innovation, offering capabilities that would have seemed impossible just a generation ago. Modern MRI systems combine powerful hardware, sophisticated pulse sequences, and intelligent software to provide comprehensive characterisation of brain structure, function, connectivity, and metabolism. The current landscape encompasses a diverse array of platforms, ranging from ultra-high-field research systems to portable, low-field devices, each serving distinct clinical and research needs. This technological diversity, coupled with ongoing innovation in acquisition and analysis methods, positions MRI as the cornerstone of modern neuroscience and neurological medicine.

The magnetic field strength of clinical MRI systems has standardised around 1.5 and 3 Tesla, with 3T systems becoming increasingly prevalent due to their superior signal-to-noise ratio and enhanced contrast resolution. These clinical workhorses provide robust, high-quality imaging for routine diagnostic applications and support advanced research protocols. Modern 3T systems feature wide-bore designs for patient comfort, silent scanning technologies to minimise acoustic noise, and compressed sensing capabilities for accelerated image acquisition. The latest generation of 3T scanners incorporates AI-driven workflow optimisation, automatic positioning and protocol selection, and real-time motion correction, significantly improving examination efficiency and image quality.

Ultra-high field MRI at 7 Tesla and above represents the cutting edge of neuroimaging technology, providing researchers with unprecedented tools for investigating brain microstructure and function (Ugurbil, 2018). These systems offer spatial resolutions approaching 100 micrometres, enabling the visualisation of cortical layers, subcortical nuclei, and substructures, as well as individual vessels, with remarkable clarity. The enhanced susceptibility contrast at 7T reveals iron distribution in deep brain nuclei with exquisite detail, while improved spectroscopic capabilities enable measurement of neurotransmitters and metabolites at concentrations previously undetectable. Several institutions worldwide have now installed 10.5T human scanners, and even higher fields are under development, promising further advances in imaging capabilities.

Parallel imaging and simultaneous multi-slice acquisition techniques have revolutionised MRI efficiency, reducing scan times by factors of three to ten without compromising quality significantly (Setsompop et al., 2012). These methods exploit the spatial encoding capabilities of multi-channel receiver coil arrays to acquire multiple slices or reduce the number of phase-encoding steps required for image formation. The widespread adoption of these acceleration techniques has enabled the acquisition of whole-brain functional MRI data with subsecond temporal resolution and high-resolution structural images in a fraction of the traditional scan time. This efficiency gain has profound implications for clinical workflow, patient throughput, and the feasibility of challenging research protocols.

Functional MRI has matured into a sophisticated tool for mapping brain networks and understanding neural dynamics. Modern fMRI protocols can capture brain activity with temporal resolutions of less than one second and spatial resolutions of 1-2 millimetres, enabling the detailed mapping of functional topography. Resting-state fMRI has emerged as a powerful approach for studying intrinsic brain networks, as it does not require task performance and reveals stable patterns of functional connectivity that are altered in neurological and psychiatric disorders. Multi-echo fMRI sequences enhance signal quality by optimally combining data acquired at different echo times, thereby improving sensitivity to neural activity while suppressing artefacts. Layer-specific fMRI techniques, enabled by ultra-high-field systems and advanced analysis methods, are beginning to reveal the laminar organisation of cortical processing.

Diffusion MRI has evolved far beyond simple diffusion tensor imaging to encompass a family of techniques capable of resolving the complex architectures of white matter. High angular resolution diffusion imaging (HARDI), diffusion spectrum imaging (DSI), and neurite orientation dispersion and density imaging (NODDI) can resolve crossing fibres and provide more detailed characterisation of tissue microstructure than traditional DTI. These advanced diffusion techniques enable more accurate tractography, quantification of axonal density and orientation dispersion, and sensitive detection of microstructural changes in disease. The development of multi-shell acquisition schemes and sophisticated analysis frameworks has transformed diffusion MRI into a quantitative tool for probing white matter integrity and connectivity at multiple spatial scales.

Quantitative MRI approaches have gained prominence as the field moves toward standardised, reproducible biomarkers. Techniques such as multi-parametric mapping, which simultaneously quantifies T1, T2, and proton density, provide tissue-specific measurements that are independent of scanner and protocol variations. Quantitative susceptibility mapping (QSM) enables the precise measurement of tissue magnetic susceptibility, which reflects the iron content, myelin density, and blood oxygenation levels. Magnetic resonance elastography (MRE) measures tissue mechanical properties, revealing changes in brain stiffness associated with ageing and various diseases. These quantitative approaches promise to transform MRI from a primarily qualitative diagnostic tool into a source of precise, quantifiable biomarkers suitable for disease monitoring and treatment evaluation. Table 1.2 illustrates the current capabilities of MRI technology and its applications.

Table 1.2. Current MRI technology capabilities and applications

Technology	Field Strength	Resolution	Key Capabilities	Primary Applications
Clinical MRI	1.5-3T	1-2 mm	Standard protocols, wide availability	Routine diagnosis, clinical trials
Advanced Clinical	3T	0.5-1 mm	Multiparametric, functional, diffusion	Complex diagnosis, presurgical planning
Ultra-high Field	7T+	0.3-0.5 mm	Microstructure, high-resolution fMRI	Research, specialised clinical
Real-time fMRI	3-7T	2-3 mm	Subsecond dynamics, neurofeedback	Cognitive neuroscience, clinical intervention
Low-field Portable	0.064-0.55T	3-5 mm	Point-of-care, accessible imaging	Emergency, resource-limited settings
Hybrid Systems	Variable	Variable	Multimodal (PET-MRI, MRI-linac)	Oncology, radiotherapy planning

Magnetic resonance spectroscopy has advanced significantly with the development of more sophisticated acquisition and analysis techniques. Single-voxel spectroscopy provides detailed neurochemical profiles from regions of interest, while spectroscopic imaging creates metabolic maps across the brain. Edited spectroscopy sequences such as MEGA-PRESS enable reliable quantification of GABA, glutamate, and glutathione, neurotransmitters and antioxidants critical for understanding brain function and dysfunction. Phosphorus spectroscopy provides insights into energy metabolism and membrane turnover, while carbon-13 imaging enables the real-time tracking of metabolic pathways. The combination of ultra-high-field systems and optimised sequences has significantly improved the sensitivity and specificity of MRS, making it an increasingly valuable complement to anatomical and functional imaging.

Multimodal neuroimaging integration represents a growing trend, combining MRI with other imaging modalities to leverage complementary information. Hybrid PET-MRI scanners enable the simultaneous acquisition of metabolic and structural-functional data, providing unprecedented insights into brain metabolism, receptor distribution, and network organisation. Concurrent EEG-fMRI combines the temporal precision of electrophysiology with the spatial resolution of MRI, allowing for the investigation of neural dynamics across multiple time scales. Integration of optical imaging, magnetoencephalography (MEG), and transcranial magnetic stimulation (TMS) with MRI creates comprehensive platforms for investigating brain structure-function relationships. These multimodal approaches are compelling for studying complex neurological conditions and cognitive processes that any single modality cannot fully characterise.

The integration of artificial intelligence into MRI workflows represents a paradigm shift with far-reaching implications. Deep learning reconstruction algorithms can reduce scan times by factors of four to eight while maintaining diagnostic image quality, addressing long-standing barriers to MRI accessibility (Hammernik et al., 2018). AI-powered quality control systems can detect motion artefacts, protocol errors, and acquisition issues in real time, enabling immediate corrections and reducing examination failures. Automated segmentation and analysis tools extract quantitative measurements with superhuman consistency, enabling large-scale studies and routine clinical quantification. Predictive models trained on large imaging datasets can aid in diagnosis, prognosis, and treatment planning, thereby augmenting radiologist expertise and potentially enhancing patient outcomes.

Portable and low-field MRI systems are emerging as a disruptive technology with the potential to democratize neuroimaging. These systems, operating at field strengths from 64 mT to 0.55 Tesla, can be deployed at the bedside, in emergency departments, or in resource-limited settings where conventional MRI is unavailable. While spatial resolution is lower than in high-field systems, these devices provide diagnostically useful information for acute neurological conditions such as stroke, haemorrhage, and hydrocephalus. The development of advanced pulse sequences and AI-enhanced reconstruction, optimised explicitly for low-field imaging, is rapidly improving image quality and expanding the clinical utility of these accessible platforms.

1.3. Clinical and Research Applications Overview

The clinical applications of MRI in neurology and neurosurgery have expanded dramatically, making it an indispensable tool for diagnosis, treatment planning, and disease monitoring across virtually all neurological conditions. In acute stroke care, MRI protocols that combine diffusion-weighted imaging, perfusion imaging, and vascular imaging can rapidly identify ischemic tissue, assess the salvageable penumbra, and detect vessel occlusions, thereby guiding critical treatment decisions within the narrow therapeutic window. Advanced vessel wall imaging techniques can differentiate between atherosclerotic disease, vasculitis, and other vascular pathologies, informing targeted interventions and treatment strategies. The ability to perform comprehensive stroke evaluation in under ten minutes using accelerated protocols has transformed acute neurological care, enabling more patients to receive time-sensitive treatments.

In neuro-oncology, multiparametric MRI has become crucial for tumour characterisation, treatment planning, and response assessment. Conventional imaging reveals tumour location, size, and mass effect, while advanced techniques provide critical insights into tumour biology and behaviour. Perfusion imaging distinguishes high-grade from low-grade tumours based on vascular characteristics, while diffusion imaging reveals cellular density and identifies invasive margins. MR spectroscopy detects metabolic signatures characteristic of specific tumour types, and molecular imaging techniques can visualise particular biomarkers. The integration of these multiple contrasts into comprehensive tumour assessment protocols enables more accurate diagnosis, better surgical planning, and more sensitive monitoring of treatment response versus tumour progression.

Neurodegenerative disease imaging has been revolutionised by advanced MRI techniques that can detect subtle structural and functional changes years before clinical symptoms emerge. In Alzheimer's disease, volumetric analysis reveals early atrophy in hippocampal and entorhinal regions, while functional connectivity analysis detects network disruptions in preclinical stages (Jack et al., 2018). Advanced techniques, such as arterial spin labelling, can measure changes in cerebral blood flow, while QSM and neuromelanin imaging reveal patterns of iron accumulation. In Parkinson's disease, neuromelanin-sensitive sequences visualise the loss of dopaminergic neurons in the substantia nigra, while diffusion imaging reveals white matter changes and alterations in structural connectivity. These imaging biomarkers are increasingly integrated into clinical trials as outcome measures and patient selection criteria, accelerating drug development for neurodegenerative conditions.

Epilepsy management has been transformed by high-resolution structural imaging and advanced post-processing techniques that can identify subtle abnormalities responsible for seizures. Protocol optimisations combining submillimetre 3D acquisitions with specific sequences for hippocampal imaging can detect mesial temporal sclerosis, cortical dysplasia, and other epileptogenic lesions that may be invisible on routine imaging. Functional MRI enables mapping of the eloquent cortex for surgical planning, while diffusion tractography reveals critical white matter pathways that must be preserved. Magnetoencephalography-informed fMRI can localise seizure foci with improved precision. These advanced imaging capabilities have significantly increased the number of patients who can be successfully treated with surgical intervention, improving outcomes in drug-resistant epilepsy.

Multiple sclerosis imaging has evolved from simple lesion detection to sophisticated techniques that can predict disease course and treatment response. Quantitative MRI measures such as brain volume loss, lesion evolution patterns, and tissue integrity metrics provide objective markers of disease activity and progression. Advanced techniques, including magnetisation transfer imaging, myelin water imaging, and diffusion kurtosis imaging, reveal subtle tissue damage in normal-appearing white and grey matter, explaining disability progression independent of focal lesions. Functional MRI and connectivity analyses demonstrate network reorganisation and compensatory mechanisms. At the same time, ultra-high-field imaging can visualise the central vein sign, which helps distinguish MS plaques from other white matter lesions. These advances enable more personalised treatment selection and monitoring in MS care. Table 1.3 shows major clinical applications of advanced MRI in neurology.

Table 1.3. Major clinical applications of advanced MRI in neurology

Clinical Condition	MRI Techniques	Key Diagnostic Features	Clinical Impact
Acute Stroke	DWI, PWI, MRA, vessel wall imaging	Ischemic core, penumbra, vessel occlusion	Treatment selection, outcome prediction
Brain Tumours	Multiparametric (T1, T2, DWI, PWI, MRS)	Tumour grade, margins, vascularity, metabolism	Diagnosis, surgical planning, and monitoring
Alzheimer's Disease	Volumetry, fMRI, ASL, QSM	Atrophy patterns, network disruption, and perfusion	Early diagnosis, progression monitoring
Parkinson's Disease	Neuromelanin, QSM, DTI	Substantia nigra changes, iron deposition	Differential diagnosis, progression tracking
Epilepsy	High-res 3D, hippocampal protocols, fMRI	Structural lesions, functional mapping	Surgical planning, outcome prediction
Multiple Sclerosis	Conventional, MTI, DTI, brain volumetry	Lesions, tissue damage, atrophy	Disease monitoring, treatment response
Traumatic Brain Injury	DTI, SWI, fMRI, MRS	White matter injury, microbleeds, network disruption	Prognosis, rehabilitation planning

Research applications of MRI have fundamentally transformed neuroscience, enabling the investigation of brain organisation and function at unprecedented scales. Large-scale brain mapping initiatives such as the Human Connectome Project have created comprehensive atlases of structural and functional connectivity in healthy individuals, providing reference frameworks for understanding individual variation and disease-related alterations. These datasets, acquired with cutting-edge protocols on advanced scanner systems, reveal the intricate network architecture underlying human cognition and behaviour. The availability of these resources to the broader scientific community has accelerated discoveries and enabled investigations that individual laboratories could not undertake.

Cognitive neuroscience has been revolutionised by the ability to map brain activity during complex mental operations with high spatial and temporal precision. Task-based fMRI studies have revealed the neural substrates of perception, attention, memory, language, decision-making, and emotion, creating detailed functional maps of cognitive processes. Multi-voxel pattern analysis and machine learning approaches can decode mental states and predict behaviour from brain activity patterns, demonstrating the information content of neural representations. Real-time fMRI enables neurofeedback paradigms where individuals learn to modulate their own brain activity, opening new possibilities for cognitive enhancement and clinical interventions. These capabilities have transformed our understanding of how the brain implements cognitive functions and how these processes can be modified.

Developmental neuroscience has leveraged advanced MRI to track brain maturation from prenatal stages through adolescence and into adulthood. Longitudinal imaging studies reveal the complex trajectories of structural brain development, including patterns of cortical thickness change, white matter maturation, and subcortical development. Functional connectivity studies demonstrate the emergence and refinement of large-scale brain networks across development, while diffusion imaging tracks the myelination and organisation of white matter tracts. These insights have profound implications for understanding neurodevelopmental disorders, optimal educational practices, and the extended period of brain maturation that continues into the third decade of life. Fetal MRI techniques enable assessment of brain development in utero, allowing early detection of congenital abnormalities and investigation of prenatal influences on brain organisation.

Psychiatric research has increasingly turned to neuroimaging to understand the neural basis of mental illness and identify biomarkers for diagnosis and treatment selection. Structural and functional MRI studies have revealed consistent brain alterations in conditions including depression, schizophrenia, bipolar disorder, and anxiety disorders, though heterogeneity within diagnostic categories remains substantial. Predictive modelling approaches that combine imaging with clinical and genetic data show promise for stratifying patients and predicting treatment response. Network-based analyses have shifted focus from individual brain regions to distributed circuits, revealing dysconnectivity patterns that may represent more fundamental pathophysiology than structural alterations. The integration of neuroimaging into precision psychiatry initiatives aims to move beyond symptom-based diagnosis toward biologically informed classification and treatment approaches.

Social and affective neuroscience has employed fMRI to investigate the neural mechanisms underlying social cognition, emotion regulation, empathy, and interpersonal behaviour. These studies have identified brain networks involved in theory of mind, emotion perception, reward processing, and social decision-making, providing insights into both typical social functioning and impairments in autism spectrum disorders, personality disorders, and other conditions that affect social behaviour. The combination of sophisticated experimental paradigms with advanced imaging and analysis techniques has revealed the complex interplay between cognitive and emotional processes in social contexts, informing both fundamental understanding and clinical interventions for social cognitive deficits.

Network neuroscience has emerged as a dominant framework for understanding brain organisation, leveraging graph-theoretical approaches to characterise brain connectivity at multiple scales. Functional connectivity analysis reveals intrinsic networks that show coherent activity patterns at rest, including the default mode network, executive control network, and salience network, among others. Structural connectivity, derived from diffusion tractography, reveals the white matter scaffolding that supports functional interactions. The integration of structural and functional connectivity provides insights into how anatomical organisation constrains and enables functional dynamics. These network-based approaches have revealed fundamental organisational principles of brain architecture, including small-world topology, modular structure, and hub regions that play crucial roles in integrating information throughout the brain.

Translational research, which bridges animal models and human studies, has been greatly facilitated by MRI's applicability across species. Comparable imaging protocols can be applied in rodents, non-human primates, and humans, enabling translation of mechanistic insights from animal models to human applications. Functional connectivity patterns, structural organisation principles, and responses to experimental interventions can be compared across species, thereby validating animal models and identifying conserved versus species-specific features of brain organisation. This translational capability accelerates the development of new treatments by enabling early-phase testing in animals with direct readout measures comparable to those used in human clinical trials.

1.4. Future Directions in MRI Neuroimaging

The future of MRI neuroimaging holds promise for transformative innovation across hardware, software, and applications. Ultra-high-field human MRI, advancing toward 14 Tesla and beyond, will provide extraordinary spatial resolution, enabling the investigation of cortical columns and layers, microscopic vessel visualisation, and the detection of currently unmeasurable metabolite concentrations. Technical challenges, including B1 field inhomogeneity, increased susceptibility artefacts, and specific absorption rate limitations, are being addressed through advanced shimming, parallel transmission, and optimised pulse sequences.

Portable and point-of-care MRI represents a disruptive innovation with the potential to change healthcare delivery fundamentally. Low-field portable systems are being refined with improved gradient performance, optimised pulse sequences, and AI-driven image enhancement, aiming for diagnostic quality. Future compact designs may enable MRI in ambulances, clinics, and remote locations, thereby democratising access and having profound global health implications.

Artificial intelligence will revolutionise every aspect of MRI, from acquisition to analysis and clinical decision support. Future AI systems may autonomously optimise scan protocols in real-time based on individual patient anatomy and clinical indications. Deep learning reconstruction will enable diagnostic-quality imaging from dramatically undersampled data, potentially reducing examination times to seconds.

Molecular MRI aims to visualise specific molecular targets and biological processes. Chemical exchange saturation transfer (CEST) imaging can detect pH changes, metabolite concentrations, and protein conformations without exogenous contrast agents. Hyperpolarised MRI enhances signal by factors of thousands to millions, enabling real-time tracking of metabolic pathways.

Connectomics and network neuroscience will evolve with sophisticated acquisition and analysis approaches, potentially achieving whole-brain cellular resolution imaging through ultra-high-field MRI combined with advanced reconstruction algorithms. The integration of structural, functional, and practical connectivity with transcriptomic and genomic data will create comprehensive models of brain organisation.

Theranostic applications combining diagnostic imaging with therapeutic interventions include MRI-guided focused ultrasound for tumour ablation, opening the blood-brain barrier, and neuromodulation. MRI-guided laser ablation provides minimally invasive epilepsy and tumour treatment.

Quantitative MRI will replace qualitative imaging, providing standardised, reproducible measurements. Multimodal integration will become seamless through hybrid systems combining MRI with optical imaging, ultrasound, and electrical recording. Convergence with genomics, proteomics, and big data analytics through large-scale biobank initiatives will reveal how biological, environmental, and experiential factors shape brain structure and function.

Conclusion

The evolution of MRI neuroimaging from its foundational principles in the 1940s to today's sophisticated multimodal platforms represents one of medicine's most transformative technological journeys. Modern neuroimaging capabilities—spanning ultra-high-field systems, functional connectivity mapping, quantitative biomarkers, and AI-enhanced analysis—have fundamentally reshaped our understanding of brain organisation and revolutionised neurological care. Clinical applications now extend across the entire spectrum of neurological and psychiatric disorders, enabling earlier diagnosis, personalised treatment planning, and objective monitoring of disease progression. Meanwhile, research applications continue to unveil the brain's intricate network architecture and cognitive mechanisms at unprecedented resolution.

Looking ahead, emerging innovations in portable systems, molecular imaging, and theranostic applications promise to democratise access further while expanding MRI's capabilities. The convergence of neuroimaging with genomics, artificial intelligence, and multimodal integration heralds a new era of precision neuroscience and neurology. As quantitative, reproducible biomarkers replace qualitative assessments, MRI will increasingly enable truly personalised medicine, fundamentally transforming how we understand, diagnose, and treat brain disorders.

Acknowledgments

The authors would like to extend our appreciation to those who offered helpful commentary during the drafting process of this manuscript. We also acknowledge the role the Nova Publishing department played in enabling the work described herein.

References

Basser, P. J., Mattiello, J., & LeBihan, D. (1994). MR diffusion tensor spectroscopy and imaging. *Biophysical Journal*, 66(1), 259-267. https://doi.org/10.1016/S0006-3495(94)80775-1.

Belliveau, J. W., Kennedy, D. N., McKinstry, R. C., Buchbinder, B. R., Weisskoff, R. M., Cohen, M. S., Vevea, J. M., Brady, T. J., & Rosen, B. R. (1991). Functional mapping of the human visual cortex by magnetic resonance imaging. *Science*, 254(5032), 716-719. https://doi.org/10.1126/science.1948051.

Bloch, F. (1946). Nuclear induction. *Physical Review*, 70(7-8), 460-474. https://doi.org/10.1103/PhysRev.70.460.

Damadian, R. (1971). Tumor detection by nuclear magnetic resonance. *Science*, 171(3976), 1151-1153. https://doi.org/10.1126/science.171.3976.1151.

Hammernik, K., Klatzer, T., Kobler, E., Recht, M. P., Sodickson, D. K., Pock, T., & Knoll, F. (2018). Learning a variational network for reconstruction of accelerated MRI data. *Magnetic Resonance in Medicine*, 79(6), 3055-3071. https://doi.org/10.1002/mrm.26977.

Jack, C. R., Bennett, D. A., Blennow, K., Carrillo, M. C., Dunn, B., Haeberlein, S. B., Holtzman, D. M., Jagust, W., Jessen, F., Karlawish, J., Liu, E., Molinuevo, J. L., Montine, T., Phelps, C., Rankin, K. P., Rowe, C. C., Scheltens, P., Siemers, E., Snyder, H. M., & Sperling, R. (2018). NIA-AA Research Framework: Toward a biological definition of Alzheimer's disease. *Alzheimer's & Dementia*, 14(4), 535-562. https://doi.org/10.1016/j.jalz.2018.02.018.

Lauterbur, P. C. (1973). Image formation by induced local interactions: Examples employing nuclear magnetic resonance. *Nature*, 242(5394), 190-191. https://doi.org/10.1038/242190a0.

Mansfield, P. (1977). Multi-planar image formation using NMR spin echoes. *Journal of Physics C: Solid State Physics*, 10(3), L55-L58. https://doi.org/10.1088/0022-3719/10/3/004.

Ogawa, S., Lee, T. M., Kay, A. R., & Tank, D. W. (1990). Brain magnetic resonance imaging with contrast dependent on blood oxygenation. *Proceedings of the National Academy of Sciences*, 87(24), 9868-9872. https://doi.org/10.1073/pnas.87.24.9868.

Setsompop, K., Gagoski, B. A., Polimeni, J. R., Witzel, T., Wedeen, V. J., & Wald, L. L. (2012). Blipped-controlled aliasing in parallel imaging for simultaneous multi-slice echo planar imaging with reduced g-factor penalty. *Magnetic Resonance in Medicine*, 67(5), 1210-1224. https://doi.org/10.1002/mrm.23097.

Ugurbil, K. (2018). Imaging at ultrahigh magnetic fields: History, challenges, and solutions. *NeuroImage*, 168, 7-32. https://doi.org/10.1016/j.neuroimage.2017.07.007.

Vaughan, J. T., Garwood, M., Collins, C. M., Liu, W., DelaBarre, L., Adriany, G., Andersen, P., Merkle, H., Goebel, R., Smith, M. B., & Ugurbil, K. (2001). 7T vs. 4T: RF power, homogeneity, and signal-to-noise comparison in head images. *Magnetic Resonance in Medicine*, 46(1), 24-30. https://doi.org/10.1002/mrm.1156.

Chapter 2

The Fundamental Principles of MRI Physics

Maajid Mohi Ud Din Malik*

Radiology and Imaging Technology, Dr. D. Y. Patil School of Allied Health Sciences, Dr. D. Y. Patil Vidyapeeth (Deemed to be University), Sant Tukaram Nagar, Pimpri, Pune, India

Abstract

Understanding the fundamental physics underlying magnetic resonance imaging (MRI) is essential for optimising imaging protocols, accurately interpreting images, and developing novel applications in neuroimaging. This chapter provides a comprehensive overview of the core physical principles that enable MRI, beginning with nuclear magnetic resonance phenomena and the behaviour of hydrogen nuclei in magnetic fields. We explore the concepts of relaxation times (T1, T2, and T2*) and their role in generating tissue contrast, examine various pulse sequences and their applications in clinical and research neuroimaging, and elucidate the principles of k-space data acquisition and image reconstruction. Signal-to-noise ratio (SNR) optimisation strategies are discussed, including factors affecting image quality and methods to enhance SNR. Recent advances in MRI physics, including parallel imaging, compressed sensing, and artificial intelligence-based reconstruction, are examined in the context of accelerated imaging and improved diagnostic capabilities. This foundational knowledge provides the framework for understanding advanced neuroimaging techniques discussed in subsequent chapters and enables informed decision-making in protocol design and image interpretation.

Keywords: nuclear magnetic resonance, relaxation times, pulse sequences, k-space, signal-to-noise ratio, SDG 9 - industry, innovation, and infrastructure

* Corresponding Author's Email: maajid.malik@dpu.edu.in

In: Recent Advances in Magnetic Resonance Imaging in Neuroimaging
Editors: Maajid Mohi Ud Din Malik, Purnachandra Kawdu Lamghare and R. S. Kuber
ISBN: 979-8-90134-244-2

Introduction

Magnetic resonance imaging represents one of the most sophisticated applications of quantum mechanics and electromagnetic theory in modern medicine. The physics underlying MRI is remarkably elegant, exploiting the magnetic properties of atomic nuclei to generate detailed images of internal anatomy without ionising radiation or invasive procedures. At its core, MRI relies on nuclear magnetic resonance, discovered independently by Felix Bloch and Edward Purcell in 1946, which describes how specific atomic nuclei behave when placed in a strong magnetic field and exposed to radiofrequency energy. The translation of these fundamental physics principles into a clinically valuable imaging modality required decades of technological innovation and theoretical refinement, ultimately producing the versatile and powerful diagnostic tool used worldwide today.

The complexity of MRI physics often poses a barrier to clinicians and researchers seeking to optimise imaging protocols or accurately interpret subtle image findings. However, a solid understanding of fundamental principles enables a more effective use of available technology and facilitates communication between imaging scientists and end users. The behaviour of nuclear spins in magnetic fields, the mechanisms of signal generation and relaxation, the strategies for encoding spatial information, and the factors affecting image quality all directly impact the diagnostic information obtainable from MRI examinations. As neuroimaging continues to advance with higher field strengths, faster acquisition methods, and more sophisticated contrast mechanisms, foundational physics knowledge becomes increasingly essential for maximising the clinical and research value of MRI scans.

This chapter systematically develops the essential physics concepts underlying MRI, progressing from basic nuclear magnetic resonance principles through relaxation phenomena, pulse sequence design, spatial encoding strategies, and signal-to-noise considerations. We emphasise the practical implications of the physical tenets for neuroimaging applications, connecting theoretical concepts to observable image characteristics and diagnostic capabilities. The chapter concludes with an examination of recent physics innovations that are transforming MRI efficiency and expanding its capabilities, providing context for the advanced techniques discussed in subsequent chapters.

2.1. Nuclear Magnetic Resonance Basics

Magnetic resonance imaging is based on the quantum mechanical property of nuclear spin, which is possessed by atomic nuclei with odd numbers of protons, neutrons, or both. The hydrogen nucleus, consisting of a single proton, is most commonly imaged due to its high natural abundance in biological tissues, particularly in water and lipid molecules, and its relatively large magnetic moment. Each hydrogen nucleus functions as a tiny magnetic dipole with associated angular momentum or spin. Without an external magnetic field, nuclear magnetic moments are randomly oriented, resulting in no net magnetisation. When biological tissue is placed in a strong external magnetic field (B_0), hydrogen nuclei align either parallel or antiparallel to the field direction, with a slight excess in the lower-energy parallel configuration (Haacke et al., 1999).

The energy difference between parallel and antiparallel spin states is approximately 10^{-5} electron volts at clinical field strengths of 1.5 to 3 Tesla. This small energy difference means the population difference between states is only about 10 parts per million at body temperature and a 3 Tesla field strength, according to Boltzmann statistics. Despite this tiny population difference, the enormous number of hydrogen nuclei—approximately 10^{19} protons per cubic millimetre of tissue—produces measurable net magnetisation vector (M_0) aligned with the external field, directly proportional to magnetic field strength B_0, hydrogen density, and the square of the gyromagnetic ratio γ. For hydrogen, γ equals 42.58 MHz/Tesla, establishing the relationship between magnetic field strength and resonant frequency.

When aligned nuclear spins are subjected to radiofrequency (RF) electromagnetic radiation at the appropriate resonant frequency, energy absorption causes transitions between spin states, thereby perturbing the equilibrium magnetisation. The resonant Larmor frequency is determined by $\omega_0 = \gamma B_0$. At 1.5 Tesla, hydrogen nuclei resonate at approximately 63.87 MHz, while at 3 Tesla, resonance occurs at 127.74 MHz. An RF energy application causes the net magnetisation vector to rotate away from its equilibrium alignment along the B_0 axis, creating a transverse-plane magnetisation component perpendicular to B_0.

Following RF excitation, perturbed magnetisation undergoes complex dynamics as the spin system returns to thermal equilibrium through relaxation phenomena. The temporal evolution of magnetisation after excitation is described by the Bloch equations, which are differential equations governing nuclear magnetisation behaviour in static and time-varying magnetic fields (Bloch, 1946). Table 2.1 shows key parameters in nuclear magnetic resonance.

Table 2.1. Key parameters in nuclear magnetic resonance

Parameter	Symbol	Definition	Typical Values	Physical Significance
Gyromagnetic Ratio	γ	Ratio of magnetic moment to angular momentum	42.58 MHz/T (^{1}H)	Determines resonant frequency
Larmor Frequency	ω_0 or f_0	Resonant precession frequency	63.87 MHz (1.5T), 127.74 MHz (3T)	Frequency for RF excitation
Magnetic Field Strength	B_0	Static magnetic field	1.5T, 3T, 7T (clinical/research)	Determines SNR and relaxation times
Net Magnetization	M_0	Equilibrium magnetisation magnitude	Proportional to B_0 and proton density	Source of the MRI signal
Flip Angle	α	Rotation angle of magnetisation	90°, 180° (common values)	Controls signal and contrast
RF Field Strength	B_1	Magnetic field from RF pulse	μT range	Determines the flip angle achieved

2.2. Relaxation Times: T1, T2, and T2*

Following RF excitation, nuclear magnetisation undergoes relaxation processes that return the spin system to thermal equilibrium with its surroundings. These relaxation phenomena occur on characteristic timescales that depend on tissue composition and magnetic field strength, providing the primary sources of contrast in MRI. Two independent relaxation processes govern the temporal evolution of magnetisation: T1 relaxation, which describes the recovery of longitudinal magnetisation along B_0, and T2 relaxation, which represents the decay of transverse magnetisation in the plane perpendicular to B_0. Understanding these relaxation mechanisms and their tissue-specific dependencies is essential for optimising image contrast and accurately interpreting signal intensity differences across various tissues and pathological conditions.

T1 relaxation, also called spin-lattice or longitudinal relaxation, characterises the recovery of magnetisation along the B_0 axis following RF excitation. When a 90-degree RF pulse rotates the equilibrium magnetisation into the transverse plane, the longitudinal magnetisation is momentarily zero. Immediately following the pulse, nuclear spins begin transferring energy to surrounding molecular structures—the "lattice" in solid-state physics terminology—allowing the spin system to return to thermal equilibrium. This process restores longitudinal magnetisation exponentially toward its equilibrium value, M_0, according to the equation: $Mz(t) = M_0(1 - e^{(-t/T1)})$, where Mz is the longitudinal magnetisation and t is the time elapsed since excitation. The T1 time constant is defined as the time required for longitudinal magnetisation to recover to approximately 63% of its equilibrium value (Bottomley et al., 1984).

T1 relaxation times vary substantially across tissue types and are strongly influenced by molecular motion at frequencies near the Larmor frequency. Efficient T1 relaxation requires molecular fluctuations that create local magnetic field variations at frequencies matching the hydrogen nuclear resonance frequency. Tissues with molecular correlation times optimally matched to the Larmor frequency exhibit short T1 values, while tissues with very rapid or very slow molecular motion have longer T1 values. Water molecules in cerebrospinal fluid exhibit rapid isotropic motion, resulting in long T1 times (approximately 4000 ms at 3T). In contrast, tissues with restricted water motion, such as white matter with its organised lipid structures, have shorter T1 times (approximately 800-1000 ms at 3T). Grey matter, with intermediate water content and cellular density, exhibits T1 values of roughly 1300-1500 ms at 3T. Significantly, T1 relaxation times increase with magnetic field strength because higher fields shift the optimal molecular motion frequency, generally moving away from the natural correlation times of biological tissues.

T2 relaxation, termed spin-spin or transverse relaxation, describes the exponential decay of transverse magnetisation following RF excitation. Unlike T1 relaxation, which involves energy exchange with the environment, T2 relaxation results from interactions among neighbouring nuclear spins that cause loss of phase coherence in the transverse magnetisation. Immediately after a 90-degree pulse, nuclear spins precess in phase, resulting in maximum transverse magnetisation. However, each nucleus experiences a slightly different local magnetic field from nearby atomic spins, causing it to precess at a slightly different frequency. This frequency dispersion causes progressive dephasing—accumulation of random phase differences among spins—that reduces the net transverse magnetisation. The decay of transverse magnetisation follows an exponential function: $Mxy(t) = M_0e^{(-t/T2)}$, where Mxy represents transverse magnetisation. The T2 time constant is the time required for transverse magnetisation to decay to approximately 37% of its initial value.

T2 relaxation times are always shorter than or equal to corresponding T1 values, as both processes contribute to the overall return to equilibrium. In biological tissues, T2 times reflect the degree of molecular organisation and the efficiency of spin-spin interactions. Highly structured tissues, such as white matter, with restricted molecular motion exhibit short T2 values (70-80 ms at 3T) due to efficient spin-spin interactions within the organised lipid environment. Cerebrospinal fluid, with its mobile water molecules that average out local field inhomogeneities, has long T2 times (approximately 2000 ms). Grey matter exhibits intermediate T2 values (80-100 ms at 3T), reflecting its cellular composition and water content. Unlike T1, T2 relaxation times exhibit a relatively modest dependence on field strength, although subtle changes occur due to alterations in molecular dynamics and susceptibility effects at different field strengths.

T2* (T2-star) relaxation represents the observed transverse magnetisation decay rate in real imaging conditions, incorporating both intrinsic T2 relaxation and additional dephasing due to static magnetic field inhomogeneities. These inhomogeneities arise from imperfect magnetic design, variations in magnetic susceptibility at tissue interfaces, and induced fields from ferromagnetic materials. The relationship between T2* and T2 can be expressed as: 1/T2* = 1/T2 + 1/T2,' where T2' represents the decay rate contribution from field inhomogeneities. Since field inhomogeneities add to intrinsic T2 dephasing, T2* is always shorter than T2, often substantially so near air-tissue interfaces or metallic implants where susceptibility-induced field gradients are large. T2* values in brain tissue at 3T typically range from 40 to 60 ms, approximately half the corresponding T2 values (Haacke et al., 1999).

The distinction between T2 and T2* has important practical implications for pulse sequence design and image contrast. T2-weighted imaging employs spin echo techniques that utilise 180-degree refocusing pulses to reverse dephasing caused by static field inhomogeneities, yielding images weighted by intrinsic T2 relaxation. In contrast, gradient-echo sequences do not refocus static-field effects, producing T2*-weighted images that are sensitive to susceptibility variations. This T2* sensitivity enables applications such as susceptibility-weighted imaging for detecting haemorrhage and iron deposition, as well as blood oxygen level-dependent functional MRI, which exploits susceptibility differences between oxygenated and deoxygenated haemoglobin. The choice between T2 and T2* weighting depends on the desired contrast mechanism and sensitivity to different tissue properties.

Relaxation mechanisms at the molecular level involve complex interactions between nuclear spins and their local magnetic environments. Several processes contribute to T1 relaxation, including dipole-dipole interactions between atomic spins and unpaired electrons, chemical exchange between different molecular environments, and interactions with macromolecular structures. The efficiency of these mechanisms depends on the spectral density of molecular fluctuations at the Larmor frequency, explaining why T1 is field-dependent. T2 relaxation mechanisms include similar dipole-dipole interactions, but also incorporate effects from chemical exchange, molecular diffusion through field gradients, and coherent interactions among multiple spins. Understanding these molecular mechanisms enables the interpretation of changes in relaxation times in pathological conditions and the development of contrast mechanisms targeting specific molecular processes.

Pathological processes typically alter tissue relaxation times in characteristic patterns, providing diagnostic information. Tissue oedema increases water content and reduces macromolecular concentration, generally prolonging both T1 and T2 relaxation times. Tumours often exhibit prolonged relaxation times due to increased water content, altered cellular density, and disrupted tissue architecture. Haemorrhage produces complex relaxation-time changes that evolve as blood breakdown products transition through different oxidation states, with the paramagnetic effects of deoxyhaemoglobin and methaemoglobin dramatically shortening T2 and T2*. Demyelination in conditions such as multiple sclerosis typically prolongs T2 due to increased water content and disruption of the myelin structure. Recognition of these patterns enables tissue characterisation and pathology detection based on alterations in relaxation times.

2.3. Pulse Sequences and Image Contrast

Pulse sequences are precisely timed combinations of radiofrequency pulses and magnetic field gradients that control how the MRI signal is generated, manipulated, and acquired. The choice and design of pulse sequences determine image contrast, spatial resolution, acquisition time, and sensitivity to different tissue properties. Understanding the fundamental pulse sequence families and their contrast mechanisms is crucial for selecting the most suitable protocols for specific clinical and research applications. The two primary pulse sequence categories—spin echo and gradient echo—form the foundation for numerous variants optimised for various applications, each exploiting relaxation phenomena and magnetic field manipulations in distinct ways to generate the desired tissue contrast and image characteristics.

Spin echo pulse sequences represent the classical approach to MRI, employing a 90-degree excitation pulse followed by one or more 180-degree refocusing pulses to generate echoes while compensating for static field inhomogeneities. The basic spin echo sequence begins with a 90-degree pulse that rotates the equilibrium magnetisation into the transverse plane, initiating both T2 relaxation and dephasing due to field inhomogeneities. After a time interval TE/2 (half the echo time), a 180-degree pulse is applied, inverting all spin phases. Spins that had accumulated a positive phase relative to the average now have a negative phase, and vice versa. As precession continues after the refocusing pulse, spins that were dephasing now rephase, returning to phase alignment at time TE after the initial 90-degree pulse, producing an echo. This spin-echo refocuses dephasing caused by static-field inhomogeneities but cannot reverse irreversible T2 relaxation, yielding true T2-weighted contrast (Hahn, 1950).

The repetition time (TR) and echo time (TE) are the primary timing parameters that control contrast in spin-echo imaging. TR, the interval between successive 90-degree excitation pulses, determines the degree of T1 recovery between excitations and thus T1 weighting. Short TR values (300-800 ms) allow insufficient time for full T1 recovery, resulting in tissues with different T1 values having substantially different longitudinal magnetisation available for the subsequent excitation, which produces T1-weighted contrast. Long TR values (2000-6000 ms) permit nearly complete T1 recovery in most tissues, minimising T1 contrast. TE controls T2 weighting by determining how much T2 decay occurs before the signal is measured. Short TE values (10-20 ms) capture signal before substantial T2 decay, minimising T2 contrast, while long TE values (80-120 ms) allow significant T2-dependent signal loss, producing T2-weighted images where tissues with long T2 appear bright and tissues with short T2 appear dark.

Standard spin-echo protocols can be categorised based on the combinations of TR and TE. T1-weighted images utilise short TR and TE values, thereby emphasising T1 differences while minimising T2 effects. These images display fat as bright, cerebrospinal fluid as dark, and grey matter as more colourful than white matter, which is helpful for anatomical delineation. T2-weighted images utilise a long TR and long TE, thereby suppressing T1 effects while maximising T2 contrast. CSF appears very bright, grey matter seems cheerful, and white matter appears intermediate in intensity, with excellent sensitivity for detecting pathology that increases tissue water content. Proton density-weighted images utilise a long TR and a short TE, thereby minimising T1 and T2 weighting and reflecting differences in hydrogen density primarily. These images show relatively balanced intensities across tissue types with moderate contrast. The flexibility to manipulate contrast by selecting the timing parameters makes spin-echo sequences versatile diagnostic tools, as shown in Table 2.2.

Table 2.2. Spin echo pulse sequence contrast mechanisms

Image Weighting	TR	TE	Contrast Basis	Tissue Appearance	Clinical Applications
T1-weighted	Short (300-800 ms)	Short (10-20 ms)	T1 recovery differences	Fat bright, CSF dark, GM > WM	Anatomy, post-contrast enhancement
T2-weighted	Long (2000-6000 ms)	Long (80-120 ms)	T2 decay differences	CSF bright, GM bright, WM dark	Oedema, inflammation, pathology
Proton Density	Long (2000-4000 ms)	Short (10-30 ms)	Hydrogen concentration	Balanced intensities	Cartilage, meniscus, intermediate contrast
FLAIR	Very long (8000-10000 ms)	Long (80-120 ms)	T2 with CSF suppression	CSF dark, lesions bright	Periventricular lesions, MS plaques

Fast spin-echo (FSE) or turbo spin-echo (TSE) sequences dramatically reduce acquisition time by acquiring multiple phase-encoding lines per TR interval, using a train of 180-degree refocusing pulses to generate various echoes. Each echo is assigned a different phase-encoding gradient, effectively acquiring multiple k-space lines in a single excitation. The echo train length—the number of echoes acquired per excitation—determines the acceleration factor, with typical values ranging from 8 to 32 for clinical brain imaging. However, multiple refocusing pulses create an effective TE that differs from the nominal TE, and different tissues may experience different effective TEs due to magnetisation transfer and relaxation during the echo train. Despite these complexities, FSE has largely replaced conventional spin echo for clinical imaging due to its substantial time savings, enabling T2-weighted imaging in 2-4 minutes rather than 10-15 minutes (Hennig et al., 1986).

Gradient-echo sequences employ a different approach to signal generation, utilising magnetic field gradients rather than 180-degree RF pulses to produce echoes. A gradient echo sequence begins with an RF excitation pulse, typically with a flip angle less than 90 degrees to preserve longitudinal magnetisation for rapid repetition. Following excitation, a gradient is applied to intentionally dephase the transverse magnetisation. The gradient polarity is then reversed, causing spin rephasing and the formation of a gradient echo. Unlike spin-echo, gradient-echo sequences do not refocus static-field inhomogeneities, yielding T2* rather than T2 weighting. The ability to use small flip angles enables very short TR values (as low as 3-10 ms), facilitating rapid acquisition and three-dimensional imaging. However, gradient-echo images are more susceptible to artefacts from field inhomogeneities, particularly near air-tissue interfaces.

Gradient-echo contrast behaviour differs fundamentally from spin-echo contrast due to T2* weighting and the use of variable flip angles. The Ernst angle, given by $\alpha = \arccos(e^{(-TR/T1)})$, represents the flip angle that maximises signal for given TR and T1 values, thereby optimising signal efficiency for rapid imaging. Gradient echo sequences with long TR and small flip angles produce T2*-weighted images that are sensitive to susceptibility effects, making them valuable for detecting haemorrhage, calcium, and iron deposition. With short TR and large flip angles, gradient-echo sequences generate T1-weighted images suitable for rapid anatomical imaging and dynamic contrast-enhanced studies. The spoiled gradient echo variant destroys residual transverse magnetisation between excitations, preventing steady-state buildup and producing clean T1 weighting. In contrast, balanced steady-state free precession (bSSFP) maintains coherent steady states, generating unique T2/T1-weighted contrast that is useful for cardiac and fetal imaging.

Inversion recovery sequences incorporate a preparatory 180-degree inversion pulse before the standard excitation and acquisition, allowing for the selective nulling of signals from specific tissues and enhanced T1 contrast. Following the inversion pulse, tissues recover toward equilibrium at rates determined by their T1 values. By acquiring the image at a specific inversion time (TI) after the inversion pulse, signals from tissues with specific T1 values can be nulled (set to zero) or emphasised. Fluid-attenuated inversion recovery (FLAIR) uses a long TI (approximately 2400 ms at 3T) to null cerebrospinal fluid signal in T2-weighted images, dramatically improving conspicuity of periventricular and cortical lesions that bright CSF might otherwise obscure. Short TI inversion recovery (STIR) nulls the fat signal, providing uniform fat suppression that is useful for musculoskeletal imaging and oedema detection. Double inversion recovery can null both CSF and white matter, thereby enhancing grey-matter contrast for the detection of cortical lesions.

Magnetisation preparation modules add another layer of contrast manipulation, applying preparatory pulse sequences before image acquisition to modulate tissue magnetisation in specific ways. Magnetisation transfer prepulses selectively saturate macromolecular protons, reducing signal from tissues with significant macromolecular content through chemical exchange and dipolar coupling. Diffusion preparation gradients impart sensitivity to molecular water diffusion, forming the basis for diffusion-weighted imaging. Arterial spin labelling utilises spatially selective inversion pulses to label arterial blood, thereby enabling magnetic non-contrast perfusion imaging. Flow preparation modules suppress or enhance signals from moving blood, either eliminating vascular signal to improve tissue visualisation or selectively imaging vessels for magnetic resonance angiography. The modular nature of modern pulse sequences, which combine excitation, preparation, contrast manipulation, and acquisition components, enables the exquisite tailoring of contrast mechanisms to specific diagnostic tasks.

2.4. K-Space and Image Reconstruction

K-space is the spatial frequency domain representation of MRI data, a mathematical construct that provides essential insights into image formation, resolution, contrast, and artefacts. Understanding k-space is crucial for optimising imaging protocols, implementing acceleration techniques, and resolving image quality issues. Each point in k-space corresponds to a particular spatial frequency component of the final image—low spatial frequencies representing broad features and overall contrast, while high spatial frequencies represent fine details and edge information. The MRI acquisition process fills k-space by applying specific combinations of magnetic field gradients during signal readout, with gradient amplitude and duration determining which k-space locations are sampled. The final image is obtained by Fourier-transforming the completed k-space data, converting spatial-frequency information into the familiar spatial-domain representation (Ljunggren, 1983).

The Fourier transform governs the relationship between k-space and image space. This mathematical operation decomposes signals into their constituent frequency components or, conversely, synthesises signals from them. In MRI, the two-dimensional Fourier transform converts k-space data into images, while the inverse transform converts images back to k-space. This reciprocal relationship has important implications: features in k-space affect global image properties, while features in image space correspond to distributed patterns in k-space. The centre of k-space contains low spatial frequency information, which determines the overall image contrast and intensity. In contrast, the peripheral regions of k-space contain high spatial frequency information, defining edges and fine details. Consequently, artefacts or data corruption in central k-space produce widespread changes in image intensity, while peripheral k-space problems cause loss of sharpness or the appearance of edge artefacts.

Gradient magnetic fields provide the mechanism for spatial encoding and k-space traversal in MRI. Three orthogonal gradient coils generate controlled linear variations in magnetic field strength along the x, y, and z directions. By modulating these gradients during signal acquisition, different spatial frequencies can be encoded into the received signal. The gradient amplitude determines how rapidly phase or frequency varies across space, corresponding to the rate of k-space traversal. Stronger gradients traverse k-space more rapidly, enabling faster imaging but requiring more powerful gradient hardware. The readout or frequency-encoding gradient remains active during signal acquisition, causing the resonant frequency to vary linearly across the imaging field of view. This frequency variation encodes spatial position along one direction, with different frequencies corresponding to different k-space columns sampled during each readout.

Phase encoding provides spatial localisation along the second dimension, perpendicular to the frequency-encoding direction. Before each signal readout, a brief phase-encoding gradient is applied, imparting a position-dependent phase shift across the imaging volume. The amplitude of this gradient varies between successive acquisitions, encoding different rows of k-space. Multiple repetitions with different phase-encoding amplitudes are required to fully sample k-space, with the number of phase-encoding steps determining spatial resolution along the phase-encode direction. This repeated-acquisition requirement makes phase encoding the primary determinant of scan time in conventional MRI, since each k-space row requires a separate TR interval. Slice selection utilises a gradient applied perpendicular to the imaging plane simultaneously with the RF excitation pulse, ensuring that only a thin slice of tissue experiences the resonant frequency and contributes to the signal.

K-space trajectory design offers substantial flexibility in data acquisition, with different trajectories providing advantages for specific applications. Cartesian sampling follows a rectangular grid pattern, acquiring data row by row in parallel lines, offering the most common and intuitive approach with simple reconstruction and high-quality images. Radial sampling traverses k-space along spokes radiating from the centre, similar to wheel spokes, providing robustness against motion and flow artefacts, but requiring more complex reconstruction with regridding to Cartesian coordinates. Spiral trajectories follow curved paths spiralling outward from the k-space centre, enabling very rapid coverage of k-space and excellent sampling efficiency. Echo-planar imaging (EPI) acquires all k-space data following a single excitation by rapidly oscillating the readout gradient while incrementing the phase-encoding gradient, enabling subsecond image acquisition critical for functional MRI and diffusion imaging (Mansfield, 1977).

Image resolution is directly related to the extent of k-space sampling, with larger k-space coverage yielding finer spatial resolution. The maximum spatial frequency sampled determines the smallest resolvable feature in the image, while the spacing between k-space samples determines the field of view. The relationship between k-space sampling and image properties follows from Fourier theory: the field of view equals the inverse of the k-space sample spacing, while resolution equals the inverse of the k-space coverage. To achieve higher resolution, either the field of view must be reduced, or more k-space lines must be acquired, the latter increasing scan time proportionally. Rectangular fields of view with different resolutions in different directions utilise asymmetric k-space coverage to reduce acquisition time when high resolution is required in only one direction, which is common in spine imaging, where superior-inferior resolution requirements differ from left-right.

Partial k-space acquisition techniques exploit conjugate symmetry properties of k-space to reduce scan time by sampling only slightly more than half of k-space, then synthesising the unacquired region through mathematical operations. For real-valued objects in the image domain, k-space exhibits Hermitian symmetry, meaning k-space values at positive and negative spatial frequencies are complex conjugates. However, phase accumulation from field inhomogeneities and motion violates perfect symmetry, necessitating the acquisition of slightly more than half k-space to enable phase correction. Partial k-space methods, including partial Fourier and half Fourier techniques, typically acquire 60-75% of k-space, reducing scan time by 25-40% while accepting modest signal-to-noise penalty and potential artefacts from phase inconsistencies. These methods are particularly valuable for diffusion imaging and rapid dynamic studies where time efficiency is critical. Table 2.3 shows K-space trajectories and their characteristics.

Table 2.3. K-space trajectories and their characteristics

Trajectory	Sampling Pattern	Advantages	Disadvantages	Primary Applications
Cartesian	Parallel lines	Simple reconstruction, high quality	Sensitive to motion between lines	Standard anatomical imaging
Radial	Spokes from the centre	Motion robust, uniform sampling	Complex reconstruction, streaking	Motion-sensitive applications, DCE
Spiral	Spiraling curves	Efficient coverage, fast	Susceptibility to off-resonance	Functional MRI, cardiac imaging
Echo-Planar (EPI)	Zigzag pattern	Ultra-fast acquisition	Geometric distortion, artefacts	fMRI, diffusion, rapid imaging
Propeller	Rotating blades	Motion correction, robust	Longer acquisition time	Pediatric, uncooperative patients

Parallel imaging exploits the spatial sensitivity information inherent in multi-channel receiver coil arrays to reduce acquisition time by undersampling k-space. Each coil in an array has a distinct spatial sensitivity profile, preferentially detecting signal from tissue near the coil while attenuating signal from distant regions. By simultaneously receiving signals with multiple coils, spatial information is encoded in the relative signal intensities across coils, supplementing the gradient-based encoding. This enables intentional undersampling of k-space—skipping some phase-encoding steps—while still retaining sufficient information to reconstruct artefact-free images by combining coil sensitivity information with acquired data. SENSE (Sensitivity Encoding) performs this reconstruction in image space, while GRAPPA (Generalised Autocalibrating Partially Parallel Acquisition) operates in k-space; however, both achieve similar acceleration factors, resulting in 2-4 times faster imaging (Pruessmann et al., 1999).

Image reconstruction from k-space data involves mathematical processing that transforms raw frequency-domain measurements into viewable images. Basic reconstruction applies the inverse Fourier transform to fully sampled k-space data, directly generating complex images with both magnitude and phase components.

Magnitude images display signal intensity without phase information, which is the standard presentation for most clinical imaging. Phase images preserve phase variations across space, making them useful for velocity and field mapping, as well as specific quantitative applications. More advanced reconstruction algorithms incorporate parallel imaging unfolding, motion correction, iterative optimisation, and regularisation to enhance image quality, minimise artefacts, and facilitate accelerated acquisition. Compressed sensing reconstruction, a recent innovation, leverages image sparsity in transformed domains to reconstruct high-quality images from highly undersampled data, achieving acceleration factors that surpass those of parallel imaging alone (Lustig et al., 2007).

2.5. Signal-to-Noise Ratio Optimisation

The signal-to-noise ratio (SNR) is a fundamental metric that quantifies MRI image quality, determines diagnostic utility, and sets practical limits on spatial, temporal, and acquisition speeds. SNR is defined as the ratio of the signal amplitude from the tissue of interest to the standard deviation of the background noise, essentially measuring how distinctly the tissue signal stands above random fluctuations. A higher SNR enables the detection of subtle tissue differences, smaller lesions, and finer structural details, whereas a low SNR obscures anatomical features and reduces diagnostic confidence. Understanding the multiple factors that affect SNR and strategies for optimisation is essential for designing imaging protocols that balance image quality, spatial resolution, temporal resolution, and patient comfort within practical scan time constraints.

The fundamental signal in MRI arises from the transverse magnetisation precessing after RF excitation, which induces a voltage in the receiver coil via electromagnetic induction. Signal strength is directly proportional to several factors: the static magnetic field strength B_0, which determines equilibrium magnetisation; voxel volume, as larger voxels contain more contributing nuclei; proton density, representing the concentration of hydrogen nuclei; and the specific pulse sequence parameters controlling how much magnetisation is converted to transverse orientation and how much decay occurs before measurement. The relationship can be approximated as Signal $\propto B_0 \times$ Voxel Volume $\times$ Proton Density $\times$ sin(flip angle) $\times e^{(-TE/T2)}$, illustrating that signal increases linearly with field strength and voxel volume, depends on tissue properties through proton density and T2, and is modulated by sequence parameters (flip angle and echo time).

Noise in MRI arises primarily from thermal fluctuations in the receiver coil and patient tissues, both of which act as electrical conductors with inherent resistance. Random thermal motion of electrons generates voltage fluctuations that are indistinguishable from the actual signal when detected by the receiver system. Patient tissues contribute noise through their electrical resistance and coupling to receiver coils, with noise magnitude depending on tissue conductivity, imaging field of view, and coil configuration. At field strengths below 1.5 Tesla, coil noise typically dominates, whereas at 3 Tesla and above, patient noise becomes increasingly significant. Electronic noise from preamplifiers and receiver chains also contributes, but is generally minimised through careful engineering. Critically, noise increases approximately linearly with magnetic field strength due to increased tissue conductivity at higher frequencies. However, signal increases linearly as well, yielding a net SNR benefit from higher fields.

The relationship between SNR and various imaging parameters can be quantified through established relationships derived from signal and noise physics. SNR increases with the square root of voxel volume, meaning doubling voxel size increases SNR by $\sqrt{2} = 1.4$ times, while halving voxel size for higher resolution decreases SNR by the same factor. SNR also increases with the square root of the number of signal averages (NEX). Therefore, acquiring the same data twice and averaging increases SNR by 1.4 times, but doubles the scan time. Bandwidth (the range of frequencies sampled during readout) affects SNR inversely as the square root. Reducing bandwidth by half increases SNR by 1.4 times, but also increases the minimum echo time and susceptibility to artefacts. Field strength provides approximately linear SNR gain, making 3T systems roughly twice as SNR-rich as 1.5T systems for similar parameters. However, this advantage diminishes for some tissues at higher fields due to T1 lengthening (Edelstein et al., 1986).

The receiver coil design has a profound impact on SNR, with the coil's sensitivity profile and configuration representing critical factors. Surface coils positioned close to the anatomy of interest provide high SNR in nearby regions but a rapid sensitivity drop-off with distance from the coil. Volume coils, such as head coils, provide more uniform sensitivity across larger regions but lower peak SNR compared to surface coils. Phased-array coils combine multiple smaller coil elements, each with localised high sensitivity, to achieve both high SNR and extended coverage. Modern head arrays may contain 20-64 elements, enabling excellent SNR throughout the brain while supporting parallel imaging acceleration. The principle of reciprocity—that receive sensitivity follows the same pattern as transmit field distribution—guides coil design, with optimal coils filling the sample volume and matching the region of interest as closely as practical.

Optimisation strategies for SNR must balance multiple competing requirements within acceptable constraints on scan time and image quality. When high spatial resolution is required, several approaches can mitigate SNR loss: increasing field strength provides linear SNR gain without time penalty; growing number of averages improves SNR as the square root of averages but proportionally increases time; reducing bandwidth improves SNR but may not be feasible if minimum TE must be maintained; and using optimized coils with high sensitivity in the region of interest maximizes achievable SNR. Conversely, when time is limited, accepting lower SNR through larger voxels, fewer averages, or higher bandwidth may be necessary. Three-dimensional acquisitions often provide superior SNR efficiency compared to multi-slice two-dimensional imaging because all acquired data contribute to every partition, effectively averaging noise while building through-plane resolution.

Parallel imaging acceleration trades SNR for acquisition speed, according to the geometry factor (g-factor), which quantifies the SNR penalty introduced by coil sensitivity encoding. Ideal parallel imaging with perfectly orthogonal coil sensitivities would maintain SNR independent of acceleration; however, real coils have overlapping sensitivity profiles, causing noise amplification during image reconstruction. The g-factor quantifies this penalty, typically ranging from 1.0 (no penalty) to 2.0 or higher, depending on acceleration factor and coil configuration. An acceleration factor R with g-factor g reduces SNR by a factor $g\sqrt{R}$ compared to a fully-sampled acquisition. Modern coil arrays with many elements minimise g-factor penalties, enabling acceleration factors of 3-4 with acceptable SNR for many applications. A strategic combination of modest resolution reduction, optimised coil selection, and parallel imaging acceleration often provides the best practical balance between speed and quality.

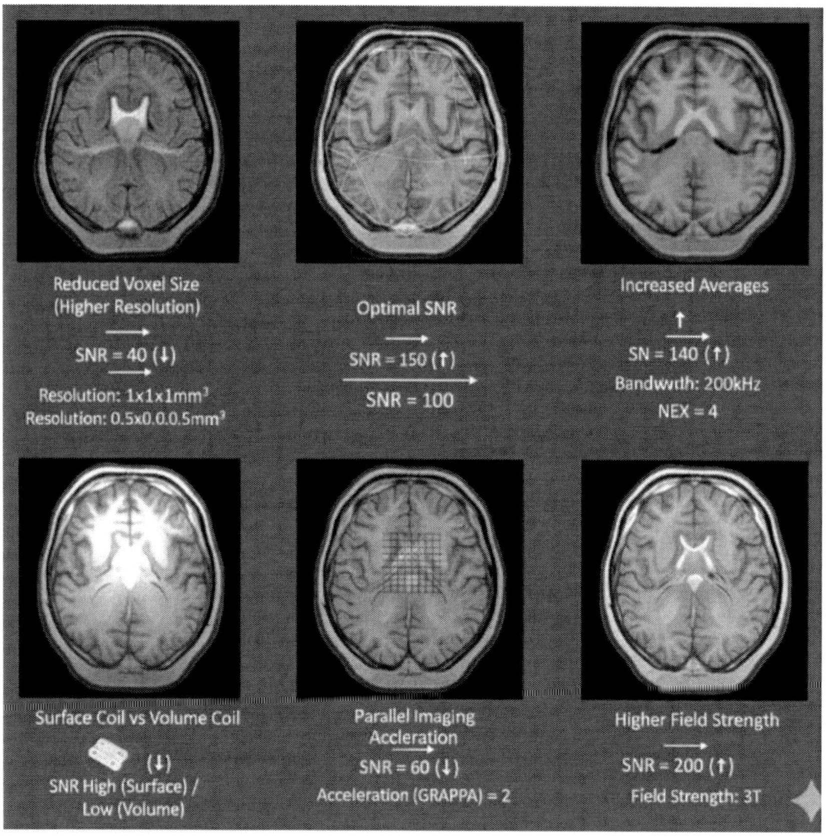

Figure 2. Factors affecting signal-to-noise ratio in MRI.

Advanced SNR optimisation techniques continue to emerge, including compressed sensing, which exploits image sparsity to enable greater acceleration than parallel imaging alone, with potentially lower SNR penalties. Denoising algorithms, particularly those based on machine learning, can retrospectively improve apparent SNR by identifying and removing noise patterns while preserving signal features. However, care must be taken to avoid obscuring real pathology. Simultaneous multi-slice imaging accelerates acquisition by exciting and acquiring multiple slices simultaneously, utilising coil sensitivity variations in the through-plane direction to separate slices during reconstruction, thereby providing time savings without a per-slice SNR penalty. Multi-band factors of 4-8 are now routinely used in functional imaging and diffusion studies, dramatically reducing examination time or enabling higher resolution within fixed time constraints.

Figure 2 shows A central brain MRI image with optimal SNR surrounded by six comparison images showing the effects of different parameter changes. The top row displays: left panel showing the impact of reduced voxel size (higher resolution, lower SNR with visible noise); middle panel showing the effect of reduced bandwidth (higher SNR but with increased geometric distortion); right panel showing the impact of increased averages (higher SNR, smoother appearance). The bottom row shows: left panel demonstrating surface coil vs volume coil SNR distribution (bright near coil, dropping with distance); middle panel illustrating parallel imaging acceleration effect (reduced SNR, potential artefacts in areas of poor coil geometry); right panel showing the benefit of higher field strength (more precise detail, improved conspicuity). Each comparison includes SNR measurements and parameter values, with arrows indicating whether SNR increases or decreases.

2.6. Recent Advances in MRI Physics

The past decade has witnessed remarkable innovations in MRI physics, fundamentally transforming imaging capabilities, efficiency, and accessibility through ultra-high-field technology, rapid imaging methods, novel contrast mechanisms, and artificial intelligence-driven acquisition and reconstruction.

Ultra-high-field MRI systems operating at 7 Tesla and above offer substantial improvements in signal-to-noise ratio and susceptibility contrast, enabling the investigation of brain microstructure at unprecedented resolution. Linear SNR increases with field strength—approximately doubling from 3T to 7T—permitting submillimetre isotropic whole-brain imaging, revealing cortical layers, small subcortical nuclei, and microvasculature previously invisible *in vivo*. Enhanced susceptibility effects significantly improve the visualisation of iron-containing structures, including the substantia nigra, subthalamic nucleus, and cortical veins. However, ultra-high field imaging presents technical challenges, including increased radiofrequency (B1) field inhomogeneity, greater susceptibility artefacts, elevated specific absorption rate (SAR), and greater complexity. Parallel transmission using multiple independent RF transmit channels addresses B1 inhomogeneity by tailoring excitation patterns spatially, enabling more uniform flip angles (Ugurbil, 2018).

Compressed sensing represents a paradigm shift in MRI acquisition, enabling dramatic acceleration by exploiting the inherent sparsity of images in transformed domains. When images are sparse in transform domains (such as wavelets, finite differences, or learned dictionaries), accurate reconstruction is possible from far fewer samples through iterative optimisation algorithms that incorporate sparsity constraints. Acceleration factors of 4-10 times have been demonstrated for parallel imaging alone (Lustig et al., 2007).

Simultaneous multi-slice (SMS) or multi-band imaging achieves remarkable acceleration by exciting and acquiring multiple slices simultaneously, exploiting coil sensitivity variations along the slice direction. Multi-band factors of 4-8 enable whole-brain coverage with subsecond temporal resolution, revolutionising functional MRI and diffusion imaging (Setsompop et al., 2012).

Artificial intelligence and deep learning are rapidly transforming the processes of MRI acquisition and reconstruction. Deep learning reconstruction networks trained on large databases learn optimal reconstruction strategies that outperform traditional algorithms, enabling higher acceleration factors with superior image quality (Hammernik et al., 2018).

Quantitative MRI approaches are advancing toward standardised, reproducible measurements that are independent of scanner hardware and protocols. Low-field portable MRI represents disruptive technology that addresses cost and accessibility needs, while novel contrast mechanisms, including chemical exchange saturation transfer (CEST) imaging, quantitative susceptibility mapping (QSM), and improved arterial spin labelling (ASL) perfusion imaging, continue to expand the imageable tissue properties and physiological processes.

Conclusion

Magnetic resonance imaging physics represents a sophisticated application of quantum mechanics, electromagnetism, and signal processing. Understanding fundamental principles—such as nuclear spin behaviour, tissue relaxation properties, pulse sequence manipulation, k-space encoding, and signal optimisation—is essential for protocol optimisation and accurate image interpretation.

T1, T2, and T2* relaxation times arise from different physical mechanisms, providing complementary tissue contrast that is selectively emphasised through pulse sequence selection. K-space mathematics and Fourier transformation underlie spatial encoding, connecting gradient fields to image resolution, field of view, and acquisition time. Signal-to-noise ratio optimisation involves balancing spatial resolution, temporal resolution, coverage, and scan time within the constraints of physics and hardware.

Recent advances are dramatically expanding MRI's capabilities. Ultra-high-field systems reveal brain microstructure at mesoscopic scales, while compressed sensing and machine learning enable unprecedented acceleration. Simultaneous multi-slice imaging has revolutionised functional and diffusion-weighted imaging studies. Portable low-field systems promise democratised access to neuroimaging. Quantitative imaging transforms MRI from qualitative diagnostics to standardised biomarkers for precision medicine. Novel contrasts, including chemical exchange saturation transfer and quantitative susceptibility mapping, expand the visualizable tissue properties. The integration of artificial intelligence throughout acquisition, reconstruction, and analysis represents the most transformative development in this field.

Future innovations combining ultra-high fields, intelligent acquisition, advanced reconstruction, and novel contrasts will enable more fine-grained spatial-temporal investigation of the brain. Standardisation will facilitate multicentre research and personalised medicine applications while upholding foundational principles of physics.

Acknowledgments

The authors would like to extend our appreciation to those who offered helpful commentary during the drafting process of this manuscript. We also acknowledge the role the Nova Publishing department played in enabling the work described herein.

References

Bloch, F. (1946). Nuclear induction. *Physical Review*, 70(7-8), 460-474. https://doi.org/10.1103/PhysRev.70.460.

Bottomley, P. A., Foster, T. H., Argersinger, R. E., & Pfeifer, L. M. (1984). A review of normal tissue hydrogen NMR relaxation times and relaxation mechanisms from 1-100 MHz: Dependence on tissue type, NMR frequency, temperature, species, excision, and age. *Medical Physics*, 11(4), 425-448. https://doi.org/10.1118/1.595535.

Edelstein, W. A., Glover, G. H., Hardy, C. J., & Redington, R. W. (1986). The intrinsic signal-to-noise ratio in NMR imaging. *Magnetic Resonance in Medicine*, 3(4), 604-618. https://doi.org/10.1002/mrm.1910030413.

Haacke, E. M., Brown, R. W., Thompson, M. R., & Venkatesan, R. (1999). *Magnetic resonance imaging: Physical principles and sequence design*. John Wiley & Sons.

Hahn, E. L. (1950). Spin echoes. *Physical Review*, 80(4), 580-594. https://doi.org/10.1103/PhysRev.80.580.

Hammernik, K., Klatzer, T., Kobler, E., Recht, M. P., Sodickson, D. K., Pock, T., & Knoll, F. (2018). Learning a variational network for reconstruction of accelerated MRI data. *Magnetic Resonance in Medicine*, 79(6), 3055-3071. https://doi.org/10.1002/mrm.26977.

Hennig, J., Nauerth, A., & Friedburg, H. (1986). RARE imaging: A fast imaging method for clinical MR. *Magnetic Resonance in Medicine*, 3(6), 823-833. https://doi.org/10.1002/mrm.1910030602.

Ljunggren, S. (1983). A simple graphical representation of Fourier-based imaging methods. *Journal of Magnetic Resonance*, 54(2), 338-343. https://doi.org/10.1016/0022-2364(83)90060-4.

Lustig, M., Donoho, D., & Pauly, J. M. (2007). Sparse MRI: The application of compressed sensing for rapid MR imaging. *Magnetic Resonance in Medicine*, 58(6), 1182-1195. https://doi.org/10.1002/mrm.21391.

Mansfield, P. (1977). Multi-planar image formation using NMR spin echoes. *Journal of Physics C: Solid State Physics*, 10(3), L55-L58. https://doi.org/10.1088/0022-3719/10/3/004.

Pruessmann, K. P., Weiger, M., Scheidegger, M. B., & Boesiger, P. (1999). SENSE: Sensitivity encoding for fast MRI. *Magnetic Resonance in Medicine*, 42(5), 952-962. https://doi.org/10.1002/(SICI)1522-2594(199911)42:5<952::AID-MRM16>3.0.CO;2-S.

Setsompop, K., Gagoski, B. A., Polimeni, J. R., Witzel, T., Wedeen, V. J., & Wald, L. L. (2012). Blipped-controlled aliasing in parallel imaging for simultaneous multislice echo planar imaging with reduced g-factor penalty. *Magnetic Resonance in Medicine*, 67(5), 1210-1224. https://doi.org/10.1002/mrm.23097.

Ugurbil, K. (2018). Imaging at ultrahigh magnetic fields: History, challenges, and solutions. *NeuroImage*, 168, 7-32. https://doi.org/10.1016/j.neuroimage.2017.07.007.

Chapter 3

Ultra-High Field MRI (7T and Beyond)

Rajesh S. Kuber[1,*]
and Maajid Mohi Ud Din Malik[2,†]

[1]Department of Radio-Diagnosis, Dr. D. Y. Patil Medical College, Hospital and Research Centre, Dr. D. Y. Patil Vidyapeeth (Deemed to be University)- Sant Tukaram Nagar, Pimpri, Pune, India
[2]Radiology and Imaging Technology, Dr. D. Y. Patil School of Allied Health Sciences, Dr. D. Y. Patil Vidyapeeth (Deemed to be University), Sant Tukaram Nagar, Pimpri, Pune, India

Abstract

Ultra-high-field magnetic resonance imaging, defined as systems operating at 7 Tesla and above, represents the cutting edge of neuroimaging technology, offering an unprecedented signal-to-noise ratio and novel contrast mechanisms that reveal brain microstructure invisible at conventional field strengths. This chapter comprehensively examines the technical foundations, advantages, challenges, and applications of ultra-high field MRI in neuroscience research and emerging clinical practice. We explore the complex interplay of increased signal strength, altered relaxation properties, enhanced susceptibility effects, and technical challenges, including radiofrequency field inhomogeneity, elevated specific absorption rate, and increased susceptibility artefacts. The improved spatial resolution achievable at 7T enables the visualisation of cortical layers, small subcortical nuclei, and microvasculature at submillimetre scales, while novel contrast mechanisms based on susceptibility, chemical exchange, and tissue microstructure provide new insights into brain organisation and pathology. Applications spanning cognitive neuroscience, disease characterisation, and basic neuroanatomy are reviewed, alongside considerations for clinical translation, including safety protocols and regulatory pathways. The chapter concludes with an examination of future developments, including 10.5 Tesla human systems that are now operational and the prospects for even higher field strengths that may redefine the limits of *in vivo* brain imaging.

* Corresponding Author's Email: rajesh.kuber@dpu.edu.in
† Corresponding Author's Email: maajid.malik@dpu.edu.in

In: Recent Advances in Magnetic Resonance Imaging in Neuroimaging
Editors: Maajid Mohi Ud Din Malik, Purnachandra Kawdu Lamghare and R. S. Kuber
ISBN: 979-8-90134-244-2

Keywords: ultra-high field MRI, 7 Tesla, susceptibility imaging, brain microstructure, parallel transmission. SDG 3 - good health and well-being

Introduction

The progression toward higher magnetic field strengths has been a defining trajectory in the development of magnetic resonance imaging (MRI) since its inception, driven by the fundamental relationship between field strength and signal-to-noise ratio. While clinical MRI has matured around 1.5 and 3 Tesla field strengths, research into ultra-high field imaging at 7 Tesla and beyond has opened entirely new dimensions in brain visualisation and characterisation. The term "ultra-high field" typically refers to human MRI systems operating at 7 Tesla or higher; however, some definitions also include advanced 3 Tesla systems with specialised capabilities. These powerful magnets generate fields approximately 140,000 times stronger than Earth's magnetic field, creating an environment where quantum-mechanical phenomena can be exploited with unprecedented precision to reveal brain structure and function at the microscopic scale.

The appeal of ultra-high-field MRI stems from both quantitative and qualitative advantages over conventional MRI systems. The approximately linear increase in signal-to-noise ratio with field strength provides the statistical power necessary for submillimetre spatial resolution across the entire brain, enabling the visualisation of anatomical details previously accessible only through histological examination of post-mortem tissue. Beyond simple SNR gains, ultra-high field imaging introduces new contrast mechanisms and sensitivity to tissue properties that are weak or absent at lower fields. Enhanced susceptibility effects reveal iron distribution in deep brain nuclei with exquisite clarity. At the same time, increased spectral dispersion in magnetic resonance spectroscopy enables the detection and separation of neurochemicals that are indistinguishable at 3T. The altered relaxation time characteristics at 7T, particularly the increased T1 values and relatively stable T2 values, modify tissue contrast in ways that can be exploited for specific applications.

However, the transition to ultra-high-field imaging is not merely about increasing magnet strength; it introduces fundamental physics challenges that require innovative engineering solutions and novel acquisition strategies. Radiofrequency wavelengths become comparable to human head dimensions at 7T, causing wave interference phenomena that produce severe B1 field inhomogeneities and spatially varying flip angles. The specific absorption rate—the rate at which RF energy is deposited in tissue—increases quadratically with field strength, necessitating careful power management to maintain patient safety. Susceptibility artefacts intensify near air-tissue interfaces, potentially causing severe geometric distortions and signal voids in echo-planar imaging. These challenges have motivated the development of parallel RF transmission, advanced shimming techniques, and novel pulse sequences specifically optimised for ultra-high-field physics. This chapter examines both the remarkable opportunities and significant challenges of ultra-high-field neuroimaging, providing a comprehensive foundation for understanding current capabilities and future directions in this rapidly evolving field.

3.1. Technical Considerations for Ultra-High Field Imaging

The engineering and physics challenges of ultra-high-field MRI depart significantly from conventional field strengths, necessitating a fundamental rethinking of system design, RF management, and acquisition strategies. The most prominent technical consideration arises from the radiofrequency wavelength at 7 Tesla, which for hydrogen protons corresponds to approximately 12 centimetres in tissue, comparable to the dimensions of the human head. This wavelength similarity gives rise to electromagnetic phenomena—interference, standing waves, and dielectric resonances—that are negligible at lower fields but dominate RF behaviour at 7T. The resulting B1 field inhomogeneity produces spatially varying flip angles across the imaging volume, resulting in intensity variations in images, particularly in the temporal lobes and cerebellum, where constructive and destructive interference effects are most pronounced (Vaughan et al., 2001).

Traditional volume RF coils, which serve as both transmitters and receivers at lower fields, perform poorly at 7T due to these wavelength effects. The standard birdcage coil design produces highly non-uniform B1 fields, characterised by central brightening and peripheral signal loss, which severely degrade image quality and compromise quantitative measurements. This limitation has driven the development of alternative coil architectures, including transverse electromagnetic (TEM) coils, microstrip line arrays, and loop arrays, which provide improved B1 homogeneity through element-specific phase and amplitude adjustments. Modern 7T systems increasingly employ separate transmit and receive coil arrays, with transmit arrays enabling parallel RF transmission. This allows multiple independent channels to simultaneously communicate with tailored amplitude and phase patterns, thereby shaping the composite B1 field and improving uniformity.

Parallel RF transmission, also known as transmit SENSE or pTx, represents the primary strategy for addressing B1 inhomogeneity at ultra-high field strengths. This approach employs multiple independent RF transmit channels, typically 8-16 for brain imaging, each driving separate coil elements with individually controlled amplitude and phase. Through careful design of RF pulse patterns across channels—termed RF shimming for static patterns or spoke pulses for dynamic patterns—the composite B1 field can be sculpted to achieve a more uniform flip-angle distribution. Static RF shimming optimises transmit channel weights for a given region and maintains these settings throughout the acquisition, providing a practical improvement with minimal sequence modification. Dynamic parallel transmission utilises time-varying, spatially tailored RF pulses calculated through optimisation algorithms that account for individual subject B1 field maps, thereby achieving excellent uniformity. However, this approach requires sophisticated pulse design and patient-specific calibration (Katscher et al., 2003).

Specific absorption rate management becomes critical at ultra-high fields because tissue power deposition increases quadratically with both field strength and RF frequency. SAR, measured in watts per kilogram, quantifies the rate of RF energy absorption by tissue, which generates heat and must be limited to prevent dangerous temperature increases. The SAR limit for head imaging is 3.2 W/kg averaged over the head for 10 minutes, with local SAR limits of 10 W/kg for small tissue volumes. At 7T, the 298 MHz resonant frequency of hydrogen means that SAR can easily exceed safe limits with conventional pulse sequences, as well as with high-speed spin-echo sequences employing trains of 180-degree refocusing pulses. SAR constraints fundamentally limit the types of sequences and acquisition parameters feasible at 7T, necessitating the development of low-SAR alternatives, including gradient-echo sequences, variable-flip-angle refocusing schemes, and VERSE (Variable-rate selective excitation) RF pulses, which reduce peak power while maintaining excitation profiles.

Magnetic field homogeneity requirements become more stringent at ultra-high fields due to increased absolute frequency variation from a given field deviation. A 0.1 parts per million field inhomogeneity corresponds to 3 Hz at 1.5T but 30 Hz at 7T, representing a proportionally greater relative difference compared to typical acquisition bandwidths. This increased sensitivity necessitates more sophisticated shimming approaches, combining passive shimming using ferromagnetic shim materials, first-order active shimming using dedicated shim coils, and potentially higher-order shimming with arrays of many small coil elements. Despite best efforts, achieving field homogeneity comparable to that of 3T in absolute frequency terms remains challenging at 7T, particularly in regions near the sinuses and ear canals, where susceptibility interfaces create strong local field gradients. Slice-specific or region-specific shimming, which optimises shim settings independently for each slice or anatomical region, provides improved homogeneity compared to whole-brain shimming; however, it adds complexity to acquisition protocols.

Gradient system specifications for ultra-high-field imaging must strike a balance among the competing requirements of strength, slew rate, and eddy-current management. Stronger gradients enable higher resolution and faster switching for advanced encoding schemes; however, the larger magnet bore of 7T systems often results in gradient coils with lower peak performance than those of state-of-the-art 3T gradients. Typical 7T systems provide gradient amplitudes of 40-80 mT/m with slew rates of 200-400 T/m/s, which are respectable but not substantially superior to those of high-performance 3T systems. Eddy current compensation becomes increasingly critical at 7T, as the higher B0 field strength makes B0 eddy currents proportionally more significant, necessitating sophisticated pre-emphasis and dynamic shim compensation. The interaction between gradient switching and the strong static field can induce mechanical vibrations and acoustic noise, necessitating robust mechanical design and potentially active acoustic noise cancellation for patient comfort.

Susceptibility effects, while providing valuable contrast, also create challenging artefacts at ultra-high magnetic fields. Magnetic susceptibility is the ability of materials to alter local magnetic fields when placed in an external magnetic field; air, bone, and tissue exhibit different susceptibility values. At interfaces between materials with different susceptibilities, such as air-filled sinuses adjacent to brain tissue, local field gradients develop that intensify linearly with the strength of the B0 field. These gradients cause geometric distortions in echo-planar imaging, signal pile-up or voids in regions of through-plane gradients, and fat-water chemical shift displacement that increases proportionally with field strength. Advanced distortion correction methods, including field-mapping-based correction, reverse-phase-encode acquisition for distortion estimation, and point-spread function mapping, mitigate these artefacts; however, some degree of distortion remains inherent to ultra-high-field echo-planar imaging near susceptibility interfaces. Table 3.1 presents technical challenges and solutions in ultra-high-field MRI.

Table 3.1. Technical challenges and solutions at ultra-high field MRI

Technical Challenge	Physical Basis	Impact on Imaging	Solutions/Mitigation Strategies
B1 Inhomogeneity	RF wavelength ≈ head size	Non-uniform flip angles, intensity variations	Parallel transmission, RF shimming, tailored pulses
Elevated SAR	Quadratic increase with frequency	Sequence limitations, heating risk	Low-SAR sequences, variable flip angles, VERSE pulses
Increased Susceptibility	Linear increase with B0	Geometric distortion, signal voids	Advanced shimming, distortion correction, optimised sequences
Chemical Shift Artefacts	Linear increase with B0	Fat-water misregistration	Higher bandwidth, fat suppression, Dixon methods
Field Inhomogeneity	Tighter absolute specs needed	Line broadening, artefacts	Multi-order shimming, slice-specific optimisation
T1 Lengthening	Field-dependent relaxation	Reduced T1 contrast, longer TR	Optimised contrast timing, MP-RAGE parameters

3.2. Advantages and Challenges of 7T MRI

The fundamental advantage of ultra-high field MRI derives from the approximately linear increase in signal-to-noise ratio with static magnetic field strength, providing roughly twice the SNR at 7T compared to 3T for similar acquisition parameters. This SNR gain translates directly into multiple beneficial trade-offs: achieving higher spatial resolution while maintaining adequate SNR, reducing acquisition time through fewer signal averages while preserving image quality, or enabling novel contrast mechanisms with inherently lower SNR that become practical only at high field. For neuroimaging applications, the SNR advantage enables whole-brain imaging at isotropic submillimetre resolution, revealing anatomical details such as cortical layer structure, small vessel architecture, and fine white matter organisation that are obscured by partial volume averaging at conventional resolutions. The ability to visualise brain microstructure *in vivo* with clarity approaching that of histological preparations represents a transformative capability for both fundamental neuroscience and the clinical investigation of focal pathologies.

Beyond simple SNR enhancement, 7T introduces qualitatively different contrast mechanisms that provide novel tissue characterisation capabilities. Susceptibility effects increase linearly with field strength, dramatically enhancing visualisation of structures with high iron content or pronounced venous vasculature. The substantia nigra, red nucleus, dentate nucleus, and basal ganglia structures exhibit a strong susceptibility contrast at 7T due to their high iron concentration, enabling precise delineation that is impossible at lower fields. Venous vasculature is prominently visible in susceptibility-weighted imaging and T2*-weighted sequences, creating detailed maps of brain venous architecture that are useful for understanding drainage patterns, identifying vascular malformations, and functional imaging applications. The enhanced susceptibility sensitivity also enables quantitative susceptibility mapping with improved precision, providing quantitative measurements of iron and myelin that are potentially useful as biomarkers in neurodegenerative diseases (Duyn et al., 2007).

Spectroscopic imaging capabilities expand significantly at 7T due to the linear scaling of chemical shift dispersion with field strength. Metabolite peaks that overlap at 3T become separated at 7T, enabling the reliable quantification of compounds such as glutamate, glutamine, GABA, glutathione, and other neurochemicals present at millimolar concentrations. The improved spectral resolution enables shorter echo times with reduced J-coupling evolution, resulting in more accurate metabolite quantification and access to resonances with short T2 relaxation times. Two-dimensional correlation spectroscopy becomes practical at 7T, providing additional spectral dimensions for resolving overlapping peaks and identifying metabolites through their correlation patterns. These spectroscopic advances enable investigation of neurotransmitter balance, metabolic dysfunction, and neurochemical alterations in psychiatric and neurological disorders with unprecedented sensitivity and specificity.

The enhanced spatial resolution achievable at 7T enables cortical layer imaging, revealing the six-layer architecture of the neocortex through differential T1, T2, and T2* properties across cortical depth. Layer-specific imaging offers insights into the distinction between feedforward and feedback processing streams, developmental maturation patterns, and layer-selective pathology in neurological diseases. Submillimetre functional MRI at 7T can resolve activation within individual cortical layers and columns, enabling investigation of cortical computation at the mesoscopic scale, linking neuronal circuits to systems-level function. High-resolution anatomical imaging reveals small structures, including individual cranial nerve nuclei, hypothalamic subnuclei, and brainstem regions, that serve critical functions but remain poorly characterised *in vivo* due to their small size and limited contrast at conventional field strengths.

However, these advantages come with significant challenges beyond the technical considerations already discussed. Image artefacts intensify at 7T, necessitating careful protocol optimisation and effective artefact mitigation strategies. Susceptibility artefacts that create subtle distortions at 3T become severe at 7T, particularly in the orbitofrontal cortex and anterior temporal regions near air-filled sinuses. Signal dropout in these regions can obscure pathology or compromise functional imaging studies of emotion, reward, and memory systems. Dielectric resonance effects create regional variations in signal intensity that, while partially addressable through parallel transmission, remain a persistent challenge for quantitative imaging that requires a uniform signal across the brain. Motion sensitivity increases at 7T due to longer scan times for sequences navigating SAR constraints and tighter phase coherence requirements in high-resolution imaging, with patient motion causing proportionally greater degradation than at lower fields.

The practical challenges of 7T imaging extend beyond physics to operational and accessibility issues. The substantially higher cost of 7T systems—typically three to five times that of clinical 3T systems—and specialised infrastructure requirements, including enhanced radiofrequency shielding and cooling systems, limit availability to a small number of research centres worldwide. The relatively small installed base means fewer pulse sequences are commercially available, less optimisation effort has been invested compared to 3T, and fewer technologists possess operational expertise. Patient claustrophobia may be exacerbated by smaller bore sizes and acoustic noise levels that exceed 3T despite mitigation efforts. These practical barriers slow clinical translation and limit the patient populations that can be studied, though ongoing technical advances and increased deployment are gradually addressing these limitations.

Quantitative imaging at 7T presents both opportunities and challenges. While improved SNR enables more precise parameter measurements, altered relaxation-time characteristics and increased B1 and B0 inhomogeneities complicate quantification. T1 relaxation times increase by 20-40% from 3T to 7T across brain tissues, necessitating longer repetition times for T1-weighted imaging and modification of inversion recovery timing for optimal contrast. T2 relaxation times remain relatively stable, but T2* values decrease substantially due to increased susceptibility effects, necessitating adjustments to echo times and careful consideration of through-plane dephasing effects. Quantitative T1, T2, and susceptibility mapping require accurate correction for B1 and B0 inhomogeneities, demanding additional calibration acquisitions and sophisticated correction algorithms. When properly implemented, these quantitative methods provide measurements with improved precision and potentially greater sensitivity to tissue microstructure than conventional field strengths.

3.3. Enhanced Spatial Resolution and Tissue Contrast

The enhanced spatial resolution achievable at ultra-high-field MRI fundamentally changes what anatomical features can be resolved *in vivo*, enabling the visualisation of brain structures at scales previously accessible only through ex vivo imaging or histology. Submillimetre isotropic-resolution imaging, routinely achievable at 7T with acquisition times of 10-15 minutes, provides voxels with volumes 8-27 times smaller than those in standard clinical protocols, dramatically reducing partial-volume effects and revealing fine anatomical details. This resolution enables the consistent visualisation of cortical layers, small subcortical nuclei, cranial nerve nuclei in the brainstem, and white matter fascicles as small as 1-2 millimetres in diameter. The combination of improved SNR and enhanced susceptibility contrast creates a synergistic effect, enabling not only the resolution of smaller structures but also the characterisation of their tissue properties with greater specificity through multiple contrast mechanisms.

Cortical layer visualisation is among the most scientifically impactful capabilities of 7T MRI, as the six-layer architecture of the neocortex underlies cortical computation and exhibits layer-specific alterations in neurological diseases. Different cortical layers can be distinguished by their unique T1, T2, T2*, and susceptibility properties, which arise from variations in neuronal density, myelin content, and vascular architecture across cortical depth. Layer IV, the primary thalamic input layer, appears as a dark band in T2*-weighted images at 7T due to high iron content in densely packed neurons, while layer V, containing large pyramidal neurons, shows distinct signal characteristics. T1-weighted imaging at an isotropic resolution of 0.3-0.4 mm reveals the alternating light- and dark-pattern corresponding to cortical layers, enabling the mapping of layer thickness, the disruption of laminar architecture in malformations of cortical development, and the investigation of layer-specific changes in neurodegenerative diseases (Duyn et al., 2007).

Deep brain nuclei visualisation benefits significantly from ultra-high field imaging, thanks to the combined effects of improved resolution and enhanced iron-based contrast. The subthalamic nucleus, a critical target for deep brain stimulation in Parkinson's disease but difficult to visualise at 3T, appears with clear boundaries at 7T in T2*-weighted and susceptibility-weighted images due to its high iron content. Direct visualisation of the subthalamic nucleus and its surrounding structures enables more precise surgical targeting, potentially improving clinical outcomes in movement disorder treatments. The substantia nigra displays clear demarcation between the iron-rich pars compacta and the pars reticulata, with neuromelanin-sensitive imaging providing complementary contrast. Other small nuclei, including the red nucleus, dentate nucleus, and various thalamic subnuclei, exhibit enhanced delineation, enabling studies of their roles in motor control, cognition, and disease processes.

Vascular architecture imaging at 7T provides unprecedented detail of the brain's microvascular network through susceptibility-based contrast mechanisms. Venous vessels as small as 100-200 micrometres can be visualised due to the paramagnetic effect of deoxyhemoglobin, allowing for detailed venograms to be created without contrast injection. This capability enables the investigation of venous drainage patterns, the identification of developmental venous anomalies, the characterisation of arteriovenous malformations, and the assessment of periventricular venous collagenosis. Time-of-flight magnetic resonance angiography at 7T offers exquisite arterial visualisation with submillimetre resolution, revealing perforating arteries, lenticulostriate vessels, and distal branch anatomy, which helps investigate stroke mechanisms and plan neurovascular surgery. The enhanced vascular contrast also complicates some imaging applications, as prominent vessels can obscure underlying parenchymal pathology or create artefacts in functional imaging.

White matter microstructure characterisation advances substantially at 7T through multiple complementary approaches. High-resolution T2-weighted imaging can resolve individual white matter fascicles in regions where numerous tracts course in proximity, such as the internal capsule, where corticospinal, thalamic, and frontopontine fibres can be separately identified. Diffusion tensor imaging at high resolution reveals crossing fibre architecture with improved angular resolution, while advanced diffusion models, including NODDI and multi-compartment fitting, benefit from improved SNR for more reliable parameter estimation. Myelin-sensitive imaging techniques, including T2* mapping, quantitative susceptibility mapping, and magnetisation transfer imaging, show enhanced sensitivity at 7T, potentially enabling the detection of subtle demyelination preceding clinical symptoms in multiple sclerosis or the visualisation of myelination patterns during development and ageing.

Grey matter microarchitecture becomes accessible through ultra-high-field imaging techniques that are sensitive to tissue anisotropy and organisation at microscopic scales. Diffusion imaging in grey matter, which is challenging at conventional fields due to low fractional anisotropy, reveals consistent patterns of preferred diffusion orientation in the cortex at 7T, likely reflecting the columnar organisation and dendritic arbour orientation. Quantitative T1 and T2 mapping at submillimetre resolution reveals laminar patterns that reflect regional variations in cellular density, dendritic arbour density, and vascular architecture. These microstructural measures provide biomarkers for cortical organisation that are potentially sensitive to developmental abnormalities, neurodegenerative changes, and functional specialisation invisible to conventional structural imaging.

Table 3.2. Anatomical structures and features resolved at 7T

Anatomical Region	Structures Visualised at 7T	Contrast Mechanisms	Clinical/Research Applications
Cerebral Cortex	Cortical layers, columnar patterns	T1, T2*, susceptibility	Cortical development, malformations, and neurodegenerative disease
Basal Ganglia	Subthalamic nucleus, GPi/GPe, substantia nigra subregions	T2*, QSM, neuromelanin	DBS targeting Parkinson's disease, movement disorders
Thalamus	Thalamic subnuclei and nuclei	T1, T2, susceptibility	Connectivity studies, pain disorders, thalamic lesions
Hippocampus	Subfields (CA1-4, DG, subiculum), internal structure	T2, high-res T1	Epilepsy, memory disorders, Alzheimer's disease
Brainstem	Cranial nerve nuclei, periaqueductal grey, raphe nuclei	T2*, T2	Brainstem lesions, pain processing, and autonomic function
Vasculature	Perforating arteries, venules, microvasculature	TOF-MRA, SWI, BOLD	Stroke mechanism, vascular malformations, perfusion
White Matter	Individual fascicles, crossing fibres	DTI, high-res T2	Fibre tracking, surgical planning, connectivity

Pathology detection and characterisation benefit from the enhanced resolution and contrast available at 7T across multiple neurological conditions. Multiple sclerosis lesions are more readily detected, particularly cortical and small periventricular plaques that are often missed at lower magnetic field strengths. Meanwhile, the central vein sign—a vein coursing through the lesion centre—can be identified in the majority of MS plaques at 7T, helping distinguish MS from vascular lesions. Minor cavernous malformations, subtle cortical dysplasias, and tiny metastases become more conspicuous through susceptibility-based detection and improved spatial resolution. Temporal lobe epilepsy patients show more precise visualisation of hippocampal internal architecture, potentially revealing subtle sclerosis or architectural distortion not apparent at 3T. These detection advantages may enable earlier diagnosis, more accurate disease characterisation, and identification of patients who might benefit from specific interventions. Table 3.2 presents anatomical structures and features resolved at 7tesla MRI.

3.4. Applications in Neuroscience Research

Ultra-high-field MRI has catalysed transformative advances in neuroscience research by enabling investigations of brain structure, function, and chemistry at unprecedented spatial and spectral resolutions. The capability to visualise and measure brain properties at mesoscopic scales—bridging the gap between microscopic cellular processes and macroscopic brain organisation—has opened up new experimental paradigms and enabled direct testing of hypotheses previously accessible only through invasive animal studies or computational modelling. Research applications encompass fundamental systems and cognitive neuroscience, disease mechanisms, brain development, and translational studies linking animal models to human brain function.

Functional MRI at 7T offers spatial resolution and sensitivity that enable the investigation of cortical organisation at the level of cortical layers and columns, the fundamental computational units of cortical processing. Layer-specific fMRI, employing submillimetreresolution and careful attention to vascular contamination, can distinguish activation in superficial layers that receive feedback inputs from deep layers that send feedforward output, providing insights into hierarchical cortical processing. Columnar-level fMRI in the early visual cortex reveals orientation, ocular dominance, and colour-selective domains with spatial organisation that matches that of invasive mapping studies in non-human primates. These capabilities enable testing cortical theories that propose layer- and column-specific computations, thereby bridging single-neuron physiology and large-scale network organisation. The enhanced BOLD sensitivity at 7T also allows detection of subtle activation differences and improved statistical power for mapping functional topography with greater precision than achievable at lower fields (Yacoub et al., 2008).

Connectivity studies benefit substantially from ultra-high-field imaging across multiple complementary approaches. High-resolution structural connectivity derived from diffusion imaging reveals the white matter architecture at a scale where individual fascicles can be tracked separately, enabling more accurate reconstruction of anatomical connectomes and resolving crossing fibre regions that confound conventional tractography. Resting-state functional connectivity at 7T exhibits an improved signal-to-noise ratio, allowing the detection of weaker correlations and a finer parcellation of functional networks, which reveals the organisation of subnetworks within canonical networks, such as the default mode network. The combination of high-resolution structural and functional connectivity enables the construction of detailed brain graphs with improved spatial specificity, advancing network neuroscience investigations of information integration, modular organisation, and hub architecture underlying cognition and consciousness.

Neurochemical imaging using high-field magnetic resonance spectroscopy offers insights into neurotransmitter systems, metabolic processes, and neurochemical alterations in disease that are not accessible through other non-invasive methods. The improved spectral resolution at 7T enables reliable measurement of GABA, the primary inhibitory neurotransmitter, and glutamate, the primary excitatory neurotransmitter, providing insights into the excitation-inhibition balance, which is critical for cortical function. Spectroscopic imaging generates spatial maps of neurotransmitter concentrations, revealing regional variations that reflect functional specialisation and disease-related alterations. Studies have demonstrated altered GABA and glutamate levels in schizophrenia, autism spectrum disorders, and epilepsy, while glutathione measurements provide markers of oxidative stress in neurodegenerative diseases. The capability to non-invasively map neurochemistry enables mechanistic studies of psychiatric medications, the investigation of neurotransmitter system development and ageing, and the identification of neurochemical biomarkers for disease diagnosis and treatment monitoring.

Cognitive neuroscience applications exploit the enhanced spatial and temporal resolution of 7T fMRI to investigate neural mechanisms underlying perception, attention, memory, decision-making, and emotion with unprecedented detail. High-resolution fMRI in the visual cortex reveals the fine-scale organisation of feature maps for orientation, spatial frequency, and object categories, thereby testing computational models of visual representation. Attention studies at 7T demonstrate layer-specific modulation of the sensory cortex by top-down signals, providing evidence in support of predictive coding theories. Memory encoding and retrieval studies reveal differential involvement of hippocampal subfields, with the dentate gyrus and CA3 involved in pattern separation. In contrast, CA1 exhibits pattern completion, a mechanism proposed by computational models but previously unverifiable in humans. Decision-making studies benefit from clear visualisation of small structures, including the subthalamic nucleus and pedunculopontine nucleus, which reveal their roles in setting the decision threshold and action selection.

Brain development and plasticity investigations leverage 7T capabilities to track structural and functional changes throughout the lifespan and in response to various experiences. High-resolution imaging reveals patterns of cortical myelination, dendritic elaboration, and synaptic pruning across childhood and adolescence, providing biomarkers of healthy development and potential indicators of neurodevelopmental disorders. Learning-induced plasticity can be tracked through changes in cortical thickness, white matter integrity, and functional connectivity at a spatial scale that matches animal models of plasticity, enabling translational studies that link cellular mechanisms to human cognitive enhancement. Ageing studies reveal patterns of iron accumulation, microstructural degradation, and network reorganisation with high sensitivity, potentially identifying early markers of pathological versus healthy ageing trajectories.

Disease mechanism investigations at 7T range from neurodegenerative disorders to psychiatric conditions, epilepsy, and cerebrovascular disease. In Alzheimer's disease, high-resolution imaging reveals patterns of cortical thinning, hippocampal atrophy, and iron accumulation, with improved sensitivity to early changes. Cortical layer analysis may also reveal layer-specific vulnerability patterns. Parkinson's disease studies demonstrate the visualisation of nigrosomes and quantification of iron in the substantia nigra, which are potential biomarkers for early diagnosis and monitoring disease progression. Epilepsy research benefits from improved lesion detection, particularly subtle focal cortical dysplasias, and from the ability to map epileptogenic networks with high spatial resolution. Psychiatric disorder investigations utilise spectroscopic imaging to assess neurotransmitter alterations, high-resolution structural imaging to detect subtle anatomical changes, and functional connectivity to map the network disruptions underlying symptoms.

Translational neuroscience, which links animal models to human brain function, benefits enormously from 7T imaging because similar field strengths are used in rodent and non-human primate research, enabling comparable contrast mechanisms and resolution relative to brain size. Functional connectivity patterns, cortical organisation principles, and responses to pharmacological or optogenetic manipulations observed in animal models can be directly compared to 7T human data, validating models and identifying conserved versus species-specific features. This translational capability accelerates the development of new treatments by enabling early-phase testing in animals with readouts directly comparable to those in human clinical trials, and by facilitating the identification of target engagement biomarkers applicable across species.

3.5. Clinical Translation and Safety Considerations

The translation of ultra-high-field MRI from research to clinical application has progressed steadily, with 7 Tesla systems achieving regulatory clearance for clinical use in multiple countries and experiencing early adoption in specialised clinical centres. Clinical implementation demands efficient protocols, robust image quality, straightforward interpretation, and clear diagnostic value compared to standard-of-care imaging. The transition is complicated by the limited worldwide availability of 7T systems, which are concentrated primarily in academic medical centres, and substantial investment requirements.

The European Union granted CE marking for clinical use in 2017, while the United States FDA provided clearance for specific systems in 2017-2019. Approvals were based on extensive safety data demonstrating that appropriately managed 7T imaging does not produce adverse health effects beyond those of conventional MRI. The approval process required adequate safety monitoring demonstration, compliance with specific absorption rate limits, and validation that clinical image quality meets diagnostic standards.

Safety considerations at 7T extend beyond those of conventional MRI due to the increased static field strength, elevated radiofrequency power deposition, and stronger gradient-field interactions. The 7 Tesla static magnetic field produces forces and torques on ferromagnetic objects approximately five times stronger than those produced by a 1.5T field, necessitating stricter screening for metallic implants. Patients with specific implanted devices, including most cardiac pacemakers, some neurostimulators, and many cochlear implants, are contraindicated for use with this device. However, MRI-conditional devices specifically tested at 7 Tesla (7 T) are emerging. Strong static fields intensify magneto-mechanical effects, including magneto-phosphenes and vertigo, which are transient and benign but can be uncomfortable for some patients (Padormo et al., 2016).

Specific absorption rate (SAR) management is the primary safety challenge, as SAR increases with the square of both the static field strength and the RF frequency. At 7T's 298 MHz hydrogen resonance frequency, moderate flip-angle imaging can approach SAR limits. Real-time SAR monitoring systems track power deposition and automatically adjust sequence parameters or pause acquisition if limits are approached.

Acoustic noise at 7T exceeds that of 3T systems due to stronger Lorentz forces, resulting in sound pressure levels of 130 dB without hearing protection. All patients must wear earplugs or noise-cancelling headphones that provide at least 30 dB of attenuation.

Emerging clinical applications span multiple neurological specialities with the most substantial evidence in epilepsy, movement disorders, and multiple sclerosis. In epilepsy, 7T detects subtle focal cortical dysplasias missed at 3T in up to 30% of patients with negative conventional imaging. Table 3.3 shows clinical applications and safety considerations for 7T MRI.

Table 3.3. Clinical applications and safety considerations for 7T MRI

Clinical Application	Diagnostic Advantage Over 3T	Evidence Level	Safety Considerations
Epilepsy Lesion Detection	Detection of subtle FCD, improved hippocampal imaging	Strong (multiple studies)	Standard 7T safety protocols are adequate
DBS Surgical Planning	Direct target visualisation, reduced atlas dependency	Moderate (small studies)	Device compatibility is critical for follow-up
Multiple Sclerosis	Cortical lesions, central vein sign specificity	Moderate (ongoing trials)	Standard protocols, potential for longitudinal tracking
Brain Tumour Characterisation	Improved delineation, microvasculature, spectroscopy	Emerging (case series)	Careful screening for surgical hardware
Neurodegenerative Disease	Iron mapping, microstructural changes, and early detection	Emerging (research)	Extended acquisitions may challenge tolerance
Vascular Malformations	Improved angiography and small AVM detection	Emerging (case reports)	Flow artefacts may be enhanced

3.6. Future Prospects: 10.5T and Higher

The frontier of ultra-high-field MRI continues to advance beyond 7 Tesla, with human whole-body 10.5 Tesla systems now operational at several sites worldwide, and development efforts underway for even higher field strengths, up to 14 Tesla and potentially beyond. These next-generation systems promise further gains in signal-to-noise ratio, spectral resolution, and susceptibility sensitivity while introducing new physics challenges that require innovative engineering solutions and may necessitate fundamental rethinking of acquisition approaches. The 10.5T systems offer approximately a 50% SNR gain over 7T systems, based solely on field strength, enabling a doubling of spatial resolution or a substantial reduction in acquisition time while maintaining a 7T-equivalent SNR. However, the progression to higher fields encounters diminishing returns in some applications and intensification of technical challenges that may ultimately define practical limits for human imaging.

The existing 10.5 Tesla systems installed at research centres, including the National Institutes of Health (USA), NeuroSpin (France), and the University of Minnesota, demonstrate the feasibility of human brain imaging at this unprecedented field strength. Early human imaging has shown remarkable anatomical detail with submillimetre resolution, revealing cortical architecture, subcortical nuclei, and white matter organisation with clarity exceeding that of 7T. Spectroscopic acquisitions demonstrate the expected improvement in spectral dispersion and sensitivity, enabling the detection of low-concentration metabolites and enhanced quantification accuracy. However, the intensified technical challenges at 10.5T, including severe B1 inhomogeneity, elevated SAR approaching the limits of gradient-echo sequences, and pronounced susceptibility artefacts, particularly in the inferior frontal and temporal regions, have necessitated extensive sequence development and optimisation efforts. Parallel transmission with up to 16 channels has proven essential for achieving acceptable B1 homogeneity, while advanced shimming and distortion correction are necessary for attaining usable image quality in artefact-prone regions.

The radiofrequency wavelength at 10.5T approaches 8 centimetres in tissue, substantially smaller than the head's dimensions, leading to even more severe interference phenomena than at 7T. Simple RF shimming proves inadequate, requiring sophisticated parallel transmission with optimisation of both magnitude and phase across multiple transmit elements. Dynamic RF shimming with slice- or even k-space-line-specific transmit patterns may be necessary for uniform excitation across the entire brain. The increased RF frequency of 447 MHz for hydrogen at 10.5T also intensifies tissue penetration challenges, with skin depth effects causing signal attenuation in central brain regions. Advanced coil designs, including dipole antennas and hybrid transmit arrays engineered explicitly for these frequencies, show promise for addressing these challenges, albeit at the cost of increased system complexity and patient setup time.

The specific absorption rate at 10.5T increases to approximately twice that at 7T for equivalent pulse sequences, severely constraining sequence options and threatening the practical utility of some applications. Even gradient echo sequences with modest flip angles can approach SAR limits when repeated at high rates for functional imaging or when 3D encoding requires many partitions. Fast spin echo imaging, which is valuable for clinical T2-weighted imaging, becomes extremely challenging due to SAR from refocusing pulse trains, necessitating alternative approaches such as GRASE (Gradient and Spin Echo), which combines gradient and spin echoes, or abandoning spin echo contrast entirely in favour of gradient echo with sophisticated susceptibility artefact management. Patient heating, while remaining within safe limits with proper sequence design, becomes more perceptible, potentially limiting examination duration and patient tolerance. Novel low-SAR excitation strategies, including transmit-array spatial encoding, adiabatic pulses with extended duration but lower peak power, and hybrid techniques combining excitation and encoding, may be necessary for practical 10.5T imaging.

Physiological noise, arising from cardiac pulsation, respiratory motion, and blood flow fluctuations, becomes the dominant noise source at 10.5T and higher fields, thereby diminishing the SNR advantage associated with increased field strength. Unlike thermal noise, which decreases with improved coil design and electronics, physiological noise is intrinsic to living tissue and cannot be eliminated; it can only be characterised and partially removed through signal processing. The SNR gain from increasing field strength scales approximately linearly at low fields, where thermal noise dominates, but transitions to a square-root dependence at high fields, where physiological noise becomes the dominant factor. This phenomenon suggests diminishing returns from further field increases beyond 10.5T for some applications, particularly in exceptionally functional imaging, where physiological fluctuations limit achievable sensitivity, regardless of hardware performance. Advanced processing techniques, including physiological noise modelling, multi-echo acquisition for optimal combination, and data-driven denoising, may partially mitigate these effects.

Susceptibility effects at 10.5T and beyond create both opportunities and challenges for neuroimaging. The enhanced iron contrast and vascular sensitivity enable exquisite visualisation of deep brain nuclei and microvasculature. At the same time, geometric distortions and signal voids intensify near air-tissue interfaces, potentially reaching unusable levels. Distortion correction becomes essential rather than optional, necessitating field mapping and retrospective correction for all applications that rely on geometric accuracy. Some brain regions, including the orbitofrontal cortex, may remain severely compromised by artefacts despite correction efforts, limiting whole-brain coverage for certain study types. Novel acquisition strategies, including multi-echo combinations for optimised T2* weighting, 3D spiral or radial trajectories with reduced susceptibility sensitivity, and ultra-high resolution, show promise for mitigating these artefacts while preserving beneficial contrast.

The scientific and clinical value proposition for 10.5T and higher field strengths necessitates careful consideration of the questions and applications that justify the substantial technical complexity and cost. For basic neuroscience investigations of cortical microarchitecture, subcortical anatomy, and white matter organisation at the finest achievable scales, the resolution advantages of 10.5T enable investigations that are impossible at lower fields, providing unique scientific value. Spectroscopic applications benefit substantially from increased chemical-shift dispersion and sensitivity, allowing the detection of compounds and the measurement of dynamics that are inaccessible at 7T. However, for many functional imaging applications, the limitations of physiological noise and technical challenges may outweigh the benefits of optimised 7T systems. The clinical translation of 10.5T faces even higher barriers than 7T, given the intensified safety considerations, the limited installed base, and the regulatory pathways yet to be established.

Development efforts for 14 Tesla human systems are underway, representing the current technological frontier for whole-body imaging. The physics challenges intensify further at 14T, with an RF wavelength of approximately 6 centimetres necessitating highly sophisticated parallel transmission, SAR approaching limits even for low-flip-angle sequences, and susceptibility effects requiring a fundamental rethinking of encoding strategies. Potential solutions under investigation include travelling-wave MRI, which exploits RF wave propagation rather than standing waves; radiative antenna arrays that provide improved penetration efficiency; and entirely novel contrast mechanisms that are less dependent on spin-echo or gradient-echo approaches. Whether 14T and higher fields prove scientifically valuable and practically feasible remains an open question, with answers depending on the successful development of enabling technologies and the identification of applications where their unique capabilities justify the extraordinary complexity.

Alternative approaches to improving imaging performance may prove more fruitful than indefinite increases in field strength, including optimised gradient systems with significantly higher performance than current systems, advanced acquisition strategies that exploit redundancy and sparsity, and machine learning approaches to image reconstruction and analysis. The combination of moderate field strength (7-10.5T) with cutting-edge gradients, parallel transmission, and AI-enhanced acquisition and reconstruction may provide better overall performance than higher fields with conventional technology. The future of ultra-high-field MRI is likely to involve parallel development along multiple pathways, with field strength increases continuing for applications where they provide clear value. At the same time, alternative innovations address limitations independent of field strength.

Conclusion

Ultra-high-field MRI at 7 Tesla and beyond represents a transformative advancement in brain imaging, offering fundamental advantages including increased signal-to-noise ratio, enabling submillimetre spatial resolution, enhanced susceptibility contrast, improved spectroscopic capabilities, and novel tissue contrast mechanisms. These capabilities allow the visualisation of cortical layers, small subcortical nuclei, microvasculature, and *in vivo* neurotransmitter quantification at scales previously accessible only through invasive methods or post-mortem examination.

Technical challenges, including radiofrequency field inhomogeneity, elevated specific absorption rate, and intensified susceptibility artefacts, have driven innovations in parallel RF transmission, advanced shimming, low-SAR pulse sequences, and sophisticated reconstruction methods. These solutions enable robust, high-quality imaging across a wide range of applications.

Research applications have transformed neuroscience, enabling layer-specific functional imaging, neurochemical mapping, and enhanced disease characterisation. Clinical translation has demonstrated clear value in epilepsy lesion detection, movement disorder surgical planning, and multiple sclerosis characterisation, though widespread adoption faces barriers related to cost, availability, and reimbursement.

Future development toward 10.5T and 14T systems continues, though diminishing returns and intensifying technical challenges require careful consideration. Integration with complementary modalities, advances in acquisition efficiency through compressed sensing and machine learning, and quantitative imaging approaches will position ultra-high-field MRI as a critical source of biomarkers for precision medicine, driving neuroimaging innovation and clinical advances in the diagnosis and treatment of neurological and psychiatric diseases.

Acknowledgments

The authors would like to extend our appreciation to those who offered helpful commentary during the drafting process of this manuscript. We also acknowledge the role the Nova Publishing department played in enabling the work described herein.

References

Duyn, J. H., van Gelderen, P., Li, T. Q., de Zwart, J. A., Koretsky, A. P., & Fukunaga, M. (2007). High-field MRI of the brain cortical substructure based on signal phase. *Proceedings of the National Academy of Sciences*, 104(28), 11796-11801. https://doi.org/10.1073/pnas.0610821104.

Katscher, U., Börnert, P., Leussler, C., & van den Brink, J. S. (2003). Transmit SENSE. *Magnetic Resonance in Medicine*, 49(1), 144-150. https://doi.org/10.1002/mrm.10353.

Padormo, F., Beqiri, A., Hajnal, J. V., & Malik, S. J. (2016). Parallel transmission for ultrahigh-field imaging. *NMR in Biomedicine*, 29(9), 1145-1161. https://doi.org/10.1002/nbm.3313.

Ugurbil, K. (2018). Imaging at ultrahigh magnetic fields: History, challenges, and solutions. *NeuroImage*, 168, 7-32. https://doi.org/10.1016/j.neuroimage.2017.07.007.

Vaughan, J. T., Garwood, M., Collins, C. M., Liu, W., DelaBarre, L., Adriany, G., Andersen, P., Merkle, H., Goebel, R., Smith, M. B., & Ugurbil, K. (2001). 7T vs. 4T: RF power, homogeneity, and signal-to-noise comparison in head images. *Magnetic Resonance in Medicine*, 46(1), 24-30. https://doi.org/10.1002/mrm.1156.

Yacoub, E., Harel, N., & Uğurbil, K. (2008). High-field fMRI unveils orientation columns in humans. *Proceedings of the National Academy of Sciences*, 105(30), 10607-10612. https://doi.org/10.1073/pnas.0804110105.

Chapter 4

Advanced Structural MRI Techniques

Purnachandra Kawdu Lamghare[1,*]
and Maajid Mohi Ud Din Malik[2,†]
[1]Department of Radio-Diagnosis, Dr. D. Y. Patil Medical College, Hospital and Research Centre, Dr. D. Y. Patil Vidyapeeth (Deemed to be University), Sant Tukaram Nagar, Pimpri, Pune, India
[2]Radiology and Imaging Technology, Dr. D. Y. Patil School of Allied Health Sciences, Dr. D. Y. Patil Vidyapeeth (Deemed to be University), Sant Tukaram Nagar, Pimpri, Pune, India

Abstract

Advanced structural MRI techniques have evolved beyond conventional anatomical imaging to provide quantitative, reproducible measurements of tissue properties that reveal microstructure, composition, and pathophysiology invisible to standard clinical sequences. This chapter examines the principles, implementations, and applications of cutting-edge structural neuroimaging methods that are revolutionising our ability to characterise brain tissue in both health and disease. High-resolution anatomical imaging approaches, enabling submillimetre visualisation of brain structures, are discussed alongside quantitative mapping techniques that measure fundamental tissue parameters, including T1, T2, and proton density, with precision and standardisation. Magnetisation transfer imaging reveals the macromolecular environment and myelin content through exchange-based contrast mechanisms. In contrast, susceptibility-weighted imaging and quantitative susceptibility mapping exploit magnetic susceptibility differences to visualise iron, calcium, venous vasculature, and haemorrhage with exquisite sensitivity. Emerging paradigms, including synthetic MRI and MRI fingerprinting, promise to revolutionise structural imaging by simultaneously quantifying multiple tissue parameters from efficient acquisitions, enabling flexible contrast generation and quantitative biomarker extraction. These advanced techniques collectively represent a transition from qualitative anatomical description to quantitative tissue characterisation, with profound implications for early disease

* Corresponding Author's Email: purnachandra.lamghare@dpu.edu.in
† Corresponding Author's Email: maajid.malik@dpu.edu.in

In: Recent Advances in Magnetic Resonance Imaging in Neuroimaging
Editors: Maajid Mohi Ud Din Malik, Purnachandra Kawdu Lamghare and R. S. Kuber
ISBN: 979-8-90134-244-2

detection, treatment monitoring, and precision medicine applications in neurology and neuroscience.

Keywords: quantitative MRI, susceptibility mapping, magnetisation transfer, MRI fingerprinting, tissue characterisation, SDG 3 - good health and well-being

Introduction

Conventional structural MRI relies primarily on qualitative assessment of signal intensity patterns and anatomical appearance, with diagnostic interpretation based mainly on pattern recognition and comparison with expected normal variants. While this approach has proven remarkably successful for detecting gross anatomical abnormalities, tumours, strokes, and inflammatory lesions, it provides limited information about subtle tissue microstructural changes, early pathological processes, and quantitative disease progression. The intrinsic contrast in standard T1-weighted, T2-weighted, and FLAIR images depends on scanner hardware, pulse sequence parameters, and acquisition protocols, resulting in measurements expressed in arbitrary units that vary across platforms and time points. This variability limits the utility of conventional imaging for detecting subtle longitudinal changes, comparing results across research sites, and establishing quantitative biomarkers for precision medicine applications.

Advanced structural MRI techniques address these limitations by providing quantitative measurements of fundamental tissue properties in standardised physical units that are, in principle, independent of scanner platform and acquisition protocol. These techniques move beyond simple signal intensity to characterise the physical, chemical, and microstructural properties underlying tissue contrast. Quantitative T1, T2, and proton density mapping provide measurements of relaxation times and hydrogen concentration that reflect tissue composition, hydration, and macromolecular content. Magnetisation transfer imaging quantifies the interaction between free water protons and macromolecular protons, providing sensitivity to myelin and other structural proteins. Susceptibility-based techniques, including susceptibility-weighted imaging and quantitative susceptibility mapping, reveal tissue magnetic properties that reflect iron content, calcium deposition, myelin organisation, and venous oxygenation. These quantitative approaches enable objective tissue characterisation, the sensitive detection of pathological changes, and standardised measurements suitable for multicentre studies and clinical trials.

Recent innovations, including synthetic MRI and MRI fingerprinting, represent paradigm shifts in the acquisition and processing of structural imaging. Rather than developing separate images with different contrast weightings, these approaches acquire rich datasets that encode tissue properties across multiple dimensions, then extract quantitative parameter maps and synthesise arbitrary contrast-weighted images retrospectively. This flexibility enables comprehensive tissue characterisation from efficient acquisitions, reduces examination time, and ensures consistency across scanning sessions. The quantitative parameters derived from these techniques offer potential biomarkers for disease diagnosis, disease progression monitoring, and treatment response assessment. This chapter systematically examines advanced structural methods, exploring their physical principles, technical implementations, clinical and research applications, and their transformative potential for the future of neuroimaging.

4.1. High-Resolution Anatomical Imaging

High-resolution anatomical MRI has evolved from qualitative visualisation to the precise delineation of brain microstructure, enabling the detection of subtle morphological changes and small pathological lesions that escape detection at conventional resolutions. The progression toward submillimetre isotropic imaging has been driven by improvements in hardware, including stronger gradients, multi-channel receiver arrays, and higher field strengths, combined with sequence optimisations and advanced reconstruction methods. Modern high-resolution structural protocols routinely achieve isotropic voxel sizes of 0.5-0.8 millimetres, with research applications pushing toward 0.3 millimetres, providing spatial detail that approaches that of ex vivo imaging while maintaining whole-brain coverage and clinically feasible acquisition times. These resolution improvements fundamentally expand the range of anatomical features that can be resolved, revealing cortical architecture, subcortical nuclear organisation, and white matter fascicular anatomy with unprecedented clarity in living human subjects.

The magnetisation-prepared rapid gradient echo (MP-RAGE) sequence has emerged as the workhorse for high-resolution T1-weighted anatomical imaging, particularly at 3 Tesla and higher field strengths. This sequence employs an inversion recovery preparation to enhance T1 contrast, followed by a rapid gradient-echo acquisition of multiple k-space lines during the optimally timed recovery period. The combination of substantial T1 weighting and efficient k-space coverage enables the acquisition of high-resolution three-dimensional datasets in 5-8 minutes, with excellent grey-white matter contrast. Optimisation of MP-RAGE parameters, including inversion time, flip angle, and repetition time for specific field strengths and clinical applications, has been extensively studied, with recommended protocols available for various platforms. At 7 Tesla and above, MP-RAGE benefits from increased SNR and prolonged T1 relaxation times, though B1 inhomogeneity necessitates careful parameter selection and potentially parallel transmission for uniform contrast (Mugler & Brookeman, 1990).

Three-dimensional T2-weighted imaging techniques, including SPACE (Sampling Perfection with Application-optimised Contrasts using different flip angle Evolutions) and CUBE sequences, provide complementary high-resolution anatomical information with sensitivity to pathological processes that increase tissue water content. These variable-flip-angle turbo spin-echo sequences maintain stable signal throughout long echo trains while managing specific absorption rate within safety limits, enabling isotropic submillimetre T2-weighted imaging in clinically acceptable scan times of 5-

10 minutes. The improved spatial resolution reveals small lesions, including cortical MS plaques, subtle hippocampal sclerosis, and tiny cavernomas that partial volume effects at standard resolution may obscure. The combination of high-resolution T1- and T2-weighted imaging provides comprehensive anatomical characterisation, suitable for detecting diverse pathologies and characterising tissue properties through multi-contrast analysis.

Cortical thickness measurement has become a standard application of high-resolution structural imaging, providing quantitative metrics of regional brain atrophy in neurodegenerative diseases, normal ageing, and neurodevelopmental disorders. Automated segmentation algorithms, including FreeSurfer, FSL, and ANTs, process T1-weighted images to identify grey-white and pial surfaces, calculating cortical thickness as the distance between these boundaries at thousands of vertices across the cortical surface. The submillimetre resolution of modern structural acquisitions enhances surface reconstruction accuracy, reduces partial volume errors, and facilitates the detection of subtle atrophic changes. Longitudinal cortical thickness analysis reveals spatiotemporal patterns of degeneration in Alzheimer's disease, frontotemporal dementia, and other conditions, with regional thinning rates serving as endpoints in clinical trials and potential biomarkers for disease staging and prognosis (Fischl & Dale, 2000).

Subcortical structure segmentation benefits significantly from high-resolution imaging, as many deep brain nuclei measure only a few millimetres in their smallest dimension and are poorly resolved at conventional 1-mm isotropic resolution. Submillimetre imaging reduces partial-volume effects and improves boundary definition between adjacent structures, enabling accurate volumetric measurements of the hippocampus, amygdala, thalamic nuclei, and basal ganglia components. Advanced segmentation approaches incorporating multi-atlas methods, shape priors, and machine learning achieve high accuracy and reliability when applied to high-resolution data. Volumetric measurements of hippocampal subfields, including CA1, CA3, dentate gyrus, and subiculum, become feasible with 0.4-0.5-millimetre resolution, providing more specific biomarkers of medial temporal pathology than whole hippocampal volume. Similarly, thalamic parcellation into constituent nuclei enables investigation of specific thalamocortical circuits in cognitive and sensory processing.

White matter architecture visualisation advances substantially with high-resolution imaging, as individual fascicles and fibre crossings become distinguishable rather than blurred together by partial-volume averaging. High-resolution T2-weighted imaging can resolve multiple tracts within the internal capsule, differentiate the numerous components of the cingulum bundle, and identify small commissural fibres, including the anterior commissure and hippocampal commissure. When combined with diffusion imaging at matched resolution, precise anatomical boundaries guide tractography and improve the specificity of structural connectivity analyses. Ultra-high-resolution imaging at 7 Tesla reveals even finer details of white matter organisation, including the stria of Gennari in the primary visual cortex, individual fibre bundles within significant tracts, and the complex crossing patterns at junctional regions that pose challenges for diffusion tractography at coarser resolutions.

Motion sensitivity increases with spatial resolution, as higher-resolution encoding requires the acquisition of higher spatial-frequency k-space data, which is more susceptible to motion-induced phase errors. Patient movement during high-resolution scans can cause ghosting artefacts, image blurring, and surface reconstruction errors, severely degrading image quality and analysis results. Prospective motion correction systems, which utilise optical tracking or navigator echoes to measure head position and dynamically update acquisition parameters in real-time, can substantially improve image quality, particularly for long, high-resolution scans and in populations with involuntary movement, such as pediatric patients and those with movement disorders. Retrospective motion correction methods, which analyse the acquired data to estimate and compensate for motion, provide complementary approaches, albeit with more limited correction capabilities. The combination of prospective and retrospective strategies, along with patient comfort measures and effective communication, maximises the successful acquisition of high-quality, high-resolution datasets. Table 4.1 shows high-resolution structural MRI sequences and applications.

Table 4.1. High-resolution structural MRI sequences and applications

Sequence Type	Typical Resolution	Acquisition Time	Primary Contrast	Key Applications	Technical Considerations
MP-RAGE	0.7-1.0 mm isotropic	5-8 min	T1-weighted	Cortical thickness, volumetry, and anatomy	B1 optimisation at high field
3D T2 TSE (SPACE/CUBE)	0.6-0.8 mm isotropic	6-10 min	T2-weighted	Lesion detection, hippocampal imaging	SAR management, long echo trains
Double Inversion Recovery	1.0 mm isotropic	8-12 min	Grey matter selective	Cortical lesions in MS	Long acquisition time
White Matter Nulled	0.8 mm isotropic	6-8 min	Subcortical contrast	Deep grey nuclei, lesions	Inversion time optimisation
Susceptibility-Weighted	0.5-1.0 mm	5-8 min	T2* + phase	Venous vasculature, haemorrhage	Unwrapping artifacts possible
Multi-echo MPRAGE	0.7-0.9 mm isotropic	10-15 min	Combined T1/T2*	Comprehensive tissue properties	Longer acquisition, registration needed

4.2. Quantitative MRI: T1, T2, and Proton Density Mapping

Quantitative MRI represents a fundamental shift from weighted imaging, where signal intensity is influenced by multiple factors in complex ways, to parametric mapping that directly measures intrinsic tissue properties in absolute physical units. T1, T2, and proton density are fundamental NMR parameters that fully characterise the MRI signal behaviour of a tissue, providing a comprehensive description of its MRI properties independent of the imaging sequence used for measurement. Accurate quantification of these parameters enables standardised measurements that are comparable across scanners, field strengths, and time points, addressing a critical limitation of conventional weighted imaging, where signal intensities are arbitrary and protocol-dependent. The clinical and research value of quantitative MRI lies in its ability to provide objective biomarkers sensitive to pathological changes, facilitate multicentre studies through measurement standardisation, and enable the synthetic generation of arbitrary contrast-weighted images from a single acquisition.

T1 mapping techniques measure the spin-lattice relaxation time, which reflects tissue composition, macromolecular content, and water content through its dependence on molecular dynamics at the Larmor frequency. The most robust T1 mapping methods acquire multiple images with different degrees of T1 weighting, then fit the signal evolution to the appropriate recovery equation to extract T1 values at each voxel. Inversion recovery methods employing multiple inversion times provide accurate T1 measurements but require long acquisition times because complete longitudinal relaxation is required between measurements. Variable-flip-angle methods, utilising spoiled gradient-echo acquisitions with different flip angles, offer faster alternatives. These methods acquire data at multiple flip angles with short repetition times and estimate T1 from signal variations. The accuracy of variable-flip-angle T1 mapping depends critically on accurate knowledge of the actual flip-angle distribution, which requires B1 mapping to correct for radiofrequency field inhomogeneities, particularly at 3T and higher fields (Deoni et al., 2005).

The Look-Locker technique and its variants provide efficient T1 mapping by acquiring multiple images at different time points following an inversion pulse, sampling the recovery curve within a single inversion recovery experiment. Modified Look-Locker inversion recovery (MOLLI) has been optimised for cardiac T1 mapping and adapted for brain applications, allowing for the generation of T1 maps in 5-10 minutes with high precision. The rapid acquisition comes at the cost of T1 underestimation, as repeated readout pulses perturb recovery and require correction factors derived from Bloch equation simulations. MP2RAGE (Magnetisation Prepared 2 Rapid Gradient Echoes) addresses this limitation by acquiring two gradient echo images at different inversion times and computing T1 from their ratio, thereby providing self-normalised T1 maps with minimal sensitivity to B1 inhomogeneity, receiver coil profiles, and proton density variations. The inherent bias field correction makes MP2RAGE particularly valuable for quantitative studies and automated segmentation applications.

T2 mapping quantifies transverse relaxation time, reflecting tissue microstructure through the efficiency of spin-spin interactions and local field inhomogeneities at the molecular scale. Multi-echo spin echo (MESE) sequences acquire multiple spin echoes with incrementing echo times following a single excitation, providing data points along the T2 decay curve for exponential fitting. Accurate T2 mapping requires a sufficient number of echoes (typically 8-32) spanning the decay curve and careful attention to stimulated echo contamination from imperfect refocusing pulses. Extended phase graph modelling accounts for complex magnetisation pathways in multi-echo sequences, thereby improving T2 quantification accuracy, particularly for tissues with short T2 components. Multi-component T2 analysis can distinguish multiple water pools with different relaxation times, identifying myelin water with T2 values of 10-40 milliseconds, distinct from intra- and extracellular water with T2 values of 80-120 milliseconds. This distinction provides myelin-specific biomarkers, as discussed further in Section 4.3.

Proton density mapping measures the concentration of mobile hydrogen nuclei contributing to the MRI signal, reflecting tissue water content and cellularity. Pure proton density imaging requires eliminating T1 and T2 weighting by using very long TR and very short TE, which is impractical for clinical imaging. Quantitative proton density mapping derives PD from multi-parameter acquisitions that simultaneously characterise T1, T2, and PD by fitting signal equations that incorporate all three parameters. The synthetic MRI approach, employing multi-echo and multi-saturation-delay acquisitions, provides quantitative maps of all three parameters from a single scan lasting 5–6 minutes. Proton density reflects tissue hydration and cellularity, with increased values in oedema, tumour, and inflammation, and decreased values in dense cellular structures and areas of tissue loss. Unlike T1 and T2, which have been extensively studied, the independent diagnostic value of quantitative PD remains under investigation, although its contribution to multi-parameter tissue characterisation shows promise.

Simultaneous multi-parameter mapping approaches acquire data with diverse T1 and T2 weightings in a single, efficient acquisition, then jointly fit all parameters to signal models. The most clinically implemented approach, commercially available as SyMRI, uses a multi-dynamic multi-echo sequence (MDME) that acquires multiple saturation delays and echo times, providing complete tissue characterisation in 5-6 minutes. The quantitative parameter maps enable the retrospective synthesis of conventional contrast-weighted images, including T1, T2, FLAIR, and STIR, with arbitrary parameters, thereby eliminating the need for separate acquisitions. More importantly, the quantitative values provide standardised measurements for comparing across time points and patients. Multi-centre studies have demonstrated good reproducibility of T1 and T2 measurements from these techniques, supporting their use as quantitative biomarkers. However, absolute values can vary between implementations and require careful validation against reference standards (Warntjes et al., 2008).

The clinical applications of quantitative relaxometry encompass the detection of subtle pathology, objective disease monitoring, and tissue characterisation in ambiguous cases. In multiple sclerosis, T1 and T2 values within lesions correlate with the severity of demyelination and axonal loss, with lower T1 and higher T2 values indicating more severe tissue destruction. Quantitative values help distinguish active inflammation from chronic gliosis, guide lesion classification, and provide objective metrics of disease progression independent of changes in lesion volume. In brain tumours, multi-parameter quantitative imaging aids in tissue characterisation, with specific T1/T2 combinations helping to distinguish tumour types, differentiate tumour from treatment effects, and identify regions of high cellularity versus necrosis. Neurodegenerative diseases exhibit characteristic patterns of T1- and T2-weighted changes in affected structures, with quantitative measurements potentially enabling earlier detection than volumetric analysis and more sensitive tracking of disease progression.

4.3. Magnetisation Transfer Imaging

Magnetisation transfer (MT) imaging exploits the exchange of magnetisation between free water protons and protons bound to macromolecules to provide contrast sensitive to tissue microstructure, particularly myelin content in white and grey matter. The technique relies on the two-pool model of tissue water, which distinguishes between mobile free water protons with narrow resonance frequencies and long T2 relaxation times, and macromolecular protons with vast resonance frequencies and very short T2 relaxation times, too short to be directly imaged. While macromolecular protons cannot directly contribute to the MRI signal, they can be selectively saturated with off-resonance radiofrequency pulses at frequencies far from the water resonance. This saturation transfers to the free water pool via chemical exchange and dipolar coupling, reducing the observed water signal in proportion to the macromolecular content and the exchange rate. The magnetisation transfer ratio (MTR), defined as the percentage reduction in signal with MT saturation relative to the signal without it, provides a semi-quantitative measure of tissue macromolecular content and organisation, with particular sensitivity to myelin in the central nervous system (Wolff & Balaban, 1989).

The physical mechanisms underlying magnetisation transfer involve both chemical exchange of labile protons between macromolecules and water, and through-space dipolar coupling between proton spins in proximity. In myelin, both mechanisms contribute, with exchange occurring at amine and hydroxyl groups on myelin proteins and lipids. At the same time, dipolar coupling arises from the highly organised lipid bilayer structure, which brings macromolecular and water protons into close spatial proximity. The broad resonance linewidth of macromolecular protons, extending from kilohertz to the water frequency, enables selective saturation without directly affecting the water. However, the exact frequency offset and saturation power must be optimised to maximise the MT effect while minimising direct water saturation. Typical MT pulse sequences employ frequency offsets of 1-2 kilohertz and saturation powers calibrated to achieve substantial MT effect without excessive specific absorption rate or direct saturation spillover.

Magnetisation transfer ratio mapping provides a semi-quantitative assessment of macromolecular content by comparing the signal obtained with and without MT saturation pulses. Images are acquired with identical parameters except for the presence or absence of the off-resonance saturation, and MTR is calculated voxel-wise as MTR $= 100\% \times (S_0 - S_{sat}) / S_0$, where S_0 is the signal without saturation and S_{sat} is the signal with saturation. Normal white matter shows high MTR values of 35-45% reflecting high myelin content, grey matter shows intermediate values of 25-35%, and cerebrospinal fluid shows near-zero MTR due to the absence of macromolecules. Pathological processes affecting myelin, including demyelination, oedema, and tissue destruction, reduce MTR, often more sensitively than conventional imaging. The technique's sensitivity to myelin makes it valuable for multiple sclerosis, where MTR decreases occur in lesions, normal-appearing white matter, and grey matter, correlating with disability and providing a potential surrogate marker of tissue integrity.

Quantitative magnetisation transfer (qMT) imaging extends beyond semi-quantitative MTR to provide estimates of biophysical parameters, including the macromolecular pool fraction, exchange rate, and T2 relaxation times of both pools. This requires the acquisition of MT-weighted images at multiple saturation powers and/or frequency offsets, followed by fitting to a two-pool exchange model that describes magnetisation transfer dynamics. The macromolecular pool fraction, which represents the relative size of the bound pool, correlates strongly with myelin content and provides more specific tissue characterisation than MTR. The exchange rate quantifies how rapidly magnetisation transfers between pools, reflecting the chemical and physical environment. While qMT offers more specific and reproducible measurements than MTR, it requires longer acquisition times for the multiple saturation conditions and more complex post-processing. Simplified qMT approaches, including selective inversion recovery and pulsed MT sequences, reduce acquisition time while retaining some quantitative advantages over simple MTR.

Myelin water imaging represents a complementary approach to assessing myelin content through multi-component T2 analysis rather than magnetisation transfer. Brain water exists in multiple compartments with different T2 relaxation times: myelin water trapped between myelin bilayers shows a very short T2 of 10-40 milliseconds, while intra-axonal and extracellular water show longer T2 of 60-100 milliseconds. Multi-echo T2 relaxation measurements with sufficient early echoes to capture the myelin water signal, combined with multi-exponential or regularised fitting algorithms, can separate these components and quantify the myelin water fraction (MWF), defined as the ratio of the myelin water signal to the total water signal. MWF correlates with histological myelin content and provides a more specific myelin biomarker than MTR, which is influenced by other macromolecular content. However, myelin water imaging requires long acquisition times for an adequate signal-to-noise ratio. It faces technical challenges in fitting the multi-exponential decay, which limits its widespread clinical adoption despite its biophysical specificity.

The clinical applications of magnetisation transfer imaging have been most extensively studied in multiple sclerosis, where MTR and qMT parameters show strong correlations with disability, disease progression, and tissue pathology. Lesion MTR decreases relate to the severity of demyelination and axonal loss, with severe MTR reduction indicating near-complete tissue destruction and modest reduction suggesting partial demyelination with potential for remyelination. Normal-appearing white matter in MS patients shows subtle decreases in MTR compared with healthy controls, reflecting diffuse microscopic pathology not visible on conventional imaging. MTR changes in grey matter, particularly in the cortex and deep nuclei, correlate with cognitive impairment and physical disability, highlighting the importance of grey matter pathology in MS. Longitudinal MTR measurements track remyelination and tissue recovery, providing potential outcome measures for trials of remyelinating therapies. Beyond MS, MT imaging shows promise in other white matter diseases and brain tumours, where MTR helps tissue characterisation, and in neurodegenerative diseases, where myelin loss contributes to pathology. Table 4.2 illustrates magnetisation transfer and myelin imaging techniques.

Table 4.2. Magnetisation transfer and Myelin imaging techniques

Technique	Measurement	Acquisition Time	Myelin Specificity	Primary Applications	Limitations
MT Ratio (MTR)	Semi-quantitative macromolecular content	5-8 min	Moderate (influenced by T1, exchange)	MS, white matter disease, screening	Protocol-dependent, not standardised
Quantitative MT (qMT)	Pool fraction, exchange rate, T2S	15-25 min	High for bound pool fraction	Research, myelin quantification	Long acquisition, complex analysis
Myelin Water Fraction	Specific myelin compartment	10-20 min	Very high (direct myelin water)	Precise myelin mapping	Long scan, fitting challenges
Inhomogeneous MT	Bound pool fraction (rapid)	5-8 min	High (improved from MTR)	Clinical qMT alternative	Newer, less validated
MT-prepared sequences	Qualitative myelin contrast	3-5 min	Moderate	Lesion conspicuity, clinical imaging	Qualitative only

4.4. Susceptibility-Weighted Imaging (SWI)

Susceptibility-weighted imaging leverages the magnetic susceptibility properties of tissues to generate contrast that is sensitive to venous vasculature, haemorrhage, iron deposition, and calcium, with exquisite sensitivity far exceeding that of conventional T2*-weighted imaging. The technique combines magnitude and phase information from high-resolution gradient-echo acquisitions, utilising phase data to create a susceptibility mask, which is then multiplied by magnitude images to enhance the contrast of susceptibility sources. This synergistic combination produces images in which paramagnetic substances, including deoxyhaemoglobin in veins, breakdown products of haemorrhage, and iron-containing structures, appear markedly hypointense, while diamagnetic calcium shows relative hyperintensity. The enhanced conspicuity of susceptibility effects makes SWI particularly valuable for detecting cerebral microbleeds, developmental venous anomalies, small cavernomas, and patterns of iron deposition characteristic of specific neurodegenerative diseases (Haacke et al., 2004).

The physics underlying susceptibility-weighted imaging relates to how materials alter local magnetic fields when placed in the strong static field of an MRI scanner. Paramagnetic substances, including deoxyhemoglobin and ferritin, possess unpaired electrons that align with the external magnetic field, resulting in small local field increases. Diamagnetic substances, including most brain tissue and calcium, have paired electrons that slightly oppose the field, resulting in small local decreases in the field. These field perturbations cause protons near susceptibility sources to precess at slightly different frequencies than those in surrounding tissue, accumulating phase differences that are proportional to the echo time, field strength, and the magnitude of the susceptibility difference. The magnitude signal shows T2* signal loss due to dephasing, while phase images directly encode local field variations. SWI processing applies phase masks derived from filtered phase images to magnitude data, typically raising the phase mask to a power (4-6) to progressively darken regions with phase differences while preserving normal tissue signal.

High-resolution gradient echo acquisition forms the foundation of SWI, typically employing long echo times of 20-40 milliseconds at 1.5T or 15-25 milliseconds at 3T to maximise phase accumulation from susceptibility effects while maintaining adequate signal-to-noise ratio. Three-dimensional acquisitions with in-plane resolutions of 0.5-1 millimetres and slice thicknesses of 1-2 millimetres provide the spatial resolution necessary to visualise small veins and microbleeds. Flow-compensation gradients minimise phase artefacts caused by blood flow, and multiple echoes can be acquired to create T2* maps alongside SWI images. The extended acquisition time of 5-10 minutes makes SWI susceptible to motion artefacts, particularly in uncooperative patients; however, modern implementations incorporate parallel imaging and compressed sensing to reduce scan time. At 7 Tesla and above, the increased susceptibility effects require shorter echo times and careful protocol optimisation to balance enhanced sensitivity against increased artefact severity.

Phase processing is a critical component of SWI, as raw phase images contain artefacts from main-field inhomogeneities, fat-water chemical shift, and phase wrapping that must be corrected to isolate susceptibility-induced phase variations. High-pass filtering removes global phase variations from field inhomogeneities, retaining local phase differences from susceptibility sources. Unwrapping algorithms correct for phase wrapping that occurs when the phase exceeds 2π, although they can fail in regions of severe susceptibility gradients. The filtered phase is then used to create a multiplicative mask, with negative phase values (indicating paramagnetic sources) darkening the corresponding magnitude voxels. Multiple-phase mask multiplication progressively enhances contrast, though excessive multiplication can introduce artefacts and obscure anatomy. Minimum-intensity projection over several slices creates the final SWI images, which exhibit dramatic venous and haemorrhage contrast, a characteristic of the technique.

Venous visualisation represents a primary strength of SWI, as the paramagnetic deoxyhemoglobin in venous blood creates strong susceptibility effects. The technique reveals venous architecture down to 100-200 micrometre diameter vessels at 3T, with even finer detail at higher magnetic field strengths. The extensive visualisation of venous structures enables the identification of developmental venous anomalies, the mapping of venous drainage patterns, and the detection of venous thrombosis or occlusion. In acute stroke, the hypointense vessel sign on SWI indicates the location of the thrombus, while prominent veins in ischemic regions reflect increased oxygen extraction. Tumours exhibit characteristic venous patterns on SWI, including abnormal tumour vasculature, tumour-associated veins, and areas of hypoxia, which create diagnostic patterns. Venous malformations, including cavernomas and arteriovenous malformations, demonstrate exquisite detail on SWI, often revealing disease extent not apparent on conventional imaging.

Haemorrhage detection is another primary application of SWI, with sensitivity to blood products far exceeding that of T2*-weighted and gradient-echo imaging. Acute haemorrhage with deoxyhemoglobin, subacute haemorrhage with methemoglobin and hemosiderin, and chronic hemosiderin deposits all demonstrate strong hypointensity on SWI due to their paramagnetic properties. Cerebral microbleeds, punctate foci of hemosiderin deposition from prior microscopic haemorrhages, appear as small hypointense spots on SWI and are detected with much higher sensitivity than gradient echo imaging. Microbleed burden correlates with cerebral amyloid angiopathy, hypertensive vasculopathy, and other small vessel diseases, providing prognostic information and bleeding risk assessment. Traumatic brain injury reveals patterns of microhemorrhage and diffuse axonal injury on SWI that are invisible on CT and often missed on conventional MRI, improving injury characterisation and potentially explaining symptoms in patients with routine standard imaging.

Iron deposition imaging utilises SWI's sensitivity to paramagnetic iron in ferritin and hemosiderin to visualise iron distribution within brain structures. The basal ganglia, red nucleus, substantia nigra, and dentate nucleus typically accumulate iron with age, appearing progressively hypointense on SWI. Abnormal iron deposition patterns characterise specific diseases, including excessive iron in the globus pallidus and substantia nigra in pantothenate kinase-associated neurodegeneration, iron accumulation in the dentate and red nuclei in superficial siderosis, and altered striatal iron in Huntington's disease. Parkinson's disease is characterised by the loss of the normal hyperintense nigrosome 1 on SWI within the substantia nigra, a finding with high diagnostic accuracy that may enable earlier detection than clinical criteria. Multiple sclerosis lesions exhibit characteristic peripheral iron rims on SWI, representing iron-laden macrophages. The presence of these rims correlates with chronic active inflammation and a progressive disease course.

4.5. Quantitative Susceptibility Mapping (QSM)

Quantitative susceptibility mapping advances beyond the qualitative susceptibility contrast of SWI to provide quantitative measurements of tissue magnetic susceptibility in absolute units, such as parts per billion (ppb) or parts per million (ppm), relative to a reference tissue. While SWI enhances visualisation of susceptibility effects, QSM solves the inverse problem of computing the underlying susceptibility distribution that generates the observed phase pattern, producing parametric maps where susceptibility values directly reflect tissue iron content, myelin density, calcium concentration, and blood oxygenation. This quantitative approach enables objective tissue characterisation, standardised measurements that are comparable across field strengths and sites, and correlation with biochemical and histological analyses. The technique has rapidly evolved from a research curiosity to a clinical and research tool, with applications spanning neurodegenerative diseases, multiple sclerosis, brain development, and tumour characterisation (Wang & Liu, 2015).

The fundamental principle of QSM derives from the relationship between tissue susceptibility and the local magnetic field perturbation it creates. A susceptibility source with magnetic susceptibility χ placed in the main magnetic field B_0 produces a dipole field pattern surrounding it, with field strength and spatial distribution determined by the susceptibility magnitude, source geometry, and orientation relative to B_0. The measured phase in gradient-echo images reflects the integral of these field perturbations, encoding susceptibility information in a complex, non-local manner in which susceptibility sources influence each voxel's phase throughout the brain. QSM reconstruction inverts this relationship to recover the underlying susceptibility distribution from the phase data. This challenging, ill-posed inverse problem requires sophisticated algorithms to achieve accurate, artefact-free results.

Phase preprocessing steps prepare the raw gradient echo phase data for QSM reconstruction by removing confounding phase contributions unrelated to susceptibility. Background field removal separates phase contributions from sources outside the brain (air-tissue interfaces, sinuses, scanner imperfections) from the local tissue field of interest, a critical step as background fields can be larger than tissue fields and vary with head position. Multiple algorithms, including SHARP (Sophisticated Harmonic Artefact Reduction for Phase), PDF (Projection onto Dipole Fields), and V-SHARP, employ different mathematical approaches to remove background fields, each with its own advantages and limitations. Brain masking defines the region of interest for QSM calculation, typically using automated skull stripping algorithms to identify brain tissue while excluding skull, fat, and air. Careful attention to phase unwrapping and brain mask definition minimises reconstruction artefacts that can propagate from errors in these preprocessing steps.

The susceptibility inversion problem is mathematically ill-posed due to fundamental ambiguities in the relationship between susceptibility and phase. The dipole field pattern depends on source orientation relative to B_0, creating orientation-dependent phase effects that cannot be uniquely inverted without additional constraints. Regions where susceptibility variations align with the main field (cone of silence) exhibit no phase change, rendering those susceptibility features invisible. Regularisation approaches constrain the solution space to enforce physical plausibility and stability, with different algorithms employing L1 minimisation for edge preservation, L2 minimisation for smoothness, or morphology-based constraints using structural priors from magnitude images. MEDI (Morphology Enabled Dipole Inversion) is a widely used approach that incorporates edge information from magnitude images to guide susceptibility reconstruction while maintaining data consistency (Liu et al., 2012).

Quantitative susceptibility values provide direct measurements of tissue magnetic properties in physically meaningful units. Normal brain tissue shows susceptibility values ranging from approximately -50 ppb for myelin-rich white matter (diamagnetic relative to CSF reference) to +150 ppb for iron-rich deep grey nuclei (paramagnetic). The quantitative nature enables objective comparison across individuals, field strengths, and time points, a fundamental advantage over weighted imaging, where intensity values are arbitrary. Susceptibility measurements correlate strongly with iron concentration, as determined by histology and biochemical assays, with reported correlations ranging from $r = 0.8$ to 0.9 across various grey matter structures. Myelin content exhibits an inverse correlation with susceptibility, as the diamagnetic lipid structure reduces the net tissue susceptibility. These correlations establish QSM as a quantitative biomarker of iron and myelin, with potential applications in diseases that affect these tissue components.

Iron quantification using QSM has emerged as a significant research and clinical application, as the technique provides the only non-invasive method for measuring brain iron concentration *in vivo*. Normal ageing is associated with progressive iron accumulation in the basal ganglia, with increases in susceptibility of 2-5 ppb per decade in the putamen and globus pallidus. Neurodegenerative diseases exhibit characteristic patterns of altered iron distribution, with increased iron in the substantia nigra and basal ganglia in Parkinson's disease, elevated iron in the motor cortex in amyotrophic lateral sclerosis, and reduced iron in specific structures in Huntington's disease, despite overall increases in iron levels. Multiple sclerosis lesions exhibit heterogeneous susceptibility, with some lesions displaying paramagnetic rims that indicate the presence of iron-laden inflammatory cells at the lesion edges. These rim lesions represent chronic active inflammation and correlate with disability progression, potentially serving as biomarkers for aggressive disease requiring escalation of therapy.

Myelin quantification via QSM leverages myelin's diamagnetic susceptibility, offering an alternative to magnetisation transfer and myelin water imaging. White matter susceptibility becomes increasingly diamagnetic (i.e., less hostile) during myelination in development, plateaus in adulthood, and may become less diamagnetic (i.e., more hostile) in ageing and demyelinating disease. The relationship between susceptibility and myelin content is complex, as iron in oligodendrocytes and myelin lipids exert opposing effects. Advanced analysis, which separates paramagnetic and diamagnetic contributions, can potentially isolate myelin effects, although this requires additional assumptions and modelling. Despite these complexities, white matter susceptibility shows promise as a myelin biomarker, with demyelinating lesions exhibiting increased (less harmful) susceptibility, and remyelination associated with susceptibility normalisation in animal models.

Clinical applications of QSM are expanding as the technique matures and becomes more widely available through commercial implementations and open-source reconstruction tools. In Parkinson's disease, nigrosome imaging using QSM reveals a loss of the normal swallow-tail appearance of the substantia nigra with high diagnostic accuracy, potentially enabling earlier diagnosis and differentiation from atypical Parkinsonism. Surgical planning for movement disorders benefits from QSM's clear visualisation of the subthalamic nucleus, globus pallidus, and surrounding structures, without the need for contrast injection, thereby improving target definition for deep brain stimulation. Multiple sclerosis monitoring incorporates QSM for lesion characterisation and the tracking of chronic active lesions via iron-rim detection. Brain tumour applications include distinguishing haemorrhage from calcification based on susceptibility (paramagnetic versus diamagnetic) and assessing tumour microvasculature via venous susceptibility measurements.

4.6. Synthetic MRI and MRI Fingerprinting

Synthetic MRI and MRI Fingerprinting represent revolutionary approaches to brain imaging that fundamentally reimagine how MRI data is acquired and processed. Rather than developing separate images optimised for specific tissue contrast, these techniques acquire rich, multidimensional datasets that encode tissue properties, extract quantitative parameter maps through advanced post-processing, and enable the retrospective generation of arbitrary contrast-weighted images with user-specified parameters. This paradigm shift offers multiple advantages: comprehensive quantitative tissue characterisation from a single, efficient acquisition; elimination of protocol selection errors and scan repetition when contrast is suboptimal; standardised measurements enabling multicentre comparisons; and flexibility to generate novel contrast weightings as new clinical needs emerge. These techniques represent perhaps the most significant innovation in structural MRI acquisition strategy since the development of fast spin-echo imaging.

Synthetic MRI, commercially implemented as SyMRI, employs multi-dynamic multi-echo (MDME) sequences that acquire multiple gradient echoes at several saturation delay times, providing data with diverse T1, T2, and proton-density weighting. The acquisition typically requires 5-6 minutes to sample multiple echo times (4-8 echoes) and saturation delays (2-4 delays) across the entire brain volume at a resolution of 1-2 millimetres. A quantitative signal model describing how the MRI signal depends on sequence parameters and tissue properties (T1, T2, PD) is fitted to the acquired data at each voxel, extracting the three fundamental tissue parameters that characterise entirely the MRI signal behaviour. These quantitative maps then serve as the basis for synthesising arbitrary contrast-weighted images by calculating the expected signal for any desired pulse sequence parameters. Users can retrospectively generate T1-weighted, T2-weighted, FLAIR, STIR, or any other linear combination of tissue contrasts, adjusting parameters such as repetition time, echo time, and inversion time to optimise the conspicuity of specific findings without repeating the acquisition (Warntjes et al., 2008).

The clinical workflow advantages of synthetic MRI are substantial and immediately apparent. A single 5–6-minute MDME acquisition can replace multiple conventional sequences totalling 15-20 minutes, significantly reducing examination time and associated costs. More importantly, retrospective contrast adjustment eliminates the common scenario where images are acquired with suboptimal parameters requiring repeat sequences, a significant source of inefficiency and patient discomfort in clinical MRI. When pathology is identified, contrast can be optimised retrospectively to enhance conspicuity without patient recall. The quantitative T1, T2, and proton density values provide objective measurements for lesion characterisation, treatment monitoring, and standardised reporting. Automated brain volumetry integrated into some synthetic MRI implementations provides a quantitative assessment of Grey matter, white matter, CSF, and lesion volumes without additional processing steps, which is valuable for monitoring neurodegenerative disease and multiple sclerosis.

MRI Fingerprinting (MRF) extends the synthetic MRI concept by employing highly varied, pseudorandom acquisition patterns that cause different tissues to produce unique signal evolution "fingerprints" determined by their T1, T2, and other properties. Rather than incrementally sampling the parameter space with regular increments, as in conventional quantitative imaging, MRF uses randomised flip angles, repetition times, and other acquisition parameters to create maximal signal variation and optimal tissue differentiation. The resulting signal evolutions are matched to a precomputed dictionary of possible tissue signatures using pattern recognition algorithms, which efficiently identify the tissue parameters that best explain the observed signals. This dictionary-matching approach enables simultaneous quantification of multiple parameters (T1, T2, proton density, T2*, and diffusion) from rapid acquisitions while remaining robust to system imperfections, including B1 and B0 inhomogeneities (Ma et al., 2013).

The technical innovation of MRF lies in its pseudorandom acquisition design and pattern-matching reconstruction. The acquisition employs rapidly varying flip angles, following a pseudorandom or optimised pattern, that maximises signal variation and discrimination between tissue types. Repetition times may also vary, and the readout trajectory (spiral, radial, or Cartesian) can be optimised for efficient k-space coverage and robustness to motion. Each voxel undergoes a unique time course of excitations and acquisitions, resulting in a signal evolution that depends on its tissue properties. The dictionary contains precomputed signal evolutions for all possible combinations of tissue parameters of interest, calculated using Bloch equation simulations that account for sequence details and system characteristics. Matching observed signals to dictionary entries involves efficient search algorithms, such as inner-product matching or machine learning, to identify the parameter combination that best reproduces the observed signals.

The advantages of MRF over conventional quantitative imaging include improved acquisition efficiency, inherent robustness to system imperfections, and the capability for simultaneous multi-parameter quantification. The pseudorandom acquisition enables efficient use of the available signal, allowing whole-brain quantitative mapping in 5-10 minutes with resolution and precision comparable to those of conventional methods that require 20-30 minutes. B1 and B0 inhomogeneities are implicitly accounted for in dictionary creation, making parameter estimates robust without the need for separate calibration scans. Multiple tissue parameters can be quantified simultaneously, with MRF implementations demonstrating T1, T2, and proton density mapping as standard, with extensions to include T2*, diffusion coefficient, perfusion, and other parameters. The flexibility of MRF enables customisation for specific applications, optimising acquisition patterns for tissues, pathologies, or clinical questions.

Clinical validation of MRF has demonstrated quantitative accuracy comparable to gold-standard measurements and repeatability suitable for longitudinal monitoring. Multi-centre studies demonstrate good reproducibility of T1 and T2 values across scanner platforms when using standardised MRF implementations, although some systematic differences between vendors persist. Pathological validation shows that MRF parameters correlate with tissue histology and conventional imaging findings, supporting their clinical utility. Early clinical applications include brain tumour characterisation, where T1/T2 combinations aid tissue typing; multiple sclerosis lesion quantification, providing objective metrics of demyelination severity; and stroke imaging, where T1/T2 maps identify tissue at risk and completed infarction. The ability to rapidly acquire comprehensive quantitative tissue characterisation is particularly valuable in pediatric imaging, where cooperation may be limited and examination time is critical.

The future development of synthetic MRI and MRI Fingerprinting includes extending to broader parameter sets, optimising for specific clinical applications, and integrating with advanced reconstruction methods. Higher-dimensional MRF, including diffusion, perfusion, and fat quantification, would provide comprehensive tissue characterisation from a single 10-minute scan, potentially replacing entire examination protocols. Machine learning approaches to dictionary generation and signal matching may improve computational efficiency and enable real-time parameter quantification. Integration with compressed sensing and parallel imaging could further reduce acquisition time or improve spatial resolution within current time constraints. Standardisation efforts through multi-vendor studies and phantom validation will be critical for establishing these techniques as clinical standards and enabling their use as quantitative biomarkers in therapeutic trials. Table 4.3 compares advanced quantitative MRI techniques.

Table 4.3. Comparison of advanced quantitative MRI techniques

Technique	Parameters Measured	Acquisition Time	Standardization	Key Advantages	Current Limitations
Synthetic MRI (SyMRI)	T1, T2, PD	5-6 min	Good (commercial)	Retrospective contrast, volumetry	Limited to 3 parameters
MRI Fingerprinting	T1, T2, PD, (T2*, D)	5-10 min	Moderate (evolving)	Multi-parameter, B1/B0 robust	Dictionary size, processing time
MP2RAGE	T1	5-8 min	Excellent	B1-independent, precise	T1 only
Multi-component relaxation	T1, T2, multi-T2 pools	15-25 min	Moderate	Myelin water fraction	Long acquisition, fitting complexity
Look-Locker variants	T1	8-12 min	Good	Whole-brain T1 maps	T1 underestimation possible
Multi-echo spin echo	T2	10-15 min	Good	Accurate T2	Long acquisition, SAR

Conclusion

Advanced structural MRI techniques have fundamentally transformed neuroimaging from qualitative anatomical assessment to quantitative tissue characterisation, providing objective biomarkers of brain microstructure, composition, and pathophysiology. High-resolution anatomical imaging routinely achieves submillimetre spatial resolution, revealing cortical architecture, subcortical nuclear organisation, and white matter fascicular anatomy with clarity comparable to ex vivo imaging. Quantitative T1, T2, and proton density mapping provide fundamental tissue parameters that reflect hydration, macromolecular content, and microstructural organisation in absolute physical units, independent of the acquisition protocol. Magnetisation transfer imaging reveals the macromolecular environment with particular sensitivity to myelin, while susceptibility-based techniques, including SWI and QSM, visualise and quantify iron, calcium, and venous vasculature with exquisite sensitivity and specificity.

Clinical impact is increasingly evident across neurological subspecialties. In multiple sclerosis, quantitative relaxometry, magnetisation transfer, and susceptibility mapping provide sensitive markers for demyelination, axonal loss, and chronic inflammation, informing prognosis and treatment decisions. Neurodegenerative disease imaging benefits from iron quantification via QSM, myelin assessment via MTI, and quantitative volumetry, enabling earlier detection and sensitive tracking of disease progression.

Synthetic MRI and MRI Fingerprinting represent the vanguard of structural imaging innovation, fundamentally reimagining data acquisition and processing. These techniques demonstrate comprehensive quantitative tissue characterisation through efficient single acquisitions with retrospective arbitrary contrast weighting generation.

Future developments include the continued integration of multiple techniques into comprehensive, multi-parametric protocols that completely characterise tissue properties. Machine learning approaches will enable automated, multi-parametric data analysis, identifying pathology-specific patterns and predicting clinical outcomes, ultimately reshaping our understanding of neurological diseases, diagnosis, and treatment.

Acknowledgments

The authors would like to extend our appreciation to those who offered helpful commentary during the drafting process of this manuscript. We also acknowledge the role the Nova Publishing department played in enabling the work described herein.

References

Deoni, S. C., Rutt, B. K., & Peters, T. M. (2005). Rapid combined T1 and T2 mapping using gradient recalled acquisition in the steady state. *Magnetic Resonance in Medicine*, 53(3), 612-619. https://doi.org/10.1002/mrm.20407.

Fischl, B., & Dale, A. M. (2000). Measuring the thickness of the human cerebral cortex from magnetic resonance images. *Proceedings of the National Academy of Sciences*, 97(20), 11050-11055. https://doi.org/10.1073/pnas.200033797.

Haacke, E. M., Xu, Y., Cheng, Y. C., & Reichenbach, J. R. (2004). Susceptibility weighted imaging (SWI). *Magnetic Resonance in Medicine*, 52(3), 612-618. https://doi.org/10.1002/mrm.20198.

Liu, T., Spincemaille, P., De Rochefort, L., Kressler, B., & Wang, Y. (2009). Calculation of susceptibility through multiple orientation sampling (COSMOS): A method for conditioning the inverse problem from measured magnetic field map to susceptibility source image in MRI. *Magnetic Resonance in Medicine*, 61(1), 196-204. https://doi.org/10.1002/mrm.21828.

Ma, D., Gulani, V., Seiberlich, N., Liu, K., Sunshine, J. L., Duerk, J. L., & Griswold, M. A. (2013). Magnetic resonance fingerprinting. *Nature*, 495(7440), 187-192. https://doi.org/10.1038/nature11971.

Mugler, J. P., & Brookeman, J. R. (1990). Three-dimensional magnetization-prepared rapid gradient-echo imaging (3D MP RAGE). *Magnetic Resonance in Medicine*, 15(1), 152-157. https://doi.org/10.1002/mrm.1910150117.

Wang, Y., & Liu, T. (2015). Quantitative susceptibility mapping (QSM): Decoding MRI data for a tissue magnetic biomarker. *Magnetic Resonance in Medicine*, 73(1), 82-101. https://doi.org/10.1002/mrm.25358.

Warntjes, J. B., Leinhard, O. D., West, J., & Lundberg, P. (2008). Rapid magnetic resonance quantification on the brain: Optimization for clinical usage. *Magnetic Resonance in Medicine*, 60(2), 320-329. https://doi.org/10.1002/mrm.21635.

Wolff, S. D., & Balaban, R. S. (1989). Magnetization transfer contrast (MTC) and tissue water proton relaxation *in vivo*. *Magnetic Resonance in Medicine*, 10(1), 135-144. https://doi.org/10.1002/mrm.1910100113.

Chapter 5

Diffusion MRI and White Matter Imaging

Rajesh S. Kuber[1,*]
and Maajid Mohi Ud Din Malik[2,†]

[1]Department of Radio-Diagnosis, Dr. D. Y. Patil Medical College, Hospital and Research Centre, Dr. D. Y. Patil Vidyapeeth (Deemed to be University)- Sant Tukaram Nagar, Pimpri, Pune, India
[2]Radiology and Imaging Technology, Dr. D. Y. Patil School of Allied Health Sciences, Dr. D. Y. Patil Vidyapeeth (Deemed to be University), Sant Tukaram Nagar, Pimpri, Pune, India

Abstract

Diffusion magnetic resonance imaging has revolutionised our ability to probe white matter microstructure and structural connectivity in the living human brain, providing unique insights into tissue organisation at the microscopic scale by measuring water-molecule diffusion. This chapter comprehensively examines diffusion MRI principles, methodologies, and applications, spanning from basic diffusion-weighted imaging to advanced techniques for characterising complex tissue architecture. We explore the physical basis of diffusion contrast, the tensor model and its derivatives, including fractional anisotropy and mean diffusivity, as well as tractography methods for reconstructing white matter pathways. Advanced techniques, including High Angular Resolution Diffusion Imaging (HARDI), Diffusion Spectrum Imaging (DSI), and Q-ball imaging, are discussed in the context of resolving crossing fibres and complex architectures that confound simple tensor models. The Neurite Orientation Dispersion and Density Imaging (NODDI) framework provides biophysically informed estimates of axonal density and orientation dispersion, thereby bridging the gap between diffusion measurements and tissue microstructure. Clinical applications across white matter disorders, including multiple sclerosis, stroke, brain tumours, and traumatic brain injury, demonstrate the diagnostic and prognostic value of diffusion imaging. These techniques collectively enable non-invasive investigation of white matter integrity, development, plasticity, and pathology with profound implications for neuroscience and clinical neurology.

* Corresponding Author's Email: rajesh.kuber@dpu.edu.in
† Corresponding Author's Email: maajid.malik@dpu.edu.in

In: Recent Advances in Magnetic Resonance Imaging in Neuroimaging
Editors: Maajid Mohi Ud Din Malik, Purnachandra Kawdu Lamghare and R. S. Kuber
ISBN: 979-8-90134-244-2

Keywords: diffusion tensor imaging, tractography, white matter, microstructure, fibre orientation, SDG 3 - good health and well-being

Introduction

The remarkable organisation of white matter, comprising billions of axons organised into coherent bundles that connect distributed brain regions, has long fascinated neuroscientists seeking to understand brain connectivity and information flow. While postmortem dissection and histological techniques have provided valuable insights into white matter anatomy, these methods cannot assess white matter integrity in living individuals, thereby limiting their application to disease investigation and treatment monitoring. Diffusion MRI exploits the thermally-driven random motion of water molecules—Brownian motion—to probe tissue microstructure at scales far below MRI's nominal spatial resolution. In isotropic media, such as cerebrospinal fluid, water molecules diffuse equally in all directions. In contrast, in anisotropic tissues, including white matter, cellular structures restrict and orient diffusion along specific directions. Measuring this directionally dependent diffusion provides exquisite sensitivity to tissue microarchitecture, fibre orientation, and structural integrity.

The development of diffusion MRI for brain imaging dates back to the pioneering work of Denis Le Bihan, Peter Basser, and their colleagues in the late 1980s and early 1990s, which demonstrated that diffusion-weighted imaging could detect acute ischemic stroke before changes appeared on conventional MRI. This transformative clinical application established diffusion imaging as essential for the diagnosis of acute stroke, where early detection enables time-sensitive interventions that can prevent permanent brain damage. The subsequent introduction of diffusion tensor imaging in 1994 by Basser, Mattiello, and Le Bihan revolutionised white matter imaging by providing a mathematical framework for characterising diffusion anisotropy and inferring fibre orientation from the directional dependence of water diffusion. Tractography algorithms, first demonstrated in the late 1990s, enabled the reconstruction of three-dimensional white matter pathways by following diffusion directions through space, thereby creating the fields of *in vivo* white matter anatomy and structural connectomics.

Contemporary diffusion MRI encompasses a rich ecosystem of acquisition and analysis methods that address the limitations of early approaches and expand applications into new domains. The tensor model, while elegant and computationally efficient, assumes Gaussian diffusion and single-fibre populations, assumptions that are violated in substantial regions of the brain where fibres cross, intersect, or fan out. Advanced techniques, including HARDI, DSI, and Q-ball imaging, acquire diffusion data from multiple directions and potentially multiple diffusion weightings, enabling the resolution of crossing fibres and complex fibre configurations. Biophysically informed models, including NODDI, parameterise diffusion in terms of tissue compartments with specific geometries and properties, providing estimates of microstructural features such as axonal density, diameter distribution, and dispersion that relate more directly to tissue biology than empirical diffusion metrics. These methodological advances, combined with improvements in gradient hardware, multi-band imaging, and denoising algorithms, have established diffusion MRI as a cornerstone of modern neuroimaging with applications spanning development, ageing, learning, psychiatric disorders, and virtually all neurological diseases affecting white or Grey matter microstructure.

5.1. Principles of Diffusion-Weighted Imaging

Diffusion-weighted imaging leverages the MRI signal's sensitivity to microscopic translational motion of water molecules, providing contrast and quantitative information on tissue microstructure, cellularity, and organisation. The physical basis lies in the random thermal motion of molecules—Brownian motion—that causes water molecules to explore their local environment over time. In free water at body temperature, molecules diffuse with a diffusion coefficient of approximately 3.0×10^{-3} mm^2/s, moving root-mean-square distances of about 17 micrometres in 50 milliseconds, which is the typical diffusion time in MRI experiments. Biological tissues restrict and orient this diffusion through cellular membranes, myelin sheaths, axonal structure, and other microanatomical features, reducing apparent diffusion coefficients to $0.7\text{-}1.0 \times 10^{-3}$ mm^2/s in brain tissue. By measuring the distance and direction of water molecule movement during a controlled diffusion time, MRI can probe tissue structure at microscopic scales far below its nominal spatial resolution (Le Bihan et al., 1986).

The Stejskal-Tanner pulsed gradient spin-echo sequence forms the foundation of diffusion MRI, employing matched pairs of intense magnetic-field gradient pulses to encode molecular position and detect displacement. The sequence begins with a 90-degree radiofrequency pulse that creates transverse magnetisation, followed by a diffusion-encoding gradient pulse of amplitude G and duration δ, applied along a specific direction. This gradient imparts a position-dependent phase to spins, with the phase being proportional to the position along the gradient direction. After a time interval Δ (the diffusion time), a second gradient pulse of equal amplitude and duration is applied, ideally refocusing spins that have not moved. However, molecules that diffuse between gradient pulses occupy different positions during the second gradient, leading to incomplete refocusing and signal attenuation. The degree of attenuation depends on the extent of molecular displacement, providing diffusion sensitivity proportional to the b-value, defined as $b = \gamma^2 G^2 \delta^2 (\Delta - \delta/3)$, where γ is the nuclear gyromagnetic ratio.

The signal attenuation in diffusion-weighted imaging follows an exponential relationship with b-value and apparent diffusion coefficient (ADC): $S = S_0 \exp(-b \times \text{ADC})$, where S is the diffusion-weighted signal, S_0 is the signal without diffusion weighting (b=0), and ADC represents the apparent diffusion coefficient along the gradient direction. This relationship enables quantitative diffusion measurement by acquiring images at multiple b-values and fitting the exponential decay. Typical clinical protocols employ b-values of 1000 s/mm^2 for brain imaging, balancing diffusion sensitivity against signal-to-noise ratio, while research applications may extend to 3000 s/mm^2 or higher to probe restricted diffusion and microstructure. The ADC reflects not proper molecular diffusion but "apparent" diffusion, hindered and limited by tissue structures, with values varying across brain regions based on tissue composition, cellularity, and organisation.

The physical mechanisms restricting diffusion in brain tissue involve multiple spatial scales and structural elements. Cell membranes present partial barriers to diffusion, with water exchange between intra- and extracellular compartments occurring on timescales comparable to those of diffusion, resulting in restricted diffusion behaviour. In white matter, myelin sheaths surrounding axons create concentric barriers that severely restrict diffusion perpendicular to fibres while permitting relatively free diffusion parallel to fibres, generating the high diffusion anisotropy characteristic of organised white matter. The tortuosity of the extracellular space, created by tightly packed cells and processes, restricts diffusion even within the extracellular compartment. In Grey matter, dendritic and axonal arbours create a complex environment with more isotropic restrictions, although subtle anisotropy exists, reflecting columnar organisation and dominant fibre orientations. These restrictions reduce apparent diffusion coefficients and create directional dependence, revealing tissue microarchitecture.

Clinical diffusion-weighted imaging protocols typically acquire images with diffusion weighting in three orthogonal directions (x, y, z) plus a b=0 reference image, enabling calculation of trace ADC maps that average diffusion in all directions and are relatively insensitive to fibre orientation. Trace-weighted images, calculated as the geometric mean of diffusion-weighted images in three orthogonal directions, provide diffusion contrast less dependent on fibre orientation than single-direction images. The exponentially weighted signal creates a strong contrast where diffusion is restricted, with high cellularity regions, including tumours, acute infarcts, and abscesses appearing bright on diffusion-weighted images and dark on ADC maps. This reverse relationship between DWI signal and ADC value can confuse; a bright signal on DWI may indicate restricted diffusion (low ADC, as in acute stroke) or T2 shine-through (elevated T2 signal contaminating DWI), distinguishable by examining the ADC map, where proper restricted diffusion shows low values (Moseley et al., 1990).

The primary clinical application of diffusion-weighted imaging remains the detection of acute ischemic stroke, where cytotoxic oedema causes a dramatic reduction in ADC within minutes of arterial occlusion, resulting in a bright signal on DWI and a dark signal on ADC maps. The mechanism involves the failure of ATP-dependent ion pumps, causing cell swelling and a reduction in extracellular space, which restricts diffusion before changes appear on T2-weighted or FLAIR imaging. The sensitivity and specificity of DWI for acute stroke exceed 95%, establishing it as the gold standard for early stroke diagnosis. The ADC value progressively decreases in the first hours after stroke, reaches a minimum around day 3-5, then pseudonormalizes as vasogenic oedema develops, and eventually increases in chronic infarction as tissue becomes cystic. This temporal evolution enables approximate age determination of strokes and detection of multiple stroke events at different time points.

Beyond stroke, diffusion-weighted imaging provides valuable diagnostic information across a wide range of pathologies. Abscesses exhibit restricted diffusion due to the high viscosity of the purulent material and high cellularity, distinguishing them from cystic or necrotic tumours, which exhibit facilitated diffusion. Highly cellular tumours, including medulloblastoma, lymphoma, and some glioblastomas, exhibit restricted diffusion, whereas lower-grade tumours and cystic lesions show facilitated diffusion, aiding in tissue characterisation and biopsy targeting. Prion diseases, including Creutzfeldt-Jakob disease, produce characteristic cortical and basal ganglia diffusion restriction. Seizures can cause transient diffusion restriction in the affected cortex, while diffusion changes help identify epileptogenic zones in temporal lobe epilepsy. Traumatic brain injury results in diffusion abnormalities in white matter, reflecting axonal injury, with ADC values correlating with injury severity and functional outcomes. Table 5.1 presents the diffusion-weighted imaging characteristics of common pathologies.

Table 5.1. Diffusion-weighted imaging characteristics in common pathologies

Pathology	DWI Signal	ADC Value	Time Course	Mechanism	Diagnostic Implications
Acute Infarct	Bright	Decreased (↓30-50%)	Minutes to hours	Cytotoxic edema	Enables hyperacute diagnosis
Abscess	Bright	Decreased	Stable	High cellularity, viscosity	Distinguishes from tumour necrosis
Cellular Tumour	Bright	Decreased	Variable	High cellularity	Suggests high-grade histology
Chronic Infarct	Dark	Increased	Weeks to years	Cystic degeneration	Indicates an old lesion
Vasogenic Edema	Variable	Increased	Hours to days	Extracellular expansion	Tumour, inflammation surrounding
Epidermoid Cyst	Bright	Decreased	Stable	Keratin debris, high viscosity	Distinguishes from an arachnoid cyst
Seizure (ictal)	Bright	Decreased	Hours to days	Cytotoxic edema	Transient, reversible

5.2. Diffusion Tensor Imaging (DTI) and Tractography

Diffusion tensor imaging extends diffusion-weighted imaging by characterising the complete three-dimensional diffusion profile through measurements of diffusion in multiple directions, enabling the quantification of diffusion anisotropy and the inference of fibre orientation. The mathematical framework models diffusion as a second-order tensor—a 3×3 symmetric matrix—that fully describes how diffusion varies with direction at each voxel. This tensor representation captures the magnitude and directionality of diffusion through six independent parameters: three eigenvalues representing diffusion coefficients along three orthogonal principal directions, and three angles specifying the orientation of these principal directions. The tensor model assumes Gaussian diffusion, meaning the diffusion-weighted signal follows a monoexponential decay with the b-value, and that a single, coherent fibre population dominates each voxel. While these assumptions are violated in regions with crossing fibres or complex tissue architecture, the tensor model offers a computationally efficient characterisation suitable for many clinical and research applications (Basser et al., 1994).

The acquisition of diffusion tensor data requires the measurement of diffusion in at least six non-collinear directions, plus a b=0 reference image, which provides sufficient information to solve for the six unknown tensor elements. Clinical protocols typically employ 20-64 directions to improve tensor estimation accuracy and signal-to-noise ratio through averaging. Higher angular resolution, with more directions, enhances the reliability of derived metrics and tractography but increases acquisition time proportionally. Modern protocols employ multi-shell acquisition schemes that measure diffusion at multiple b-values, providing additional information about the diffusion regime and enabling more sophisticated analysis beyond the tensor model. The choice of b-value significantly impacts DTI metrics: lower b-values (700-1000 s/mm^2) emphasise hindered diffusion, which is sensitive to tissue spacing and tortuosity, while higher b-values (2000-3000 s/mm^2) probe restricted diffusion, which is sensitive to barriers and compartment sizes.

The eigendecomposition of the diffusion tensor yields three eigenvalues (λ_1, λ_2, λ_3) and corresponding eigenvectors representing the principal diffusion directions. The primary eigenvector corresponds to the largest eigenvalue and indicates the predominant direction of diffusion, typically aligned with the fibre orientation in white matter. The eigenvalues quantify the magnitude of diffusion along each principal direction, with λ_1 representing diffusion parallel to fibres (axial diffusivity) and the mean of λ_2 and λ_3 representing diffusion perpendicular to fibres (radial diffusivity). From these parameters, numerous scalar metrics can be derived that quantify different aspects of diffusion. Mean diffusivity (MD), the average of the three eigenvalues, represents the orientation-independent magnitude of diffusion, analogous to the trace of the ADC. Fractional anisotropy (FA), ranging from 0 (isotropic diffusion) to 1 (diffusion in a single direction only), quantifies the degree of diffusion directionality, with values of 0.7-0.9 in significant white matter tracts, 0.1-0.3 in Grey matter, and near 0 in cerebrospinal fluid.

Fractional anisotropy has emerged as the most widely used DTI metric, providing a sensitive yet nonspecific marker of white matter integrity. The mathematical definition $FA = \sqrt{[3/2]} \times \sqrt{[(\lambda_1\text{-MD})^2 + (\lambda_2\text{-MD})^2 + (\lambda_3\text{-MD})^2]} / \sqrt{[\lambda_1^2 + \lambda_2^2 + \lambda_3^2]}$ creates a normalised measure of how much diffusion deviates from isotropic. High FA in white matter reflects coherent fibre organisation, with restricted diffusion perpendicular to fibres and relatively free diffusion parallel to them. Numerous pathological processes reduce FA through different mechanisms: demyelination increases radial diffusivity by removing the restrictive myelin barrier; axonal loss reduces axial diffusivity by eliminating the coherent directional structure; oedema increases both axial and radial diffusivity by expanding extracellular space; and crossing fibres create apparent isotropy by introducing multiple diffusion directions. This lack of specificity limits the interpretation of FA without additional metrics or prior knowledge; however, its sensitivity to white matter integrity makes FA valuable for detecting abnormalities and tracking changes (Pierpaoli & Basser, 1996).

Axial and radial diffusivity provide complementary information about the nature of white matter alterations. Axial diffusivity (AD = λ_1) measures diffusion parallel to the primary fibre direction, sensitive to axonal integrity, with decreases potentially indicating axonal damage or loss. Radial diffusivity (RD = mean[λ_2, λ_3]) measures diffusion perpendicular to fibres, is sensitive to myelin integrity, and increases may potentially indicate demyelination. The mechanistic interpretation of these metrics is derived from animal studies, where specific pathologies produce characteristic patterns: demyelination increases RD while preserving AD; axonal injury reduces AD, while RD remains stable or increases; combined pathology affects both. However, translating these patterns to human disease is complicated by complex, heterogeneous pathology, crossing fibres that violate tensor assumptions, and the long-time scales over which human pathology evolves. Despite these caveats, AD and RD have proven valuable for characterising white matter changes in development, ageing, and disease.

Tractography algorithms reconstruct three-dimensional white matter pathways by integrating local fibre orientations to trace connections between brain regions. Deterministic tractography begins at seed points and follows the primary eigenvector direction, stepping small distances (typically 0.5-1 mm) and updating direction at each step based on the local tensor orientation. Streamlines continue until reaching target regions, exiting the brain mask, entering low-anisotropy regions (suggesting Grey matter or crossing fibres), or exceeding angular thresholds (indicating implausible sharp turns). Deterministic tracking is fast and intuitive, but it struggles to represent uncertainty in fibre orientation and tends to terminate prematurely in low-anisotropy regions. Probabilistic tractography addresses these limitations by treating fibre orientation as uncertain and sampling from orientation distributions at each step, thereby generating many candidate streamlines whose spatial distribution represents the connectivity probability rather than definite fibre pathways (Behrens et al., 2003).

Tractography applications span presurgical planning, where mapping eloquent white matter pathways helps neurosurgeons avoid damage to motor, language, or visual pathways; connectomics research, which constructs brain graphs with nodes representing brain regions and edges representing structural connections; and the investigation of connectivity changes in development, learning, ageing, and disease. The validation of tractography remains challenging, as gold-standard methods for human white matter anatomy are limited to post-mortem dissection in small samples or tracer studies in animals. Comparison studies reveal both strengths and significant limitations: tractography successfully reconstructs major pathways. Still, it exhibits high false-positive rates (reconstructing non-existent connections) and false-negative rates (missing known connections), particularly for long-range and small pathways. These limitations motivate the development of advanced techniques, including constrained spherical deconvolution tractography, global tracking that optimises entire configurations rather than individual streamlines, and the combination with functional data to validate anatomical reconstructions.

5.3. High Angular Resolution Diffusion Imaging (HARDI)

High Angular Resolution Diffusion Imaging represents a family of techniques that acquire diffusion data in many directions (typically 60-256) at one or more b-values, enabling reconstruction of the orientation distribution function (ODF) and resolution of complex fibre architectures, including crossing, kissing, and fanning fibres that violate the tensor model's single-fibre assumption. Crossing fibres affect approximately 60-90% of white matter voxels at typical clinical resolutions, creating apparent isotropy in tensor-based analyses where multiple coherent fibre populations exist. HARDI methods reconstruct the angular distribution of diffusion or fibre orientations, representing how much diffusion or how many fibres point in each direction, which enables the identification of multiple fibre peaks within a single voxel. This capability significantly improves tractography accuracy in complex regions, including the centrum semiovale, where the corona radiata and corpus callosum fibres intersect; the brainstem, where multiple ascending and descending tracts intermingle; and association fibre crossings throughout the hemispheric white matter (Tuch et al., 2002).

The physical basis of HARDI lies in the recognition that diffusion-weighted signals from complex fibre configurations exhibit directional variations that the tensor model cannot capture. When fibres cross at 90 degrees with equal volume fractions, the tensor model produces isotropic diffusion (FA≈0), losing all information about fibre orientations present. HARDI acquisitions sample the angular space densely enough to resolve the directional variation caused by each fibre population, allowing for decomposition into constituent orientations. The orientation distribution function represents the probability or magnitude of diffusion in each direction on the unit sphere, with peaks indicating fibre orientations. Various mathematical frameworks reconstruct ODFs from HARDI data, including Q-ball imaging using spherical harmonic decomposition, diffusion spectrum imaging employing Fourier transformation, and constrained spherical deconvolution, which assumes specific fibre response functions. Each framework has distinct assumptions, computational requirements, and performance characteristics.

Q-ball imaging, introduced by Tuch and colleagues, provides model-free ODF estimation by transforming diffusion-weighted signals sampled on a spherical shell in q-space (the reciprocal space of the diffusion encoding vectors). The technique utilises spherical harmonic basis functions to represent the variation in diffusion-weighted signals across different directions. Then, it applies the Funk-Radon transform to yield the ODF, which displays the angular fibre density. Q-ball requires acquisition on a single shell (constant b-value) with many directions, typically 60-128, enabling relatively fast scanning compared to multi-shell methods. The ODF peaks indicate fibre orientations, with peak heights corresponding to the volume fractions of the fibres. Higher-order spherical harmonics (typically order 4-8) enable sharper ODF peaks and better angular resolution but require more gradient directions and are more sensitive to noise. Q-ball imaging successfully resolves up to three fibre orientations per voxel in well-conditioned scenarios, substantially improving tractography through crossing regions compared to DTI.

Constrained spherical deconvolution (CSD) employs a signal model assuming that the diffusion-weighted signal is generated by the convolution of a fibre orientation distribution with a single-fibre response function characterising the signal from a perfectly aligned fibre population. By deconvolving the observed signal with this response function, estimated from high-anisotropy voxels that presumably contain single-fibre populations, CSD recovers the fibre orientation distribution (FOD), indicating the extent to which fibres point in each direction. The constrained optimisation ensures non-negativity of the FOD, preventing spurious negative peaks that can arise in unconstrained deconvolution. CSD typically produces sharper peaks than Q-ball with better angular resolution and improved specificity to fibre orientations rather than total diffusion. Multi-shell CSD variants that utilise data across multiple b-values further enhance performance by capturing diffusion information at different length scales. The technique has become widely adopted for research tractography due to excellent performance and availability in popular software packages (Tournier et al., 2004).

The clinical translation of HARDI methods faces barriers, including increased acquisition time, complex processing, and limited validation of clinical utility beyond DTI. Acquiring 60-128 directions rather than 20-30 for DTI increases scan time proportionally, which challenges patient cooperation and limits throughput. Processing HARDI data requires specialised software and expertise beyond the clinical routine, although user-friendly tools are emerging. The improved tractography accuracy in crossing regions, as clearly demonstrated in research studies, has not yet been widely adopted in clinical practice, partly because clinical decision-making often succeeds with DTI-based tractography despite its known inaccuracies. Applications where HARDI clearly provides clinical value include the precise delineation of the optic radiation trajectory in epilepsy surgery planning, where crossing fibres from multiple pathways complicate DTI tractography, and the differentiation of tumour infiltration versus displaced fibres, where multiple fibre orientations help distinguish these scenarios.

Multi-shell diffusion imaging acquires data at multiple b-values, typically 2-4 shells with b-values spanning 700-3000 s/mm^2, providing information about diffusion at multiple spatial scales. Lower b-values probe hindered diffusion in the extracellular space, while higher b-values become increasingly sensitive to restricted diffusion in cellular compartments. This multi-scale information enables more sophisticated analysis, including the separation of isotropic and anisotropic diffusion components, the estimation of axonal water fraction, and the fitting of biophysical models that require data at multiple diffusion weightings. Multi-shell protocols are increasingly adopted as the standard for advanced diffusion imaging, providing a rich dataset that supports multiple analysis approaches, from DTI (using only the low-b-value shell) to HARDI to microstructural modelling. The optimal shell placement and direction distribution remain active areas of investigation, balancing angular resolution per shell with the number of shells for characterising the diffusion regime.

Advanced tractography using HARDI data substantially improves reconstruction accuracy by better handling crossing regions and reducing premature termination. Deterministic tracking using CSD-derived fibre orientation distributions follows the peak nearest the incoming direction at each step, successfully navigating through crossings by maintaining the correct fibre population across the junction. Probabilistic tracking samples from the FOD at each step, generating distributions of connectivity that better represent uncertainty than DTI-based probabilistic tracking. Global tractography methods optimise entire tractogram configurations to explain observed diffusion data best while satisfying anatomical and geometric constraints, showing promise for reducing false-positive connections. Quantitative evaluation using tract density imaging and comparison to histological fibre orientations reveals clear improvements over DTI tractography. However, substantial challenges remain in reliably reconstructing small, long-range, and bilateral pathways. Table 5.2 compares advanced diffusion MRI acquisition methods.

Table 5.2. Comparison of advanced diffusion MRI acquisition methods

Method	Gradient Directions	B-values	Acquisition Time	Key Advantages	Limitations	Primary Applications
DTI	20-64	1 (1000 s/mm²)	3-8 min	Fast, established, metrics available	Single fibre assumption	Clinical, screening, basic research
Q-ball (HARDI)	60-128	1 (1000-3000)	8-15 min	Resolves crossings, model-free	Single shell, lower angular resolution	Research tractography
Constrained SD	45-90	1-3 shells	10-20 min	Sharp FODs, multi-shell option	Requires a response function	Advanced tractography
Diffusion Spectrum	200-500	Multiple (many b)	30-60 min	Most complete, true ODF	Very long acquisition	Research, validation
Multi-shell (NODDI)	30-60 per shell	2-3 shells	12-20 min	Microstructure modeling	Model-dependent	Microstructure quantification

5.4. Diffusion Spectrum Imaging and Q-Ball Imaging

Diffusion Spectrum Imaging represents the most comprehensive approach to characterising diffusion, acquiring diffusion-weighted data across a Cartesian grid in q-space—the reciprocal space of displacement—enabling direct reconstruction of the ensemble-average propagator (EAP) via Fourier transformation. The EAP represents the probability distribution of molecular displacements over the diffusion time, a complete description of diffusion behaviour from which all other diffusion metrics and orientation information can be derived. DSI requires no assumptions about the number of fibre populations or the diffusion model, providing model-free characterisation limited only by the spatial and angular resolution achievable within practical scan time constraints. The technique samples q-space at multiple points (typically 203-515) at b-values ranging from 8000 to 10000 s/mm², capturing both angular variation, indicating various fibre orientations, and radial variation, reflecting restricted diffusion and compartmentalisation. From the reconstructed EAP, the orientation distribution function is extracted by radial integration, revealing fibre orientations with high angular resolution (Wedeen et al., 2005).

The acquisition requirements of DSI—several hundred diffusion-weighted images at high b-values—result in examination times of 30-60 minutes for whole-brain coverage, which limits clinical applicability and often exceeds patient cooperation limits. However, the complete diffusion characterisation provided by DSI establishes it as a gold standard for validating more efficient methods and for research applications where acquisition time is not a limiting factor. The high b-values employed in DSI enhance angular resolution by emphasising restricted diffusion effects that create sharper directional variations, but require strong gradients (up to 300 mT/m in human systems) and substantially reduce the signal-to-noise ratio. Advanced denoising and reconstruction methods, including compressed sensing and radial sampling schemes, minimise acquisition time by 2-4 times while maintaining acceptable quality, thereby improving the practicality of DSI for research studies. The technique has been applied primarily in research settings to map detailed connectional anatomy and validate other diffusion methods.

Q-ball imaging, previously discussed in the context of HARDI, warrants a detailed examination as a practical alternative to DSI, offering similar orientation resolution with substantially reduced acquisition time. The mathematical elegance of Q-ball lies in its model-free estimation of ODFs, which utilises only single-shell data and analytical transformations, thereby avoiding iterative optimisation and extensive sampling. The technique begins by expanding the diffusion-weighted signal in spherical harmonics, an orthogonal basis set for functions on the sphere analogous to a Fourier series for periodic functions. Typically, 4th, 6th, or 8th order spherical harmonics are employed, requiring a minimum of 15, 28, or 45 gradient directions, respectively, to avoid underdetermination. The Funk-Radon transform, applied to the spherical harmonic representation, yields the ODF analytically. This transformation integrates the signal over great circles perpendicular to each direction, extracting the component of diffusion pointing in that direction.

The ODF peaks in Q-ball imaging indicate fibre orientations; however, the relationship between peak height and fibre volume fraction is complex and influenced by multiple factors, including fibre coherence, diameter distribution, and diffusion characteristics. Quantitative anisotropy metrics can be derived from ODFs, including generalised fractional anisotropy (GFA), which quantifies the extent to which the ODF deviates from isotropy, analogous to fractional anisotropy in DTI. Peak directions and amplitudes enable sophisticated tractography that respects multiple fibre orientations in each voxel. The quality of Q-ball reconstruction depends critically on sampling density and distribution, with uniform coverage of the sphere providing optimal angular resolution. Optimisation of gradient direction sets using electrostatic repulsion or spherical codes ensures uniform sampling, improving ODF reconstruction quality and reducing artefacts from non-uniform sampling.

The analytical Q-ball was further refined through several methodological enhancements, thereby improving accuracy and robustness. Constrained estimation approaches enforce non-negativity and smoothness constraints, thereby reducing spurious peaks caused by noise and enhancing anatomical plausibility. Assuming multi-exponential rather than single-exponential decay enables better handling of crossing fibres with different diffusion characteristics. Combining solid angle corrections improves the quantitative accuracy of peak heights, thereby better preserving volume fraction information. Despite these refinements, Q-ball remains fundamentally limited to single-shell acquisitions, potentially missing information from multi-scale diffusion characterisation available with multi-shell protocols. This limitation motivated the development of generalised Q-ball and multi-shell extensions that maintain the model-free character while exploiting multi-shell data.

Comparison studies between DSI, Q-ball, and tensor-based methods reveal trade-offs between information content, acquisition efficiency, and clinical practicality. DSI provides the most complete characterisation, successfully resolving up to four fibre orientations and characterising complex geometries, including fanning and bending; however, it requires impractically long acquisition times for clinical use. Q-ball achieves similar orientation resolution with 3-4 times faster acquisition, reliably resolving two to three fibre orientations, making it more practical for research studies with limited scan time. Both substantially outperform DTI across regions while showing similar performance in single-fibre areas. For clinical applications requiring efficient whole-brain coverage, multi-shell protocols with 60-90 total directions across 2-3 shells provide an attractive compromise, enabling both HARDI analysis and microstructural modelling from a single 10–15-minute acquisition.

Advanced applications of DSI and Q-ball imaging extend beyond tractography to the investigation of microstructural properties and tissue characterisation. The mean-squared displacement derived from the EAP quantifies the average molecular displacement, providing complementary information to ADC about the diffusion regime and restriction. The return-to-origin probability, which represents the likelihood of molecules returning to their starting location, increases in more restricted environments and correlates with cellularity. The non-Gaussian diffusion characteristics, quantified by metrics such as kurtosis and higher-order moments, reflect tissue complexity and may serve as specific biomarkers for pathological processes. These microstructural metrics, derived from comprehensive diffusion characterisation, show promise for distinguishing tumour types, grading gliomas, and assessing treatment response, although clinical validation remains limited.

5.5. Neurite Orientation Dispersion and Density Imaging (NODDI)

Neurite Orientation Dispersion and Density Imaging represents a biophysical modelling framework that relates diffusion MRI measurements to specific microstructural tissue properties through a mechanistic multi-compartment model. Rather than empirically describing diffusion through metrics like FA or MD, NODDI estimates physiologically-meaningful parameters, including intracellular volume fraction (neurite density), orientation dispersion (how parallel neurites are), and isotropic diffusion fraction (free water), parameters that relate more directly to tissue biology and potentially provide more specific biomarkers of pathology. The technique employs practical multi-shell acquisitions, which can be obtained in 10-15 minutes, making it clinically feasible while providing microstructural specificity beyond DTI. NODDI has been applied to investigate brain development, where neurite density and organisation change dramatically; neurodegenerative diseases, characterised by axonal loss and disorganisation; and psychiatric disorders, where subtle microstructural alterations may underlie symptoms (Zhang et al., 2012).

The NODDI model partitions tissue water into three compartments with distinct diffusion characteristics: intracellular water within neurites (axons and dendrites), exhibiting highly restricted diffusion; extracellular water between neurites, showing hindered diffusion; and cerebrospinal fluid, exhibiting free, isotropic diffusion. The intracellular compartment is modelled as sticks—infinitely thin cylinders with zero radius—restricting diffusion perpendicular to the neurite orientation but allowing free diffusion parallel to the neurites. Neurite orientations follow a Watson distribution characterised by a dispersion parameter describing how tightly oriented neurites are around a principal direction. The extracellular compartment is modelled as anisotropic Gaussian diffusion, with perpendicular and parallel diffusivities determined by geometric constraints from neurite packing. The CSF compartment exhibits isotropic Gaussian diffusion with fixed diffusivity of free water. The model includes three fitted parameters: neurite density index (NDI), which represents the intracellular volume fraction; orientation dispersion index (ODI), which quantifies the spread of neurite orientations; and isotropic volume fraction (f_{iso}), which represents CSF contamination.

Neurite density index provides an estimate of intracellular volume fraction ranging from 0 (no neurites) to 1 (all water intracellular), though biological neurite density typically ranges from 0.3-0.8 across Grey and white matter. NDI increases during development as axons myelinate and dendrites elaborate, plateaus in adulthood, and may decrease in neurodegenerative conditions involving axonal loss or dendritic pruning. In white matter, NDI correlates with axonal packing density measured histologically, while in Grey matter, it reflects the combined density of axons, dendrites, and dendritic spines. The metric shows high values in densely packed white matter tracts, such as the corpus callosum and corticospinal tract, intermediate values in less dense association fibres, and lower values in Grey matter, where neurite density is lower and orientation is more dispersed. Importantly, NDI is relatively independent of fibre orientation and crossing fibre geometry, providing more specific microstructural information than FA, which conflates density, orientation coherence, and geometry.

The orientation dispersion index quantifies the angular variance of neurite orientations, ranging from 0 (perfectly parallel) to 1 (isotropically distributed), and captures aspects of tissue organisation that are complementary to density. ODI remains low (0.05-0.2) in coherent white matter tracts where fibres are well-aligned, increases at crossing regions where multiple fibre populations create apparent dispersion (though this violates the single-orientation-distribution assumption), and reaches high values (0.5-0.9) in Grey matter where dendritic arbours extend in multiple directions, creating intrinsic dispersion. During brain development, ODI may decrease in white matter as axons align and organise into coherent bundles, and increase in Grey matter as dendritic arbours mature and elaborate. In pathology, ODI increases may reflect disorganisation from demyelination, inflammation, or degeneration. The combination of NDI and ODI provides richer tissue characterisation than FA alone, potentially enabling more specific identification of pathological processes and developmental patterns.

The practical implementation of NODDI requires multi-shell diffusion data with at least two shells at different b-values (typically 700 and 2000 s/mm^2) plus b=0 images, with 30-60 gradient directions distributed across shells. Higher b-value data are critical for estimating the intracellular fraction, as restricted diffusion becomes more apparent at higher b-values, whereas lower b-values constrain extracellular diffusion properties. The fitting procedure employs non-linear optimisation to find parameter values that minimise the difference between model predictions and observed signals, typically requiring several minutes per voxel on standard hardware. Accelerated fitting using lookup tables or neural networks reduces processing time to seconds per voxel, enabling practical whole-brain analysis. The model makes several simplifying assumptions, including negligible effects of axonal diameter, fixed intrinsic diffusivities, and a single predominant orientation per voxel. These assumptions may be violated in some tissues, but enable practical parameter estimation from clinically feasible acquisitions.

Applications of NODDI have demonstrated sensitivity to development, ageing, and disease processes across multiple neurological and psychiatric conditions. In brain development, NDI increases and ODI decreases in white matter from infancy through adolescence, reflecting ongoing myelination and axonal organisation, whereas grey matter exhibits more complex patterns. Ageing studies reveal decreased NDI in white matter, suggesting progressive axonal loss, and increased ODI, potentially reflecting disorganisation or increased crossing fibres resulting from selective degeneration. Multiple sclerosis is characterised by reduced NDI within lesions, which correlates with axonal loss. Normal-appearing white matter exhibits subtle alterations that precede focal lesion development. Alzheimer's disease is characterised by decreased NDI in affected cortical regions and connecting white matter tracts, consistent with neuronal loss and synaptic degeneration. Schizophrenia and autism spectrum disorder studies report altered NDI and ODI in the specific areas, though findings are heterogeneous across studies and patient populations.

Extensions and alternatives to NODDI address model limitations and expand capabilities. NODDI-DTI combines NODDI compartments with tensor-based modelling, enabling the resolution of crossing fibres while maintaining biophysical interpretation. Multi-compartment microscopic diffusion imaging (MC-MDI) employs more detailed compartment models, including finite axon diameters and multiple fibre populations. WMTI (white matter tract integrity) derived from diffusion kurtosis imaging provides related microstructural metrics from more widely available single-shell high-b-value data. ActiveAx and AxCaliber techniques estimate axon diameter distributions from very high b-value data with strong gradients, although they require specialised hardware and long acquisitions. The choice between these approaches depends on available acquisition time, gradient strength, the specific microstructural questions, and tolerance for model assumptions. NODDI's practical acquisition requirements and robust parameter estimation have made it the most widely adopted biophysical diffusion model to date.

5.6. Clinical Applications in White Matter Disorders

Diffusion MRI has become indispensable for the clinical evaluation of white matter disorders, providing sensitive detection of microstructural abnormalities, objective quantification of disease severity, and prognostic information that is often unavailable from conventional imaging. Multiple sclerosis is the most extensively studied white matter disease using diffusion imaging, where DTI metrics reveal pathology in both focal lesions visible on T2-weighted imaging and in normal-appearing white matter that appears unremarkable on conventional sequences. Within acute MS lesions, mean diffusivity increases due to oedema and inflammation, while FA decreases, reflecting disrupted tissue architecture. Chronic lesions exhibit more pronounced FA reduction, accompanied by variable changes in MD, depending on the balance between demyelination, axonal loss, and gliosis. Normal-appearing white matter demonstrates subtle but measurable DTI abnormalities in MS patients compared to healthy controls, with reduced FA and increased MD, suggesting diffuse microscopic pathology. These metrics correlate with disability and predict disease progression, providing potential biomarkers for treatment monitoring and clinical trial endpoints (Ciccarelli et al., 2008).

The clinical value of diffusion imaging in MS extends to predicting conversion from clinically isolated syndrome to definite MS, where baseline DTI abnormalities in normal-appearing brain tissue are associated with higher conversion rates. Longitudinal DTI tracking of disease progression reveals that white matter tract integrity, as assessed through tract-based spatial statistics or tractometry, declines over time at varying rates, depending on the tract and disease phenotype. Progressive MS shows more pronounced DTI abnormalities than relapsing-remitting disease, consistent with greater axonal loss in progressive forms. Advanced diffusion techniques, including NODDI and multi-compartment models, provide more specific tissue characterisation, distinguishing between axonal loss, demyelination, and inflammation, and potentially enabling more targeted treatment selection. Diffusion imaging of Grey matter, particularly cortex and deep nuclei, reveals pathology correlating strongly with cognitive impairment, highlighting the importance of Grey matter involvement in MS disability.

Stroke imaging leverages diffusion's exquisite sensitivity to cytotoxic oedema for the hyperacute diagnosis and treatment planning of strokes. The dramatic ADC reduction in ischemic tissue—appearing within minutes of arterial occlusion and preceding changes on all other MRI sequences—enables identification of acute infarction in the critical time window when thrombolytic therapy can prevent permanent damage. The combination of diffusion and perfusion imaging defines the ischemic penumbra—tissue with perfusion deficit but preserved diffusion, representing salvageable brain at risk. The diffusion-perfusion mismatch guides treatment decisions, including thrombolysis and thrombectomy, with larger mismatch ratios indicating greater potential for tissue salvage by reperfusion. Post-treatment diffusion imaging assesses infarct volume, predicts functional outcomes, and detects hemorrhagic transformation or delayed infarct growth. Chronic infarcts demonstrate dramatically elevated ADC reflecting cystic transformation, enabling age estimation, and distinguishing old from new infarcts in patients with multiple stroke events.

Traumatic brain injury produces diffuse white matter damage—diffuse axonal injury—that may be invisible on CT and conventional MRI but readily detectable through diffusion-weighted MRI. Acute DAI exhibits reduced FA and variable ADC changes, reflecting cytotoxic oedema, axonal swelling, and disrupted axonal architecture. The spatial pattern and extent of white matter injury correlate with injury severity, as assessed by the Glasgow Coma Scale, and predict functional outcomes, including return to work, cognitive recovery, and persistent disability. Mild traumatic brain injury—concussion—often appears normal on conventional imaging but shows subtle DTI abnormalities in frontal and temporal white matter, corpus callosum, and brainstem, correlating with post-concussive symptoms. Longitudinal DTI in TBI tracks recovery and persistent changes, with some abnormalities improving as acute oedema resolves, while others persist or progress, reflecting ongoing degeneration. Advanced techniques, including NODDI, offer a more precise assessment of axonal versus myelin damage, potentially informing rehabilitation and prognosis.

Brain tumour diffusion imaging aids diagnosis, grading, treatment planning, and monitoring. Tumour cellularity correlates inversely with ADC, with highly cellular tumours, including medulloblastoma, lymphoma, and high-grade gliomas, showing restricted diffusion. In contrast, low-grade gliomas and metastases exhibit more variable ADC values, depending on cellularity and necrosis. ADC values help distinguish tumour types when imaging appearance is ambiguous, such as differentiating between high-grade glioma and CNS lymphoma or metastasis. The minimum ADC within tumours predicts histological grade and prognosis in gliomas, with lower values indicating a higher grade and worse outcomes. Fractional anisotropy (FA) around tumours helps distinguish infiltrating tumour from displaced white matter: reduced FA suggests infiltration, while preserved FA indicates displacement. This information is valuable for surgical planning and radiotherapy targeting. Post-treatment diffusion changes help differentiate tumour progression from treatment effects, including pseudoprogression and radiation necrosis, with recurrent tumours showing lower ADC values than treatment effects.

White matter tract integrity in neurodegenerative diseases exhibits characteristic patterns that reflect the selective vulnerability of specific systems. Amyotrophic lateral sclerosis demonstrates prominent corticospinal tract degeneration with reduced FA and increased MD in the motor cortex, internal capsule, cerebral peduncles, and spinal cord, correlating with disease severity and predicting survival. Primary lateral sclerosis shows similar patterns with more upper motor neuron-predominant changes. Alzheimer's disease reveals early changes in temporal lobe white matter, particularly the cingulum bundle and fornix connecting to the hippocampus, with FA reduction correlating with cognitive impairment and predicting conversion from mild cognitive impairment. Frontotemporal dementia is characterised by prominent white matter changes in the frontal and temporal regions, with relative sparing of the posterior areas, distinguishing it from the pattern seen in Alzheimer's disease. Progressive supranuclear palsy involves the brainstem and the superior cerebellar peduncle. At the same time, multiple system atrophy shows changes in the pontocerebellar and middle cerebellar peduncles, patterns that aid in the differential diagnosis of Parkinsonian disorders.

Pediatric applications of diffusion imaging span congenital malformations, inherited metabolic disorders, hypoxic-ischemic injury, and brain maturation. Hypoxic-ischemic encephalopathy in neonates shows diffusion restriction in affected territories with prognostic value, as the extent and pattern of abnormality predict neurodevelopmental outcomes. Congenital brain malformations, including polymicrogyria, heterotopia, and dysplasias, exhibit altered white matter organisation detectable through DTI, while agenesis of the corpus callosum demonstrates aberrant fibre pathways. Inherited leukodystrophies produce characteristic patterns: metachromatic leukodystrophy shows confluent white-matter abnormalities with elevated MD; Krabbe disease affects subcortical U-fibres and corticospinal tracts; and X-linked adrenoleukodystrophy demonstrates posterior-predominant changes. Developmental diffusion changes in healthy children reveal progressive increases in FA and decreases in MD in white matter, reflecting myelination and axonal organisation, and providing normative references for detecting abnormal development. Table 5.3 shows diffusion MRI findings in common white matter disorders.

Table 5.3. Diffusion MRI findings in common white matter disorders

Disorder	Affected Regions	FA Changes	MD/ADC Changes	Specific Features	Clinical Utility
Multiple Sclerosis	Lesions, NAWM, tracts	↓↓ in lesions, ↓ in NAWM	↑ in lesions and NAWM	Grey matter involvement	Disease monitoring, prognosis
Acute Stroke	Vascular territory	↓	↓↓ (first week)	Mismatch with perfusion	Treatment decision, outcome prediction
Traumatic Brain Injury	Corpus callosum, frontal WM	↓	Variable (acute ↓ or ↑)	DAI in the deep/brainstem	Injury severity, prognosis
High-Grade Glioma	Tumour core, infiltration	↓↓ in core, ↓ in infiltration	↓ in cellular regions	Perilesional changes	Grading, surgical planning
Alzheimer's Disease	Temporal WM, cingulum, fornix	↓	↑	Correlates with cognition	Early detection, progression
ALS	Corticospinal tract	↓	↑	Motor pathway selective	Diagnosis support, prognosis
Leukodystrophy	Diffuse white matter	↓↓ confluent	↑↑ in active disease	Pattern varies by type	Diagnosis, monitoring

Conclusion

Diffusion magnetic resonance imaging provides non-invasive access to tissue microstructure at scales below the MRI's nominal resolution, enabling the investigation of white matter integrity, organisation, and connectivity. The diffusion tensor model, although limited by assumptions of single fibre populations, provides clinically valuable metrics, including fractional anisotropy and mean diffusivity—sensitive markers of white matter integrity across various diseases. Tractography enables the reconstruction of three-dimensional white-matter pathways, establishing the field of structural connectomics and providing essential tools for neurosurgical planning.

Tensor model limitations in regions with crossing fibres have motivated the development of high-angular-resolution techniques, including Q-ball imaging and constrained spherical deconvolution, which successfully resolve multiple fibre orientations and improve tractography accuracy. Multi-shell acquisition strategies provide an optimal compromise, supporting advanced tractography and biophysical modelling from scans as short as 10-15 minutes.

Biophysical modelling approaches, such as NODDI, relate diffusion measurements to specific microstructural properties via multi-compartment models, thereby estimating neurite density, orientation dispersion, and free-water fractions for physiologically meaningful tissue characterisation.

Clinical applications span stroke diagnosis, multiple sclerosis monitoring, traumatic brain injury assessment, tumour characterisation, and neurodegenerative disease evaluation. The technique detects pathology before conventional imaging abnormalities appear.

Future advances include ultra-strong gradients for improved compartment characterisation, machine learning for enhanced processing, integration with complementary microstructural methods, and development as quantitative biomarkers for precision medicine, guiding individualised treatment based on tissue microstructure.

Acknowledgments

The authors would like to extend our appreciation to those who offered helpful commentary during the drafting process of this manuscript. We also acknowledge the role the Nova Publishing department played in enabling the work described herein.

References

Basser, P. J., Mattiello, J., & LeBihan, D. (1994). MR diffusion tensor spectroscopy and imaging *Biophysical Journal*, 66(1), 259-267. https://doi.org/10.1016/S0006-3495(94)80775-1.

Behrens, T. E., Woolrich, M. W., Jenkinson, M., Johansen-Berg, H., Nunes, R. G., Clare, S., Matthews, P. M., Brady, J. M., & Smith, S. M. (2003). Characterization and propagation of uncertainty in diffusion-weighted MR imaging. *Magnetic Resonance in Medicine*, 50(5), 1077-1088. https://doi.org/10.1002/mrm.10609.

Ciccarelli, O., Catani, M., Johansen-Berg, H., Clark, C., & Thompson, A. (2008). Diffusion-based tractography in neurological disorders: concepts, applications, and future developments. *Lancet Neurology*, 7(8), 715-727. https://doi.org/10.1016/S1474-4422(08)70163-7.

Le Bihan, D., Breton, E., Lallemand, D., Grenier, P., Cabanis, E., & Laval-Jeantet, M. (1986). MR imaging of intravoxel incoherent motions: application to diffusion and perfusion in neurologic disorders. *Radiology*, 161(2), 401-407. https://doi.org/10.1148/radiology.161.2.3763909.

Moseley, M. E., Cohen, Y., Mintorovitch, J., Chileuitt, L., Shimizu, H., Kucharczyk, J., Wendland, M. F., & Weinstein, P. R. (1990). Early detection of regional cerebral ischemia in cats: comparison of diffusion- and T2-weighted MRI and spectroscopy. *Magnetic Resonance in Medicine*, 14(2), 330-346. https://doi.org/10.1002/mrm.1910140218.

Pierpaoli, C., & Basser, P. J. (1996). Toward a quantitative assessment of diffusion anisotropy. *Magnetic Resonance in Medicine*, 36(6), 893-906. https://doi.org/10.1002/mrm.1910360612.

Tournier, J. D., Calamante, F., Gadian, D. G., & Connelly, A. (2004). Direct estimation of the fiber orientation density function from diffusion-weighted MRI data using spherical deconvolution. *NeuroImage*, 23(3), 1176-1185. https://doi.org/10.1016/j.neuroimage.2004.07.037.

Tuch, D. S., Reese, T. G., Wiegell, M. R., Makris, N., Belliveau, J. W., & Wedeen, V. J. (2002). High angular resolution diffusion imaging reveals intravoxel white matter fiber heterogeneity. *Magnetic Resonance in Medicine*, 48(4), 577-582. https://doi.org/10.1002/mrm.10268.

Wedeen, V. J., Hagmann, P., Tseng, W. Y., Reese, T. G., & Weisskoff, R. M. (2005). Mapping complex tissue architecture with diffusion spectrum magnetic resonance imaging. *Magnetic Resonance in Medicine*, 54(6), 1377-1386. https://doi.org/10.1002/mrm.20642.

Zhang, H., Schneider, T., Wheeler-Kingshott, C. A., & Alexander, D. C. (2012). NODDI: practical *in vivo* neurite orientation dispersion and density imaging of the human brain. *NeuroImage*, 61(4), 1000-1016. https://doi.org/10.1016/j.neuroimage.2012.03.072.

Chapter 6

Functional MRI:
Blood Oxygen Level Dependent (BOLD) Imaging

Maajid Mohi Ud Din Malik*
Radiology and Imaging Technology, Dr. D. Y. Patil School of Allied Health Sciences,
Dr. D. Y. Patil Vidyapeeth (Deemed to be University), Sant Tukaram Nagar, Pimpri, Pune, India

Abstract

Functional magnetic resonance imaging, based on blood oxygen level-dependent contrast, has revolutionised cognitive neuroscience and systems neuroscience by enabling non-invasive mapping of human brain activity with millimetre spatial resolution and sub-second temporal resolution. This chapter provides a comprehensive examination of BOLD fMRI principles, methodologies, and applications spanning task-based activation studies, resting-state connectivity analysis, and emerging real-time applications. We explore the neurophysiological basis of BOLD contrast, including the neurovascular coupling mechanisms that link neural activity to hemodynamic responses, as well as the biophysical foundations of susceptibility-based detection of changes in deoxyhemoglobin concentration. Task-based fMRI paradigms, including block designs, event-related designs, and parametric manipulations, are examined in the context of cognitive process mapping and clinical applications. Resting-state fMRI has revealed intrinsic brain networks and functional connectivity architecture underlying cognition and consciousness, with implications for understanding psychiatric and neurological disorders. Advanced acquisition methods, including multi-band imaging, have dramatically accelerated data collection, enabling whole-brain coverage with sub-second temporal resolution. Real-time fMRI and neurofeedback applications demonstrate therapeutic potential through learned self-regulation of brain activity. These techniques collectively establish BOLD fMRI as a cornerstone methodology for investigating human brain function, with continuing evolution toward higher spatiotemporal resolution and expanded clinical applications.

---

* Corresponding Author's Email: maajid.malik@dpu.edu.in

In: Recent Advances in Magnetic Resonance Imaging in Neuroimaging
Editors: Maajid Mohi Ud Din Malik, Purnachandra Kawdu Lamghare and R. S. Kuber
ISBN: 979-8-90134-244-2

Keywords: BOLD fMRI, neurovascular coupling, resting-state networks, functional connectivity, brain mapping, SDG 3 - good health and well-being

Introduction

The ability to visualise human brain activity non-invasively represents one of neuroscience's most transformative capabilities, enabling the investigation of cognitive processes, consciousness, and brain disorders that were previously accessible only through invasive methods or inferred from lesion studies. Functional magnetic resonance imaging, based on blood oxygen level-dependent contrast, emerged in the early 1990s as a revolutionary technique that exploits the intrinsic magnetic properties of haemoglobin to detect neural activity-related changes in blood oxygenation. The discovery by Seiji Ogawa and colleagues that deoxyhemoglobin acts as an endogenous contrast agent whose concentration varies with neural activity provided the foundation for non-invasive functional brain imaging. The first human BOLD fMRI studies, published independently by multiple groups between 1991 and 1992, demonstrated the robust detection of sensorimotor and visual cortex activation during simple tasks, establishing the technique's feasibility and igniting an explosion of applications across cognitive, clinical, and basic systems neuroscience.

BOLD fMRI's impact on neuroscience has been profound and multifaceted, transforming how brain function is investigated and understood. The technique enables the localisation of cognitive processes to specific brain regions with spatial precision far exceeding that of other non-invasive methods, including positron emission tomography and electroencephalography, while providing whole-brain coverage unlike focal recording techniques. The non-invasive nature permits repeated measures within individuals, enabling longitudinal studies of development, learning, and disease progression. The widespread availability of MRI scanners and the standardisation of fMRI protocols have democratised functional neuroimaging, making it accessible to research groups worldwide and fostering large-scale collaborative studies. The accumulated knowledge from thousands of fMRI studies has created detailed functional atlases of human brain organisation, identified canonical brain networks that support cognition, and revealed principles of brain architecture, including hierarchical organisation, distributed processing, and dynamic network interactions.

The evolution of BOLD fMRI methodology has been characterised by continuous innovation, addressing initial limitations and expanding its capabilities. Early studies employed block designs with extended activation periods to maximise signal detection, while event-related designs, enabling single-trial analysis, were developed to investigate transient cognitive processes. Resting-state fMRI, discovered serendipitously through observation of spontaneous BOLD fluctuations, revealed intrinsic brain networks with remarkable consistency across individuals and provided tools for investigating connectivity without requiring task performance. Advanced acquisition methods, including multi-band imaging, high-resolution fMRI, and ultra-high-field applications, have pushed spatial and temporal resolution toward the limits of hemodynamic detection. Real-time fMRI, which provides immediate feedback on brain activity, has enabled therapeutic applications through neurofeedback training. This chapter comprehensively examines these developments, providing both a foundational understanding of BOLD physiology and practical knowledge of experimental design, analysis methods, and applications across cognitive and clinical neuroscience.

6.1. Principles of BOLD Contrast

Blood oxygen level-dependent contrast arises from the magnetic susceptibility difference between oxygenated and deoxygenated haemoglobin, enabling the detection of neural activity through hemodynamic changes that affect blood oxygenation. The fundamental principle exploits the fact that deoxyhemoglobin is paramagnetic due to unpaired electrons on iron atoms, creating local magnetic field inhomogeneities that cause signal loss in T2*-weighted MRI. In contrast, oxyhemoglobin is diamagnetic and creates minimal field distortion. Neural activity triggers a sequence of hemodynamic responses, including increased cerebral blood flow, blood volume, and oxygen metabolism, that collectively alter the local deoxyhemoglobin concentration. Counterintuitively, despite increased oxygen consumption by active neurons, the increase in cerebral blood flow substantially exceeds metabolic demand, resulting in a net reduction in deoxyhemoglobin concentration in venous blood draining active tissue. This "overcorrection" produces the BOLD signal increase—reduced T2* signal loss—that underlies functional imaging (Ogawa et al., 1990).

The coupling between neural activity and the hemodynamic response—known as neurovascular coupling—involves complex signalling cascades that link synaptic activity, astrocytic function, and vascular smooth muscle regulation. Neuronal activity, particularly synaptic activity and associated ion pumping, rather than action potential generation, triggers the release of vasoactive substances, including nitric oxide, adenosine, and prostaglandins, from neurons and astrocytes. These molecules signal to nearby arterioles, causing smooth muscle relaxation and vasodilation that increases local blood flow. The spatial specificity of hemodynamic responses, extending approximately 2-3 millimetres from sites of peak neural activity, stems from the spatial scale of vascular architecture and diffusion-limited signalling. The temporal characteristics reflect the sluggish vascular response, with BOLD signal changes lagging neural activity onset by 2-3 seconds, reaching peak 4-6 seconds post-stimulus, and returning to baseline over 10-15 seconds following brief neural activation. This hemodynamic response function (HRF) exhibits remarkable consistency across individuals and brain regions, though subtle variations occur with age, disease, and baseline physiology.

The canonical hemodynamic response follows a characteristic temporal profile, beginning with an initial slight dip that potentially reflects early oxygen extraction before blood flow increases, although this component is often undetectable. The primary positive BOLD response follows, indicating an increase in blood flow that exceeds oxygen consumption. Following sustained activation, the signal may exhibit adaptation or habituation as the hemodynamic response reaches a steady state. After stimulus offset, the signal undershoots below baseline before recovering, potentially reflecting changes in venous compliance or sustained metabolic demand with normalised blood flow. Understanding the HRF shape is critical for experimental design and analysis, as the slow hemodynamic response limits temporal resolution and necessitates accounting for temporal dynamics in data modelling. Individual and regional HRF variability can affect analysis sensitivity and interpretation, particularly in populations with vascular disease or when comparing regions with different vascular properties.

The biophysical basis of BOLD contrast has been extensively characterised through theoretical modelling and experimental validation. The BOLD signal magnitude depends on multiple factors, including baseline blood volume, baseline oxygen saturation, the magnitude of blood flow change, and magnetic field strength. At 3 Tesla, typical BOLD signal changes range from 1-5% for robust activation, while at 1.5 Tesla, changes are approximately half as large, and at 7 Tesla, they are double or more. The signal originates primarily from intravascular effects in small vessels and capillaries at lower fields, transitioning to the extravascular impacts that dominate at higher fields, where susceptibility gradients around vessels affect larger tissue regions. The vessel size sensitivity varies with field strength and pulse sequence, with gradient echo sequences preferentially sensitive to large vessels at low fields but increasingly sensitive to microvasculature at high fields. Spin-echo sequences provide greater microvascular specificity but lower overall sensitivity.

Quantitative BOLD modelling relates observed signal changes to underlying physiological parameters, including blood flow, blood volume, and oxygen metabolism. The Balloon model, introduced by Buxton and colleagues, conceptualises the venous compartment as an expandable balloon whose volume and oxygenation respond to arterial flow changes with characteristic time constants. The Davis model relates the BOLD signal to cerebral blood flow and cerebral metabolic rate of oxygen consumption by calibrating against hypercapnia or hyperoxia challenges that independently modulate blood flow and oxygenation. These quantitative approaches enable the extraction of physiological parameters from BOLD data, although they require additional measurements and assumptions. For most applications, the qualitative relationship between the BOLD signal and neural activity is sufficient, with signal changes interpreted as proportional to the underlying neural activity intensity, without the need for explicit modelling of intermediate hemodynamic steps (Buxton et al., 1998).

The relationship between the BOLD signal and neural activity is fundamentally indirect and probabilistic rather than deterministic. BOLD primarily reflects input to a region—such as synaptic activity and local field potentials—rather than spiking output, creating complex relationships between electrophysiological measures and BOLD. The energetic demands of synaptic transmission, neurotransmitter recycling, and ion pump activity drive metabolic and hemodynamic responses, with inhibitory activity potentially eliciting BOLD responses similar to those of excitatory activity. This complexity means that increases in BOLD signal indicate enhanced processing in a region, but don't specify whether the activity is excitatory or inhibitory, or whether spiking output increases. Combined electrophysiology-fMRI studies in animals have revealed strong correlations between BOLD and local field potentials, reflecting synaptic activity; moderate correlations with multi-unit spiking activity; and temporal coupling, in which BOLD follows electrophysiological changes with a characteristic hemodynamic lag. These relationships support BOLD's validity as a proxy for neural activity, while acknowledging its indirect nature.

Physiological noise from cardiac pulsation, respiration, and spontaneous fluctuations in blood pressure and CO_2 creates signal variations that can mimic or obscure task-evoked responses. Cardiac pulsation causes vessel pulsation and cerebrospinal fluid flow, producing oscillations at heart rate frequency (typically 1-1.5 Hz). Respiration influences CO_2 levels, affecting cerebrovascular tone and creates motion-related signal changes at respiratory frequency (0.2-0.3 Hz). These physiological fluctuations are particularly prominent in large vessels and near ventricles, often exceeding task-evoked signal changes in magnitude. Advanced preprocessing, including physiological noise correction using cardiac and respiratory recordings, or data-driven approaches such as independent component analysis, substantially improves sensitivity to task activation by identifying and removing physiological artefacts. The recognition that low-frequency (<0.1 Hz) spontaneous fluctuations contain meaningful information about brain organisation rather than merely representing noise led to the development of resting-state fMRI. Table 6.1 illustrates the physiological and technical factors that affect the BOLD signal.

Table 6.1. Key physiological and technical factors affecting BOLD signal

Factor	Effect on BOLD	Mechanism	Implications for Interpretation
Neural Activity	↑ signal (1-5% at 3T)	Increased CBF, reduced deoxyhemoglobin	Primary signal of interest
Magnetic Field Strength	Signal scales with the field	Enhanced susceptibility effects	7T provides ~2× signal vs 3T
Baseline Physiology (caffeine, CO_2)	Alters baseline tone	Changes vascular reactivity	Can affect group comparisons
Vascular Pathology	Reduced or absent response	Impaired neurovascular coupling	Limits the interpretation of the disease
Age	Reduced amplitude, slowed HRF	Vascular and metabolic changes	Requires age-matched controls
Medications (vasodilators)	Altered hemodynamic response	Changed vascular reactivity	Can confound pharmacological studies
Task Difficulty	Larger signals for more complex tasks	Increased neural recruitment	Enables parametric manipulation

6.2. Task-Based fMRI Paradigms

Task-based functional MRI employs carefully designed experimental paradigms that manipulate cognitive, sensory, or motor processes while measuring brain activity, thereby enabling the localisation of function and the investigation of neural mechanisms underlying behaviour. The fundamental approach contrasts brain activity across task and control conditions, identifying regions where activity differs significantly between conditions and inferring their involvement in the cognitive process of interest. Experimental design critically determines what questions can be addressed and with what sensitivity, requiring careful consideration of psychological subtraction logic, control conditions, timing parameters, and statistical power. The evolution of fMRI paradigm design, from simple sensorimotor localisation to sophisticated multi-factorial manipulations that investigate complex cognitive processes, reflects both methodological maturation and increasingly ambitious scientific questions about human brain function.

Block design paradigms, employed in early fMRI studies and still widely used, involve alternating extended periods of task performance with rest or control conditions, with each block typically lasting 15-30 seconds. Multiple repetitions of task and control blocks, often 4-8 cycles, provide statistical power through temporal averaging. The extended activation periods maximise BOLD signal accumulation and simplify analysis through a high temporal signal-to-noise ratio, making block designs powerful for localising brain regions involved in task performance. The alternating on-off pattern creates a clear temporal structure, facilitating visual inspection and simple statistical analysis. Applications include sensorimotor mapping for presurgical planning, language lateralisation assessment, and initial localisation of cognitive processes before more sophisticated designs probe mechanistic details. Limitations include the inability to separate closely spaced events, susceptibility to habituation and expectation effects resulting from predictable timing, and the mixing of transient and sustained neural processes within blocks (Amaro & Barker, 2006).

Event-related fMRI designs present discrete, brief trials, enabling the analysis of individual events or trial types. This provides flexibility to investigate transient cognitive processes, separate correct from incorrect trials, and employ unpredictable timing. The development of event-related fMRI in the late 1990s represented a significant methodological advance, enabling experimental paradigms common in cognitive psychology that were previously incompatible with the sustained activation requirements of block designs. Trials can be temporally separated, minimising overlap of hemodynamic responses and enabling precise estimation of individual trial responses, or they can be rapidly presented with overlapping responses, requiring more sophisticated analysis via deconvolution. The inter-trial interval varies from 2 to 4 seconds in rapid designs to 10 to 15 seconds in slow designs, with statistical efficiency considerations favouring faster presentation when sustained attention is not a problem. Trial types can be intermixed unpredictably, allowing for surprise manipulations, post-hoc classification based on behavioural performance, and investigation of adaptation effects (Dale & Buckner, 1997).

Parametric designs systematically vary task parameters across conditions or trials, allowing for the investigation of how brain activity relates to stimulus properties, cognitive demands, or behavioural performance. Unlike categorical designs that compare discrete conditions, parametric approaches examine continuous relationships between task variables and brain activity via regression analysis. Examples include varying stimulus intensity, memory load, response deadline, reward magnitude, or emotional valence across graded levels. The resulting parametric modulation reveals regions where activity increases or decreases in response to the manipulated variable, often providing more sensitive detection and stronger theoretical inference than categorical comparisons. Parametric designs enable the testing of computational models that predict specific relationships between psychological variables and neural activity, thereby connecting neuroimaging to formal cognitive theories. The approach requires the careful selection of parameter levels that span the range of interest, without floor or ceiling effects.

Mixed designs combine aspects of block and event-related paradigms to examine both sustained and transient processes, or to separate state-related from item-specific activity. For example, a working memory study might employ blocks of high versus low memory load (sustained state) with individual items as events (transient, item-specific processing), enabling the separation of load maintenance from item encoding/retrieval. Mixed designs offer a richer characterisation of task-related activity, albeit at the cost of increased design complexity and analysis requirements. The separation of sustained and transient responses requires careful modelling that accounts for overlapping hemodynamic responses and ensures sufficient temporal separation for reliable estimation. Applications include investigating interactions between cognitive control and stimulus processing, emotion regulation studies that separate sustained regulation from emotional responses to stimuli, and attention studies that distinguish sustained attention states from transient orienting responses.

The choice of baseline or control condition has a fundamental impact on what cognitive processes are isolated and how the results are interpreted. Active control conditions that match perceptual, motor, and attentional demands while differing only in the process of interest provide more specific localisation than rest baselines, following the logic of psychological subtraction. However, perfect control conditions are often impossible to design, as manipulating one cognitive process inevitably affects others. Multiple control conditions can bracket the process of interest, with convergent evidence from different contrasts strengthening conclusions. The default mode network, ironically, was discovered through consistent deactivations relative to the rest baseline, illustrating how the choice of control condition shapes findings. Considerations in control design include matching difficulty, engagement, emotional valence, and sensory stimulation, while recognising that perfect matching is a theoretical ideal rarely achieved in practice.

Statistical analysis of task-based fMRI typically employs the general linear model, which relates observed BOLD time courses to predicted responses based on the experimental design. Task timing is convolved with the hemodynamic response function to create regressors that represent expected BOLD responses for each condition. Parameter estimates (beta weights) quantify how strongly each voxel's activity relates to each regressor, with statistical tests comparing betas across conditions identifying regions showing differential activity. Mass univariate analysis testing thousands of voxels requires multiple comparisons correction through methods such as family-wise error rate control using random field theory or permutation testing, or false discovery rate control, which accepts specified proportions of false positives. Cluster-based inference identifies contiguous regions of significant voxels, exploiting spatial smoothness to alleviate the burden of multiple comparisons. More sophisticated approaches, including multivariate pattern analysis, decode information content from distributed activity patterns, often detecting condition differences where univariate analysis reveals no significant voxels.

6.3. Resting-State fMRI and Brain Connectivity

Resting-state functional MRI examines spontaneous brain activity fluctuations in the absence of explicit tasks, revealing intrinsic functional networks and connectivity architecture through correlated low-frequency BOLD fluctuations across distributed brain regions. The 1995 discovery by Biswal and colleagues that spontaneous motor cortex fluctuations are highly correlated between hemispheres established that resting BOLD fluctuations contain meaningful information about functional brain organisation, rather than merely being noise (Biswal et al., 1995). Advantages include no task performance requirement, making the method applicable to diverse populations, including young children and clinical patients who are unable to perform tasks, as well as efficiency in characterising whole-brain connectivity from short acquisitions. Resting-state fMRI has revealed consistent functional networks including default mode, dorsal attention, ventral attention, frontoparietal control, and sensorimotor networks.

The default mode network comprises the medial prefrontal cortex, posterior cingulate cortex, the precuneus, and the lateral parietal cortex, showing high activity during rest and consistent deactivation during attention-demanding tasks. Proposed functions include self-referential processing, episodic memory retrieval, theory of mind, mind-wandering, and internal mentation. The network shows disrupted connectivity in Alzheimer's disease, schizophrenia, depression, and autism spectrum disorder.

Task-positive networks, including the dorsal and ventral attention networks and the frontoparietal control network, exhibit anticorrelated activity with the default mode network, indicating a functional opposition between externally and internally directed cognition. The dorsal attention network supports goal-directed attention, while the ventral attention network supports stimulus-driven attention and reorienting. The frontoparietal control network flexibly couples with other networks implementing cognitive control functions.

Functional connectivity analysis quantifies statistical dependencies between BOLD time series using measures such as Pearson correlation, partial correlation, coherence, or information-theoretic measures. Approaches include seed-based analysis, independent component analysis, and graph-theoretical methods that represent the brain as networks of nodes and edges.

Dynamic functional connectivity extends static connectivity by examining how network organisation changes over time using sliding window approaches, Hidden Markov models, and time-frequency analysis. Clinical applications have expanded with evidence for network alterations in neurological and psychiatric disorders.

Methodological considerations include head motion management, physiological noise removal, and long acquisition durations (10 minutes or longer) for reliable connectivity estimation. Table 6.2 presents the significant characteristics of the resting-state functional framework.

Table 6.2. Major resting-state functional networks and their characteristics

Network	Key Regions	Proposed Functions	Task Modulation	Clinical Relevance
Default Mode	mPFC, PCC, precuneus, lateral parietal	Self-referential processing, memory, and mind-wandering	Deactivates during tasks	Alzheimer's, depression, and autism
Dorsal Attention	Superior parietal, FEF	Goal-directed attention, orienting	Activates for attention tasks	Attention deficits, neglect
Ventral Attention	TPJ, ventral frontal	Stimulus-driven attention, reorienting	Activates for salient stimuli	Neglect, spatial attention
Frontoparietal Control	DLPFC, lateral parietal	Cognitive control, flexible coupling	Task-dependent activation	Schizophrenia, ADHD
Salience	Anterior insula, ACC	Error detection, autonomic arousal	Activates for salient events	Anxiety, addiction
Sensorimotor	Primary motor/sensory cortex	Motor control, sensation	Activates during movement/sensation	Stroke, movement disorders
Visual	Occipital cortex, ventral/dorsal streams	Visual processing	Activates for visual stimuli	Visual cortex damage

6.4. Event-Related fMRI Design

Event-related functional MRI design principles enable the investigation of transient cognitive processes, trial-by-trial analysis, and flexible experimental paradigms that were previously impossible with block designs. The fundamental advance enabling event-related fMRI was the recognition that individual hemodynamic responses can be estimated even when trials are closely spaced, through statistical modelling that accounts for hemodynamic response timing and overlap. This capability transformed fMRI from a technique restricted to sustained processes into one that enables trial-by-trial analysis, comparable to electroencephalography and event-related potentials, but with superior spatial resolution. The methodology enables post-hoc classification of trials by behavioural performance, allowing for surprise manipulations that are not possible with predictable block designs. It also facilitates the investigation of adaptation and repetition effects, as well as temporal-ordering manipulations that probe time-dependent processes. Event-related designs have become a standard approach in cognitive neuroscience for investigating attention, memory, decision-making, emotion, and other processes where trial-level analysis is crucial.

Optimal spacing of trials in event-related designs balances statistical efficiency, favouring closely spaced trials, against the need to separate hemodynamic responses for precise estimation. When trials are separated by 12-15 seconds, individual responses are clearly distinguishable, allowing for simple analysis through averaging. As spacing decreases below 8 seconds, hemodynamic responses increasingly overlap, requiring more sophisticated analysis through deconvolution to separate contributions of successive trials. Rapid event-related designs with 2-4 second inter-trial intervals maximise statistical efficiency by collecting more trials per unit time. However, they require careful analysis and are susceptible to attention and habituation effects when presented very rapidly. The optimal spacing depends on the research question; investigations of transient responses favour slower spacing, as it enables more precise response estimation. In comparison, studies requiring many trials per condition favour faster spacing, despite the increased complexity of analysis. Jittering of inter-trial intervals by adding random variation improves the temporal resolution of hemodynamic response estimation by sampling the response at different relative phases.

Deconvolution analysis estimates individual trial responses from data with overlapping hemodynamic responses by solving the linear system that relates the observed signal to trial timing, convolved with the HRF. When trials are spaced irregularly, different portions of the hemodynamic response contribute to the signal at other times, providing information that enables the separation of overlapping reactions. The general linear model framework with trial-specific regressors implements deconvolution, with each trial type modelled as a separate regressor. Finite impulse response models estimate the hemodynamic response at multiple time points post-stimulus without assuming a specific HRF shape, providing flexibility but requiring more parameters. Basis function approaches, including canonical HRF plus temporal derivatives, balance flexibility and efficiency. The estimation quality depends on design efficiency, which is determined by the timing of the trial. Rapidly varying trial sequences enable better estimation than regular or blocked sequences. Design optimisation using genetic algorithms or simulated annealing identifies trial sequences that maximise efficiency for specific contrasts of interest.

Trial sorting and post-hoc analysis represent powerful capabilities unique to event-related designs, enabling the classification of trials by behavioural performance, response time, or other measured variables, and then examining brain activity differences between trial classes. For example, memory encoding studies can distinguish between subsequently remembered and subsequently forgotten items, identifying regions where encoding-phase activity predicts later memory success. Correct versus incorrect trials can be contrasted to identify brain activity associated with successful performance. Response time can be used as a continuous variable in parametric modulation analysis to identify regions where activity relates to processing speed or difficulty. These analyses directly connect brain activity to behavioural outcomes, providing stronger inferences about function than simple task-versus-rest contrasts. Limitations include the potential for confounding differences in attention, arousal, or other factors correlated with performance, as well as reduced power due to fewer trials per condition after splitting.

Mixed designs that combine event-related and blocked elements enable the investigation of both transient and sustained processes within unified frameworks. A memory study might employ blocks of encoding versus retrieval (sustained task sets) with individual items as events (transient item processing), enabling separate estimation of task-set maintenance from item-specific processing. Attention studies might use sustained attention versus distraction blocks with targets as events, thereby separating sustained attention state from transient target-detection responses. The analysis requires modelling both sustained block-related and transient event-related responses, typically through GLM with separate regressors for blocks and events. The separation of sustained and transient responses requires sufficient power to detect both, often necessitating longer scans than those used in pure event-related or block designs. Applications demonstrate that processes that appear as a single unified response in block designs usually segregate into distinct sustained and transient components with different neural substrates when examined in mixed designs.

Parametric modulation extends event-related analysis by examining how brain activity varies continuously with trial-level variables, revealing regions where activity scales with stimulus properties, cognitive demands, or behavioural metrics. Rather than categorical trial sorting, parametric analysis includes trial-level variables as continuous regressors, testing for linear or non-linear relationships between brain activity and the variable. Examples include stimulus intensity, emotional valence or arousal, reward magnitude, memory strength, or response conflict. Significant parametric effects indicate regions involved in representing or processing the modulated dimension. Parametric designs offer more sensitive detection than categorical comparisons and enable the testing of computational models that predict specific activity-behaviour relationships. Multiple variables can be modulated simultaneously, though this increases analysis complexity and requires careful attention to collinearity between variables. The approach has been particularly fruitful in investigations of reward processing, where activity in ventral striatum and orbitofrontal cortex scales with reward magnitude and prediction error as predicted by reinforcement learning models.

6.5. Multi-Band and Simultaneous Multi-Slice Imaging

Multi-band or simultaneous multi-slice imaging represents a significant acquisition innovation, enabling the dramatic acceleration of fMRI data collection by simultaneously exciting and acquiring multiple slices, thereby fundamentally expanding the temporal and spatial resolution achievable within practical scan times. The technique employs multi-band radiofrequency pulses to excite various slices simultaneously, then separates overlapping signals during reconstruction using coil sensitivity information from multi-channel receiver arrays, analogous to parallel imaging acceleration. Multi-band factors of 4-8 enable whole-brain coverage with subsecond temporal resolution—as fast as 400 milliseconds—or high-resolution data acquisition impractical with conventional slice-by-slice methods. The development and dissemination of the Human Connectome Project have transformed fMRI capabilities, enabling the investigation of fast neural dynamics, improving statistical power through increased temporal sampling, and facilitating high-resolution studies that resolve fine spatial structure (Feinberg et al., 2010).

Multi-band imaging physics relies on creating RF pulses that simultaneously excite multiple spatially separated slices, which overlap in frequency space. Multi-band pulses are produced by summing single-slice pulses for each desired slice, yielding composite pulses with various frequency components. SENSE-based reconstruction leverages the spatial encoding inherent in multi-channel coil arrays, where each coil has a distinct sensitivity profile across the imaging volume. Slice separation quality depends on coil sensitivity differences between slice positions, which are quantified through a slice geometry factor analogous to the parallel imaging g-factor.

Implementation requires careful acquisition parameter optimisation. Multi-band factors must consider slice separation; larger separations enable higher factors before g-factor penalties become prohibitive. Typical implementations use factors of 4-8 with slice separations of 3-5 slices. Blipped-CAIPI, employing minor gradient blips during echo-planar readout to shift slices in k-space, substantially improves g-factor by reducing slice overlap in coil sensitivity space, enabling higher multi-band factors (Setsompop et al., 2012).

Applications leverage increased temporal sampling or spatial resolution. Fast sampling at 400-600 millisecond TR enables the investigation of temporal dynamics at scales approaching neural response times and improves neural-physiological noise separation through temporal filtering. High-resolution fMRI at 1.5-2 millimetres isotropic resolution, covering the whole brain in under 2 seconds, enables the investigation of delicate spatial structures, including cortical layers and small subcortical nuclei.

Resting-state connectivity analysis benefits from increased temporal sampling, which improves frequency resolution and noise characteristics. Task-based fMRI employing multi-band acceleration increases statistical power, reduces scan time, or enables paradigms that require acceptable temporal resolution, thereby improving presurgical mapping and clinical workflow.

6.6. Real-Time fMRI and Neurofeedback

Real-time functional MRI processes and displays brain activity information during ongoing scanning, enabling immediate feedback to subjects about their brain states and creating opportunities for neurofeedback training, in which individuals learn to modulate their brain activity voluntarily. The technical implementation requires rapid data transfer from the scanner to external computing hardware, online preprocessing that includes motion correction and artefact removal, and statistical analysis or pattern recognition to identify relevant brain states or activation levels, all of which are completed within seconds of data acquisition. The results are displayed to subjects through visual feedback, including thermometers that show activity levels, continuous tracking plots, or more naturalistic displays, enabling subjects to attempt volitional regulation. After training sessions where subjects experiment with mental strategies while observing feedback, many individuals develop the ability to significantly modulate target brain region activity, with emerging evidence that learned regulation can produce therapeutic benefits for clinical conditions including depression, anxiety, chronic pain, and addiction (Weiskopf et al., 2007).

The methodology of real-time fMRI requires a careful selection of target brain regions, a suitable feedback presentation method, a well-defined training protocol, and appropriate outcome measures. Region selection considers several criteria: a theoretical rationale connecting the area to symptoms or processes of interest; demonstrable activation or connectivity patterns in independent localizer scans that establish that target signals are reliably measurable in individual subjects; and anatomical precision sufficient for real-time targeting, given individual variation. Common targets include the amygdala for emotion regulation, the anterior cingulate cortex for pain modulation, the ventral striatum for reward processing and addiction, the supplementary motor area for motor control, and the prefrontal regions for cognitive control. The target can be individual regions, contrasts between areas, or connectivity measures, with single-region approaches more straightforward but potentially missing important distributed dynamics. Whole-brain pattern classifiers using multivariate methods can provide insights into distributed brain states, but they require more sophisticated real-time analysis.

Training protocols typically employ multiple sessions over days or weeks, with each session including periods of upregulation attempts (increasing target activity), downregulation attempts (decreasing target activity), or both. Control conditions might include counting, non-target brain region feedback, or sham feedback to distinguish specific learned regulation from general effects of training and expectation. Instructions can be explicit, directing subjects to use specific mental strategies, or minimal, encouraging subjects to discover effective strategies through trial and error. Many protocols begin with explicit instructions, then transition to self-discovery as subjects develop an individualised, practical approach. Transfer tests, which examine whether learned regulation transfers to conditions without feedback, assess whether skills generalise beyond the training context. Follow-up assessments, conducted weeks to months post-training, evaluate whether regulatory ability and clinical benefits persist, which is critical for therapeutic applications.

Clinical applications of neurofeedback have shown promise in treating several conditions, although controlled studies with appropriate controls and sufficient sample sizes are still emerging. Depression treatment involving the upregulation of positive emotion-related regions, including the ventral striatum and ventromedial prefrontal cortex, has shown symptom reduction in small trials, with effects comparable to those of established treatments in some studies. Anxiety disorder treatment targeting amygdala downregulation has demonstrated reduced anxiety symptoms and altered amygdala responses to emotional stimuli, suggesting successful learned emotion regulation. Chronic pain treatment using downregulation of pain-related activity in the anterior cingulate cortex and insula has produced clinically meaningful pain reduction, lasting weeks post-training, in preliminary studies. Addiction treatment targeting craving-related brain activity shows reduced cravings and improved treatment outcomes in pilot studies of substance use disorders. These promising initial results require replication in larger, randomised controlled trials, the identification of predictors of treatment response, and the optimisation of training protocols for clinical efficiency.

Mechanisms underlying successful neurofeedback learning remain incompletely understood, with multiple non-exclusive possibilities. Operant conditioning, where immediate feedback reinforces mental strategies that produce desired changes in brain activity, represents one framework consistent with animal studies of neural operant conditioning. Motor learning models suggest that neurofeedback facilitates the acquisition of a novel cognitive-neural skill through practice with feedback, similar to the acquisition of motor skills. Awareness and cognitive strategy development, where feedback enables subjects to identify effective mental strategies they can subsequently deploy, may contribute, particularly when subjects report using specific techniques, such as imagery or attention control. Placebo and expectation effects may account for some benefits, emphasising the importance of rigorous controls. Multiple mechanisms likely operate across subjects and protocols, with individual differences in learning ability potentially related to baseline brain structure and connectivity, as well as psychological factors such as self-efficacy and motivation.

Technical advances continue to improve real-time fMRI capabilities and accessibility. Cloud-based platforms enable real-time analysis on external servers, reducing hardware requirements at scan sites. Improved artefact detection and correction algorithms enhance the reliability of real-time measures. Multivariate pattern analysis, enabling whole-brain state decoding, provides richer feedback on distributed brain states. Integration with other modalities, such as simultaneous EEG, provides complementary information about brain activity. Closed-loop stimulation, in which feedback drives transcranial magnetic stimulation or other interventions, creates hybrid approaches that are potentially more powerful than feedback alone. Portable, real-time fMRI systems that bring technology into clinical settings rather than requiring research environments will be critical for translation. Standardised protocols and training procedures would facilitate multi-site studies and eventual clinical implementation, requiring consistency across providers.

The future of real-time fMRI and neurofeedback is likely to involve personalisation based on individual differences in brain organisation, connectivity, and learning capacity. Advances in understanding which individuals benefit most from neurofeedback training will enable targeted neurofeedback application, maximising benefits. Combination with other treatments, including pharmacotherapy and psychotherapy, may produce synergistic effects that exceed those of individual interventions. Extension to populations including children, the elderly, and severely impaired patients requires protocol adaptations but could dramatically expand therapeutic applications. The ultimate potential depends on continued rigorous research that demonstrates efficacy, elucidates mechanisms, and optimises protocols—challenges shared with any novel therapeutic approach. As the field matures, real-time fMRI may become a valuable tool in the therapeutic arsenal for conditions characterised by dysfunctional brain activity patterns.

Conclusion

Blood-oxygen-level-dependent functional MRI has transformed neuroscience by providing noninvasive access to human brain activity with unmatched spatial resolution and whole-brain coverage. Exploiting magnetic susceptibility differences between oxygenated and deoxygenated haemoglobin enables the detection of neural activity through hemodynamic responses, creating detailed functional atlases of brain organisation, canonical networks, and principles of distributed processing.

Task-based fMRI paradigms, employing block and event-related designs and parametric manipulations, have localised cognitive processes to specific regions and tested theories of the neural mechanisms underlying perception, attention, memory, language, emotion, and decision-making. Clinical applications include presurgical language and motor mapping as standard of care.

Resting-state fMRI reveals highly organised spontaneous brain activity, characterised by consistent functional networks, including the default mode network and task-positive networks. The technique applies to populations that are unable to perform tasks, thereby expanding the scope of functional neuroimaging. Clinical applications investigating network disruptions have shown potential for identifying diagnostic biomarkers and predicting treatment responses.

Multi-band simultaneous multi-slice imaging enables whole-brain coverage with sub-second temporal resolution, revolutionising fMRI capabilities. Real-time fMRI and neurofeedback represent transformative interventional applications, enabling volitional brain activity regulation with emerging therapeutic benefits in depression, anxiety, chronic pain, and addiction.

Future developments include higher magnetic fields, multimodal integration with PET and MEG, machine-learning analysis approaches, and a transition to individual-level precision mapping for personalised medicine applications.

Acknowledgments

The authors would like to extend our appreciation to those who offered helpful commentary during the drafting process of this manuscript. We also acknowledge the role the Nova Publishing department played in enabling the work described herein.

References

Amaro, E., & Barker, G. J. (2006). Study design in fMRI: Basic principles. *Brain and Cognition*, 60(3), 220-232. https://doi.org/10.1016/j.bandc.2005.11.009.

Biswal, B., Yetkin, F. Z., Haughton, V. M., & Hyde, J. S. (1995). Functional connectivity in the motor cortex of the resting human brain using echo-planar MRI. *Magnetic Resonance in Medicine*, 34(4), 537-541. https://doi.org/10.1002/mrm.1910340409.

Buxton, R. B., Wong, E. C., & Frank, L. R. (1998). Dynamics of blood flow and oxygenation changes during brain activation: The balloon model. *Magnetic Resonance in Medicine*, 39(6), 855-864. https://doi.org/10.1002/mrm.1910390602.

Dale, A. M., & Buckner, R. L. (1997). Selective averaging of rapidly presented individual trials using fMRI. *Human Brain Mapping*, 5(5), 329-340. https://doi.org/10.1002/(SICI)1097-0193(1997)5:5<329::AID-HBM1>3.0.CO;2-5.

Feinberg, D. A., Moeller, S., Smith, S. M., Auerbach, E., Ramanna, S., Glasser, M. F., Miller, K. L., Ugurbil, K., & Yacoub, E. (2010). Multiplexed echo planar imaging for sub-second whole brain FMRI and fast diffusion imaging. *PLoS ONE*, 5(12), e15710. https://doi.org/10.1371/journal.pone.0015710.

Ogawa, S., Lee, T. M., Kay, A. R., & Tank, D. W. (1990). Brain magnetic resonance imaging with contrast dependent on blood oxygenation. *Proceedings of the National Academy of Sciences*, 87(24), 9868-9872. https://doi.org/10.1073/pnas.87.24.9868.

Setsompop, K., Gagoski, B. A., Polimeni, J. R., Witzel, T., Wedeen, V. J., & Wald, L. L. (2012). Blipped-controlled aliasing in parallel imaging for simultaneous multislice echo planar imaging with reduced g-factor penalty. *Magnetic Resonance in Medicine*, 67(5), 1210-1224. https://doi.org/10.1002/mrm.23097.

Weiskopf, N., Scharnowski, F., Veit, R., Goebel, R., Birbaumer, N., & Mathiak, K. (2004). Self-regulation of local brain activity using real-time functional magnetic resonance imaging (fMRI). *Journal of Physiology-Paris*, 98(4-6), 357-373. https://doi.org/10.1016/j.jphysparis.2005.09.019.

Chapter 7

Advanced fMRI Techniques

Purnachandra Kawdu Lamghare[1,*]
and Maajid Mohi Ud Din Malik[2,†]
[1]Department of Radio-Diagnosis, Dr. D. Y. Patil Medical College, Hospital and Research Centre, Dr. D. Y. Patil Vidyapeeth (Deemed to be University), Sant Tukaram Nagar, Pimpri, Pune, India
[2]Radiology and Imaging Technology, Dr. D. Y. Patil School of Allied Health Sciences, Dr. D. Y. Patil Vidyapeeth (Deemed to be University), Sant Tukaram Nagar, Pimpri, Pune, India

Abstract

Advanced functional MRI techniques have expanded beyond conventional blood oxygen level-dependent imaging to provide complementary measures of brain physiology, increased spatial specificity, and more sophisticated analysis of brain organisation and function. This chapter examines cutting-edge methodologies that are expanding the capabilities and applications of functional neuroimaging. Arterial spin labelling enables quantitative cerebral blood flow measurements without exogenous contrast agents, enabling perfusion mapping in clinical diagnosis and the calibration of BOLD responses. Layer-specific fMRI resolves activity across cortical depth at ultra-high field, revealing laminar patterns of feedforward and feedback processing that connect cellular neuroscience to systems function. Hypercapnia and hyperoxia mapping characterise cerebrovascular reactivity and enable calibrated fMRI to quantify metabolic changes underlying BOLD signals. Advanced functional connectivity approaches, including dynamic connectivity analysis, reveal time-varying network reconfigurations that reflect cognitive states and brain flexibility. Multivariate pattern analysis decodes information content from distributed activity patterns, detecting representations invisible to conventional univariate analysis. These sophisticated techniques are transforming functional neuroimaging from qualitative brain mapping to quantitative physiology, from static activation to dynamic network interactions, and from regional activity to distributed information processing. The integration of these advanced methods promises to significantly enhance our understanding of brain function in both healthy and diseased states.

---

* Corresponding Author's Email: purnachandra.lamghare@dpu.edu.in
† Corresponding Author's Email: maajid.malik@dpu.edu.in

In: Recent Advances in Magnetic Resonance Imaging in Neuroimaging
Editors: Maajid Mohi Ud Din Malik, Purnachandra Kawdu Lamghare and R. S. Kuber
ISBN: 979-8-90134-244-2

Keywords: arterial spin labelling, laminar fMRI, cerebrovascular reactivity, multivariate pattern analysis, dynamic connectivity, SDG 3 - good health and well-being

Introduction

The evolution of functional MRI has been characterised by continuous methodological innovation, extending capabilities beyond blood oxygen level-dependent contrast. While BOLD fMRI revolutionised cognitive neuroscience, limitations, including indirect neural activity relationships through neurovascular coupling, qualitative measurements, and spatial blurring from venous contributions, motivated the development of complementary techniques. Advanced techniques include arterial spin labelling for quantitative perfusion imaging without gadolinium contrast, ultra-high field layer-specific fMRI revealing cortical computation across depth, calibrated fMRI approaches quantifying metabolic contributions to hemodynamic responses, sophisticated connectivity analyses characterising brain network organisation and dynamics, and multivariate pattern analysis detecting distributed neural representations. These techniques represent the maturation of functional neuroimaging from exploratory brain mapping to the mechanistic investigation of neural computation and information processing, transforming our understanding from localised function to distributed systems and interactions.

7.1. Arterial Spin Labelling (ASL) Perfusion Imaging

Arterial spin labelling provides a quantitative measurement of cerebral blood flow by magnetically labelling arterial blood water as it flows toward the brain, then detecting the labelled blood as it perfuses the tissue, eliminating the need for exogenous contrast agents while enabling repeated measurements without safety concerns. The technique exploits the same radiofrequency principles underlying MRI, applying inversion or saturation pulses to blood in feeding arteries, and then acquiring images after a delay that allows labelled blood to flow into tissue capillaries and exchange with tissue water. The signal difference between labelled and control acquisitions reflects the amount of labelled blood delivered to the tissue, which, with appropriate modelling, can be converted to absolute cerebral blood flow in physiological units of millilitres per 100 grams of tissue per minute. This quantitative capability distinguishes ASL from BOLD fMRI's qualitative signal changes, enabling comparisons across individuals, time points, and scanners without the confounds that affect BOLD interpretation (Detre et al., 1992).

The fundamental principle of ASL involves creating a difference between the inflowing arterial blood magnetisation and static tissue magnetisation, with the resulting signal change proportional to the blood flow rate. Pulsed ASL employs a brief inversion or saturation pulse in a thick slab proximal to the imaging volume, instantaneously labelling blood passing through the slab. After a post-labelling delay, allowing blood to flow into imaging slices, images are acquired, showing reduced signal where labelled blood has perfused the tissue. Continuous ASL continuously inverts blood flowing through a labelling plane over several seconds, creating steady-state labelling with a higher signal-to-noise ratio than pulsed methods, but requiring special hardware for prolonged off-resonance inversion. Pseudo-continuous ASL combines the advantages of both approaches by employing a train of short pulses that mimics continuous inversion, using standard hardware, and is therefore the recommended clinical implementation. Each approach has distinct advantages in terms of efficiency, robustness, and multi-slice capability; however, pseudo-continuous ASL has emerged as the preferred method for most applications.

Quantification of cerebral blood flow from ASL data requires modelling the kinetics of labelled blood delivery, exchange with tissue water, and T1 relaxation, which gradually eliminate the labelling. The general kinetic model relates the perfusion signal to blood flow, labelling efficiency, arterial transit time from the labelling region to the tissue, and blood and tissue T1 relaxation times. Arterial transit time variation across brain regions and individuals complicates quantification, as the label arrives at different times in different areas. Multi-delay ASL acquires data at several post-labelling delays, enabling the estimation of both flow and transit times through model fitting, thereby improving quantification accuracy at the cost of longer acquisition times. Background suppression pulses applied before acquisition suppress the static tissue signal, dramatically improving sensitivity to the perfusion signal by reducing physiological noise and motion sensitivity. Calibration using cerebrospinal fluid or tissue with known T1 and an assumed blood-water content converts arbitrary signal differences into absolute flow values in millilitres per 100 grams per minute.

Normal cerebral blood flow values measured with ASL show Grey matter flow of 50-80 ml/100g/min and white matter flow of 15-25 ml/100g/min, with regional variation reflecting metabolic demands and vascular density. The grey-white contrast in ASL images is excellent, with sharp delineation of the cortical ribbon and subcortical nuclei. Age-related changes include progressive reduction in blood flow in older people, potentially reflecting vascular changes, neuronal loss, or altered metabolic demands. Individual variation in baseline flow is related to hematocrit, blood pressure, vascular anatomy, and physiological state, including caffeine intake and stress. This natural variation emphasises the importance of within-subject comparisons for detecting pathology and the advantages of longitudinal designs in research studies. Normative databases spanning age ranges enable identification of abnormal perfusion patterns suggesting pathology.

Clinical applications of ASL span diverse neurological conditions where perfusion abnormalities provide diagnostic or prognostic information. Acute stroke often exhibits hypoperfusion in the affected territory, which is typically larger than the diffusion restriction, identifying the penumbra as potentially salvageable through reperfusion. Chronic infarcts exhibit absent perfusion, distinguishing them from tumours or demyelination. Moyamoya disease demonstrates a characteristic pattern of reduced distal flow with increased collateral circulation. Brain tumours show elevated perfusion in high-grade gliomas, correlating with vascularity and grade, whereas metastases and primary CNS lymphomas exhibit distinct perfusion patterns. Alzheimer's disease demonstrates temporoparietal hypoperfusion preceding atrophy, with perfusion deficits predicting cognitive decline. Epilepsy shows interictal hypoperfusion and ictal hyperperfusion in seizure foci, guiding surgical planning. ASL provides these diagnostic insights without the need for gadolinium contrast, which is valuable for patients with renal dysfunction or concerns about gadolinium deposition, and enables repeated monitoring that is impossible with contrast-enhanced perfusion.

Functional ASL combines perfusion quantification with task-based or resting-state paradigms, providing an alternative to BOLD fMRI with distinct advantages and limitations. Task-evoked flow increases are directly proportional to metabolic demands, rather than reflecting the complex interplay of flow, volume, and oxygen extraction that determines the BOLD signal, potentially providing more interpretable physiological measurements. The quantitative nature enables direct comparison of activation magnitude across sessions, subjects, and studies. However, ASL sensitivity is lower than BOLD for equivalent scan time due to small perfusion signal changes (1-2%) and noise from subtraction. The temporal resolution is limited to several seconds due to the need for a post-labelling delay and signal-to-noise requirements. Applications include studies where a quantitative comparison is critical, populations with abnormal neurovascular coupling that affect BOLD interpretation, and combinations with BOLD where flow information disambiguates the origin of the BOLD signal. Simultaneous ASL-BOLD acquisition using single-shot schemes enables the efficient collection of both contrasts, providing complementary information on perfusion and oxygenation. Table 7.1 shows a comparison of ASL and BOLD functional MRI techniques.

Table 7.1. Comparison of ASL and BOLD functional MRI techniques

Feature	BOLD fMRI	ASL Perfusion fMRI	Advantages/Disadvantages
Signal Source	Deoxyhemoglobin concentration	Magnetically labelled blood water	BOLD: indirect; ASL: direct flow
Quantification	Relative (% signal change)	Absolute (ml/100g/min)	ASL enables cross-session comparison
Sensitivity	High (3-5% at 3T)	Lower (1-2%)	BOLD superior for group studies
Temporal Resolution	High (seconds)	Moderate (>3 seconds)	BOLD is better for fast dynamics
Spatial Specificity	Mixed micro/macrovascular	More specific to microvasculature	ASL is a more accurate localisation
Clinical Applications	Limited quantitative	Stroke, tumours, perfusion disorders	ASL provides diagnostic perfusion
Contrast Agent	None (endogenous)	None (endogenous)	Both avoid exogenous contrast

7.2. Layer-Specific fMRI

Layer-specific or laminar functional MRI exploits the six-layer architecture of the neocortex, visible at ultra-high field strengths, to investigate cortical computation at the mesoscopic scale, thereby linking cellular neuroscience to systems function. Different cortical layers have distinct cellular compositions, receive specific inputs, and send characteristic outputs, with laminar activity patterns revealing feedforward versus feedback processing, local computation versus long-range communication, and hierarchical organisation of cortical information processing. Layer IV, the primary thalamic input layer, predominantly receives feedforward sensory input. Superficial layers (II/III) receive feedback from higher cortical areas and project to other cortical regions. Deep layers (V/VI) send output to subcortical structures and other cortical areas. Measuring activity across cortical depth, therefore, provides insights into cortical processing streams and computational mechanisms that are invisible to conventional fMRI averaging across layers. The technique requires ultra-high-field systems (7T or higher), which provide sufficient signal-to-noise ratio for submillimeter resolution. It also utilises specialised sequences that minimise vascular contamination from surface vessels, as well as careful analysis that accounts for cortical curvature and depth-dependent vascular architecture (Polimeni et al., 2010).

The technical implementation of layer-specific fMRI employs gradient-echo or spin-echo sequences with in-plane resolutions of 0.4-0.8 millimetres and thin slices oriented perpendicular to the cortical surface within regions of interest. Gradient echo provides better sensitivity but also includes contributions from both microvasculature and large draining veins on the cortical surface, which can obscure laminar patterns. Spin echo reduces the contribution from large vessels through diffusion weighting during the refocusing pulse, providing a more specific microvascular signal at the cost of reduced sensitivity. The choice between approaches depends on whether sensitivity or specificity is more critical for the application. Acquisition typically focuses on small regions of interest rather than the whole brain to achieve the required resolution within an acceptable scan time, though multi-band acceleration enables greater coverage. Post-processing includes careful alignment with high-resolution anatomical images, cortical surface reconstruction, and sampling of activity across cortical depth, defined relative to the Grey-White boundary and pial surface. Analysis must account for depth-dependent partial volume effects, varying vascular contributions across depth, and individual variations in layer thickness.

Cortical depth-dependent BOLD responses exhibit characteristic patterns that reflect laminar physiology and vascular architecture. In the primary sensory cortex, stimulus-evoked responses typically show peaks in the middle cortical layers, corresponding to layer IV input zones, with secondary peaks in the superficial and deep layers. The exact laminar profile varies with stimulus parameters, attentional state, and task demands, revealing the dynamic engagement of different cortical layers. Feedback modulation is characterised by enhanced activity in the superficial layer, whereas feedforward drive exhibits stronger responses in the middle layer. The relative timing of responses across depth can indicate whether processing proceeds feedforward (from deep to superficial) or involves feedback (from superficial to deep). However, the sluggish hemodynamic response limits temporal precision. Comparison of laminar profiles across the cortical hierarchy reveals systematic changes that reflect hierarchical processing, with higher areas showing relatively greater activation in the superficial layer, suggesting increased feedback influence.

Applications of layer-specific fMRI span basic neuroscience questions about cortical computation and clinical investigations of layer-selective pathology. In visual neuroscience, laminar fMRI has revealed orientation, ocular dominance, and feature maps across cortical depth, confirming and extending findings from animal electrophysiology. Attention studies demonstrate layer-specific modulation: top-down attention preferentially enhances superficial layer activity, while stimulus-driven attention modulates middle layers, supporting theories of attention as a feedback signal. Predictive coding models propose that feedback conveys predictions, while feedforward signals carry prediction errors. These models predict specific laminar patterns, which are testable with layer-specific fMRI, with emerging evidence supporting these predictions. Memory studies show layer-specific patterns during encoding and retrieval, suggesting distinct contributions of input, processing, and output layers to memory formation.

Clinical applications remain in early stages but show promise for investigating layer-selective pathology in neurological and psychiatric disorders. Schizophrenia theories propose dysfunction of superficial layer inhibitory interneurons, potentially testable through abnormal laminar activation patterns. Alzheimer's disease pathology begins in specific cortical layers before spreading, and layer-specific fMRI may potentially enable earlier detection. Epilepsy may show abnormal laminar activity in seizure foci detectable before conventional imaging abnormalities appear. Multiple sclerosis cortical lesions affect specific layers, which can be potentially characterised through laminar fMRI. However, clinical translation requires solving the challenges of long scan times, patient motion, and the need for ultra-high-field systems. As methods become more efficient and high-field systems become more available, clinical applications may expand.

Challenges and limitations of layer-specific fMRI include the demanding acquisition and analysis requirements, sensitivity to motion and physiological noise, and ambiguity in relating BOLD laminar profiles to underlying neural activity due to depth-dependent vascular effects and limited spatial coverage, which restricts studies to small cortical regions. The draining vein problem, in which surface veins collect blood from all layers, can obscure or distort actual laminar patterns, a problem partially addressed by spin-echo imaging but not eliminated. Individual variation in cortical folding, thickness, and layer proportions complicates group analysis and comparison to animal studies. Despite these limitations, the unique insights into cortical computation afforded by laminar fMRI—directly connecting human neuroimaging to cellular-level organisation investigated in animal models—make it a powerful technique for mechanistic investigation of cortical processing.

7.3. Hypercapnia and Hyperoxia Mapping

Hypercapnia and hyperoxia challenges involve the controlled manipulation of inhaled gas composition to independently modulate cerebral blood flow and blood oxygenation, enabling calibration of the BOLD response and mapping of cerebrovascular reactivity. Hypercapnia—elevated blood CO2 levels induced by CO2-enriched gas inhalation—causes cerebral vasodilation and increased blood flow without directly affecting oxygen metabolism, providing a tool for measuring vascular reactivity and calibrating BOLD responses. Hyperoxia—high-oxygen-concentration inhalation—increases blood oxygenation and causes mild vasoconstriction without directly altering metabolism. By comparing BOLD signal changes during gas challenges with task-evoked responses, calibrated fMRI approaches separate metabolic and vascular contributions to the BOLD signal, potentially yielding quantitative cerebral metabolic rate of oxygen consumption (CMRO2) measures (Davis et al., 1998).

Hypercapnia's physiological basis involves CO2 acting as a potent cerebral vasodilator through its impact on vascular smooth muscle, mediated by changes in extracellular pH. Inhalation of 5% CO2 increases arterial CO2 partial pressure by approximately 10 mmHg, resulting in cerebral blood flow increases of 30-50% and corresponding BOLD signal increases of 2-4% at 3 Tesla. Hyperoxia increases arterial oxygen partial pressure and haemoglobin saturation, reducing deoxyhaemoglobin concentration and increasing the BOLD signal through enhanced oxygenation.

Cerebrovascular reactivity mapping utilises hypercapnia challenges to assess the amplitude of vascular responses across the brain, providing clinically valuable information on vascular health and reserve capacity. Applications include stroke risk assessment and hemodynamic impairment evaluation from carotid stenosis or moyamoya disease.

Calibrated BOLD approaches utilise hypercapnia or hyperoxia data to calibrate the BOLD signal-oxygen metabolism relationship, thereby enabling the estimation of CMRO2 changes during task performance. The Davis model relates the BOLD signal change to cerebral blood flow and CMRO2 changes via a proportionality constant (M parameter), which represents the maximum possible BOLD signal change with complete deoxyhemoglobin washout (Hoge et al., 1999).

Applications include investigating variations in neurovascular and neurometabolic coupling across brain regions, cognitive processes, development, ageing, and disease. Table 7.2 shows gas challenge techniques in advanced fMRI.

Table 7.2. Gas challenge techniques in advanced fMRI

Gas Challenge	Physiological Effect	Typical BOLD Change	Primary Applications	Advantages	Limitations
Hypercapnia (5% CO2)	Vasodilation, ↑CBF 30-50%	+2-4% at 3T	CVR mapping, calibrated fMRI	Flow-selective, validated	Subject discomfort
Hyperoxia (100% O2)	↑Arterial O2, mild vasoconstriction	+1-2%	Oxygenation mapping, tumour hypoxia	Safe, well-tolerated	Smaller signal, complex effects
Breath-hold	↑CO2 from apnea	+1-3%	CVR mapping, no equipment needed	Simple, accessible	Variable tolerance, less control
Combined CO2/O2	Both flow and oxygenation	Variable	Complete vascular characterisation	Comprehensive	Complex protocol

7.4. Functional Connectivity and Network Analysis

Functional connectivity analysis characterises the statistical relationships between brain region activity time courses, revealing networks of regions that exhibit coordinated activity patterns, suggesting functional interactions. The basic approach calculates correlation, coherence, or other measures of dependence between BOLD time series from different brain locations, with high connectivity indicating that regions tend to activate and deactivate in tandem. Network analysis extends pairwise connectivity to characterise whole-brain organisation using graph theory, representing the brain as a network of nodes (regions) and edges (connections), enabling the quantification of organisational properties, including modularity, hubs, small-world architecture, and efficiency. These approaches have revealed fundamental principles of brain network organisation: brains exhibit small-world topology, balancing local clustering and global integration; segregate into modules that support specialised functions while maintaining integrative hubs; and show hierarchical organisation, ranging from primary sensory-motor systems through the association cortex. The network perspective has transformed neuroscience from a focus on individual regions to an emphasis on distributed systems and their interactions (Bullmore & Sporns, 2009).

Methodological approaches to functional connectivity vary in their assumptions, computational demands, and sensitivity to different aspects of brain organisation. Seed-based connectivity defines one or more regions of interest and calculates connectivity between the seeds and all brain voxels, producing maps showing networks connected to the seed regions. This directed approach tests specific hypotheses about areas but requires a priori region selection, which may miss unexpected network organisation. Independent component analysis decomposes whole-brain data into maximally independent spatial components, representing networks and automatically identifying major networks without requiring prior knowledge of seeds. Still, it does demand component number selection and interpretation. Dictionary learning and related methods employ sparse representations, clustering identifies similar connectivity patterns across voxels, and graph-based approaches characterise network topology. The choice of method depends on whether exploratory network identification or hypothesis-driven connectivity testing is the primary goal, the computational resources available, and the type of network organisation being studied.

Graph-theoretical analysis quantifies brain network organisation through mathematical measures that characterise network structure and function. Modularity quantifies how well the network segregates into communities of densely interconnected nodes, with high modularity indicating the presence of specialised subsystems. Hubs are nodes with high connectivity, high betweenness centrality (lying on many shortest paths between other nodes), or high participation coefficient (connecting across modules), playing critical roles in integration. The brain exhibits consistent hub regions, including the posterior cingulate cortex, precuneus, and lateral parietal regions within the default mode network, as well as prefrontal and temporal regions. Small-world architecture, characterised by high local clustering similar to that of regular lattices, combined with short path lengths identical to those of random networks, describes the organisation of the healthy brain, enabling efficient local processing and global integration. Efficiency measures quantify how effectively the network transfers information, with global efficiency reflecting integration and local efficiency reflecting segregation. These metrics reveal organisational principles underlying brain function and show alterations in neurological and psychiatric disorders.

Network dynamics extend static connectivity by examining how network organisation changes over time, recognising that brains dynamically reconfigure to meet changing task demands. Sliding-window approaches compute connectivity within temporal windows that are stepped through the scan, revealing fluctuations in network strength, topology, and module assignment. State-based methods, including hidden Markov models and clustering, identify discrete brain states that recur over time and exhibit characteristic connectivity patterns, with transitions between states potentially reflecting cognitive state changes. Time-frequency methods investigate whether connectivity is modulated at specific frequencies, revealing frequency-specific networks potentially reflecting different communication mechanisms. Dynamic network flexibility—how readily nodes change their module assignment—varies across regions and individuals, potentially relating to cognitive flexibility and learning. Regions with high flexibility may implement adaptive control, while stable core networks provide consistent information processing.

Clinical applications of connectivity analysis have proliferated as relationships between network alterations and clinical symptoms are established. Alzheimer's disease shows disrupted connectivity within the default mode network preceding widespread atrophy, with connectivity deficits correlating with cognitive impairment and predicting conversion from mild cognitive impairment. Schizophrenia demonstrates reduced connectivity between the prefrontal cortex and distributed cortical regions, consistent with dysconnectivity theories, plus altered thalamo-cortical connectivity potentially explaining positive symptoms. Depression exhibits increased connectivity within the default mode network and between the default mode and subgenual cingulate, as well as reduced connectivity in frontoparietal networks, patterns that potentially predict treatment response. Autism spectrum disorder exhibits reduced long-range connectivity and increased local connectivity, with the underconnectivity theory suggesting that poor long-range integration underlies social and communication deficits. Brain injury produces widespread connectivity disruptions correlating with clinical outcomes, with connectivity metrics showing promise for prognosis in traumatic brain injury and stroke.

Methodological considerations in connectivity analysis include numerous sources of artefacts and confounds that require careful preprocessing and analysis. Head motion creates spurious correlations through signal displacement, which is partially addressed through motion regression but requires sophisticated approaches, such as scrubbing high-motion volumes or ICA-based denoising. Global signal regression—regressing the mean brain signal across all voxels—remains controversial: it increases anticorrelations and may introduce artefacts, but it also removes physiological noise. Physiological correction using cardiac and respiratory recordings or data-driven approaches improves specificity. The choice of brain parcellation into nodes significantly impacts results, as different schemes yield distinct network properties. Statistical testing of connectivity differences requires careful attention to dependence structure and multiple comparisons. Despite these challenges, carefully implemented connectivity analysis provides valuable insights into brain organisation and disease-related alterations.

7.5. Dynamic Functional Connectivity

Dynamic functional connectivity examines temporal variations in brain network organisation, moving beyond the assumption of static connectivity and its stable network structure across scans to reveal how brains flexibly reconfigure as cognitive demands, attentional states, and arousal fluctuate. The recognition that connectivity patterns change over timescales of seconds to minutes, rather than remaining constant, has transformed the understanding of brain network function, revealing flexibility and adaptation as fundamental features of brain function. Dynamic connectivity approaches employ sliding temporal windows, computing connectivity within each window as it moves through the data. These approaches identify recurring connectivity states through clustering or hidden Markov modelling, or examine frequency-specific modulation of connectivity. The biological interpretation of observed dynamics remains debated, with some dynamics reflecting actual network reconfiguration while others may arise from sampling variability, edge-of-stability fluctuations, or non-stationarity. Nonetheless, mounting evidence suggests that dynamic connectivity metrics are related to cognitive performance, consciousness states, development, ageing, and clinical conditions, supporting their functional significance beyond methodological artefacts (Hutchison et al., 2013).

Sliding-window correlation represents the most straightforward approach to dynamic connectivity, computing connectivity within temporal windows of 30-120 seconds, stepping through the scan at intervals of single TRs or several TRs. Each window yields a connectivity matrix that captures the network organisation during that period, with the sequence of matrices revealing how connectivity evolves. The window length trades temporal resolution against reliability of correlation estimates, with shorter windows capturing rapid dynamics but increasing noise. Measures extracted from windowed connectivity include the variance of connectivity across windows, which quantifies temporal variability, transitions between high and low connectivity states, and correlations between connectivity time courses, indicating whether region pairs exhibit similar connectivity dynamics. Pattern analysis can identify recurring connectivity configurations by clustering connectivity matrices, revealing a repertoire of network states the brain visits. Statistical testing of dynamic connectivity differences between groups or conditions requires addressing temporal autocorrelation and variability in window characteristics.

Brain-state identification via clustering or hidden Markov models provides a discrete characterisation of network configurations and their temporal dynamics. Clustering approaches, such as k-means, can be applied to windowed connectivity matrices to identify centroids that represent prototypical connectivity patterns. The sequence of cluster assignments reveals state sequences and transition frequencies, while state occupancy quantifies the amount of time spent in each configuration. Hidden Markov models explicitly model state sequences as Markov chains, inferring hidden states from observed data and providing probabilistic state assignments. The resulting states often exhibit interpretable functional organisation, such as states with strong within-network connectivity, states that emphasise integration across networks, or states that reflect task-related network configurations. State dynamics, including dwell times, transition probabilities, and state occurrence patterns, differ across task conditions, consciousness levels, and clinical populations, revealing the functional significance of network reconfiguration.

Time-frequency analysis investigates whether connectivity is modulated at specific frequencies, potentially revealing distinct communication mechanisms at different timescales. Coherence and phase synchrony quantify frequency-specific coordination between regions, with different frequencies potentially supporting various types of information transfer. Low frequencies (<0.1 Hz) dominate resting-state connectivity, while higher frequencies may reflect more direct neural coupling. Wavelet coherence enables time-frequency analysis, revealing how connectivity at specific frequencies fluctuates over time. Some studies suggest that connectivity transiently increases at specific frequencies during cognitive events, consistent with coherence-based communication theories, which propose that neural populations coordinate by synchronising oscillations. However, the hemodynamic filtering of neural activity limits interpretation of high-frequency BOLD connectivity, and the relationship between fMRI-observed connectivity dynamics and underlying neural oscillations remains incompletely understood.

The biological basis and functional significance of dynamic connectivity remain active research areas with ongoing debates. Simulations demonstrate that specific dynamic connectivity patterns can arise from stationary networks with noise, cautioning against over-interpretation. However, studies showing relationships between dynamics and behaviour, task performance, or clinical symptoms argue for a functional significance beyond artefact. Proposed mechanisms include genuine network reconfiguration driven by neuromodulatory systems, edge-of-stability dynamics in which networks operate near critical points, producing natural variability; attentional fluctuations that modulate connectivity; and changes in arousal state that affect global brain organisation. Combined EEG-fMRI studies reveal that some fMRI connectivity dynamics correlate with electrical signatures of cognitive states, supporting neural origins. The time constants of observed dynamics—seconds to minutes—match attention and arousal fluctuations more closely than millisecond-scale neural communication, suggesting that dynamics may reflect slower state changes rather than trial-by-trial neural synchronisation.

Clinical applications of dynamic connectivity have demonstrated altered flexibility and state dynamics in various disorders. Schizophrenia shows reduced dynamic range with less variability in connectivity patterns, potentially reflecting reduced flexibility in network reconfiguration underlying cognitive deficits. Autism spectrum disorder demonstrates atypical connectivity dynamics with altered state transition probabilities. Depression exhibits increased time in states dominated by default mode connectivity, consistent with excessive self-focus. Attention-deficit hyperactivity disorder (ADHD) exhibits more variable connectivity, potentially reflecting fluctuations in attention. Epilepsy studies reveal altered dynamics near seizure onset, with potential for predicting seizures from connectivity state evolution. Traumatic brain injury disrupts normal connectivity dynamics, leading to a reduction in the complexity of state sequences. These clinical applications demonstrate that connectivity dynamics capture clinically relevant brain dysfunction, complementing static connectivity measures and supporting their value in understanding disease mechanisms and potentially guiding treatment.

7.6. Multivariate Pattern Analysis (MVPA)

Multivariate pattern analysis represents a paradigm shift in fMRI data analysis, moving from asking where in the brain processes occur to asking what information is described. This approach utilises pattern classification, representational similarity analysis, and encoding models to decode neural representations from distributed activity patterns. Unlike conventional univariate analysis, which tests each voxel independently, MVPA jointly considers patterns across multiple voxels, enabling the detection of information encoded in subtle, distributed patterns that are invisible to mass-univariate approaches. The technique can decode stimulus categories, cognitive states, task rules, and even the content of thoughts from brain activity patterns, demonstrating that behaviorally relevant information is distributed across neural populations rather than localised to single regions. MVPA connects neuroimaging to information theory and computational neuroscience by quantifying representational content, testing neural coding hypotheses, and enabling reading out of mental states. The approach has revealed unanticipated representations in regions that show no univariate activation, demonstrating that information is often encoded in patterns across seemingly homogeneous areas. This has provided tools for testing computational models of cognition (Haxby et al., 2001; Norman et al., 2006).

Classification analysis trains machine learning algorithms to distinguish between conditions based on spatial activity patterns, then tests whether the classifier generalises to held-out data. Successful decoding demonstrates that conditions are associated with distinguishable neural patterns. Support vector machines are the most commonly used classifier, finding optimal hyperplanes that separate conditions in high-dimensional voxel space. However, other methods, including logistic regression, naive Bayes, and neural networks, are also employed. The standard approach uses cross-validation: training is performed on data from all but one run, and testing is conducted on the held-out run, repeating this process for all runs and averaging the accuracies. Accuracy significantly above chance indicates decodable information, with the voxel pattern weights revealing which voxels contribute most to discrimination. Classification can distinguish stimulus categories, task conditions, behavioural responses, or any conditions that differ across trials. The approach is compelling for decoding information from regions where conditions produce no detectable mean activity differences, revealing information coding in relative patterns across neural populations.

Representational similarity analysis (RSA) characterises neural representations by computing the pattern similarity between all pairs of conditions, creating a representational dissimilarity matrix (RDM) that captures the representational geometry. The RDM shows which conditions produce similar neural patterns and which produce distinct patterns, revealing the representational structure. RDMs can be compared between brain regions to test whether regions use similar representational schemes, between subjects to assess individual differences, or between brain data and computational models to test neural coding hypotheses. Model-based RSA correlates brain RDMs with model predictions, identifying regions whose representations match model predictions. For example, comparing brain RDMs to semantic similarity models tests whether regions represent semantic features, while comparing to visual appearance models tests visual coding. RSA provides richer characterisation than classification, revealing representational structure rather than just discriminability, and naturally handles many conditions without requiring extensive training data per condition (Kriegeskorte et al., 2008).

Encoding models predict neural responses from stimulus features or cognitive variables, complementing decoding approaches by explicitly modelling representational content. The model specifies how stimulus features map to predicted activity, with parameters fitted to observed data, then tested on held-out stimuli. For example, visual encoding models predict V1 activity from local oriented edge features, semantic encoding models predict higher cortical activity from semantic features, and motor encoding models predict motor cortex activity from movement parameters. Successful prediction demonstrates that the model captures representational content, with model comparison revealing which feature spaces best explain neural responses. Encoding models enable the testing of computational theories by comparing predictions from competing models, extrapolating to novel stimuli outside the training set, and generating explicit hypotheses about the tuning properties of neural populations. The approach has revealed a hierarchical organisation of the visual cortex, with receptive field size and feature complexity increasing along the ventral stream, semantic organisation in the temporal cortex, and motor planning representations in frontal-parietal networks.

Searchlight analysis offers a whole-brain approach to MVPA by repeatedly applying classification or RSA to small spherical neighbourhoods of voxels, thereby creating maps that show where information is decodable in the brain. Each searchlight—typically 3-6 voxel radius—represents a local neural population, with classification or RSA performed using only voxels within the sphere. The procedure is repeated, centring on each brain voxel, to produce a map where values reflect decoding accuracy or RSA correlation at each location. This data-driven approach identifies regions containing information without requiring a priori region selection; however, spatial smoothing due to searchlight size limits localisation precision. Searchlight analysis has revealed information distributed across areas that do not show univariate activation, demonstrated the anterior-posterior organisation of semantic representations, and identified multiple cortical regions encoding task rules. The computational demands of searchlight analysis are substantial, as it requires repeating MVPA thousands of times; however, parallelisation makes whole-brain searchlight analysis practical.

Applications of MVPA span cognitive domains and have yielded surprising insights into information representation. Visual neuroscience applications demonstrate that object category information is distributed across the ventral temporal cortex with partially overlapping representations. Early visual areas contain high-level information about object categories and semantics, extending beyond low-level features, and attention modulates not only response amplitude but also the pattern of representation. Memory research indicates that retrieval involves reinstating encoding patterns, with the precision of reinstatement predicting the vividness of memory. Different patterns distinguish between remembering and familiarity, and false memories can be decoded, showing that they involve real neural representations. Language studies reveal semantic representations in the anterior temporal cortex, syntactic structure in frontal regions, and cross-modal semantic representations shared across reading and listening. Decision neuroscience has decoded choice predictions from prefrontal patterns, confidence from medial frontal patterns, and strategy from frontal-parietal patterns.

Clinical applications of MVPA are emerging but show promise for identifying biomarkers and mechanisms in neurological and psychiatric disorders. Classification of patients versus controls based on whole-brain activity patterns achieves high accuracy in some disorders, potentially providing diagnostic biomarkers. Altered representational geometry in patient populations reveals disrupted representations, such as reduced category selectivity in ventral temporal cortex in autism or altered emotional representations in depression. Decoding symptom severity from neural patterns could provide objective measures that complement clinical assessment. Brain-computer interface applications utilise real-time MVPA to decode intended movements or communication from neural patterns in patients with paralysis. However, clinical translation requires validation in large independent samples, standardisation across sites, and demonstration that MVPA-derived measures provide information beyond existing assessments. Despite these challenges, the ability to read out information content from brain activity patterns offers transformative potential for understanding and treating brain disorders.

Conclusion

Advanced functional MRI techniques expand neuroimaging capabilities beyond conventional BOLD contrast, offering quantitative physiological measurements and enhanced spatial specificity. Arterial spin labelling enables the quantitative measurement of cerebral blood flow without the use of contrast agents, providing clinically valuable perfusion information for the diagnosis and monitoring of vascular disorders. Multi-delay approaches and improved acquisition efficiency position ASL to complement or replace BOLD when quantitative comparisons are critical.

Layer-specific fMRI at ultra-high field reveals cortical computation at mesoscopic scales, demonstrating distinct laminar signatures: feedforward processing drives middle layers, feedback modulates superficial layers, and output originates from deep layers, thereby validating theories of cortical hierarchical organisation.

Hypercapnia and hyperoxia mapping characterise cerebrovascular reactivity, enabling calibrated fMRI to extract quantitative metabolic information from hemodynamic responses. This addresses ambiguities in the contributions of vascular and neural systems to differences in activation.

Functional connectivity and network analysis have revolutionised our understanding of brain organisation, revealing consistent networks, including the default mode, attention, control, and sensory-motor systems, that exhibit small-world architecture and a modular-hierarchical structure. Dynamic functional connectivity extends this by revealing flexible network reconfiguration over seconds to minutes, with transitions associated with cognitive states and clinical conditions.

Multivariate pattern analysis enables the investigation of what information is represented, rather than merely where processes occur, by decoding stimulus categories, cognitive states, and mental content from distributed activity patterns.

The future integration of multiple advanced techniques—combining quantitative perfusion, laminar specificity, calibrated metabolism, network dynamics, and information decoding—will provide comprehensive characterisation of brain function, transforming both fundamental neuroscience and clinical applications.

Acknowledgments

The authors would like to extend our appreciation to those who offered helpful commentary during the drafting process of this manuscript. We also acknowledge the role the Nova Publishing department played in enabling the work described herein.

References

Bullmore, E., & Sporns, O. (2009). Complex brain networks: Graph theoretical analysis of structural and functional systems. *Nature Reviews Neuroscience*, 10(3), 186-198. https://doi.org/10.1038/nrn2575.

Davis, T. L., Kwong, K. K., Weisskoff, R. M., & Rosen, B. R. (1998). Calibrated functional MRI: Mapping the dynamics of oxidative metabolism. *Proceedings of the National Academy of Sciences*, 95(4), 1834-1839. https://doi.org/10.1073/pnas.95.4.1834.

Detre, J. A., Leigh, J. S., Williams, D. S., & Koretsky, A. P. (1992). Perfusion imaging. *Magnetic Resonance in Medicine*, 23(1), 37-45. https://doi.org/10.1002/mrm.1910230106.

Haxby, J. V., Gobbini, M. I., Furey, M. L., Ishai, A., Schouten, J. L., & Pietrini, P. (2001). Distributed and overlapping representations of faces and objects in ventral temporal cortex. *Science*, 293(5539), 2425-2430. https://doi.org/10.1126/science.1063736.

Hoge, R. D., Atkinson, J., Gill, B., Crelier, G. R., Marrett, S., & Pike, G. B. (1999). Investigation of BOLD signal dependence on cerebral blood flow and oxygen consumption: The deoxyhemoglobin dilution model. *Magnetic Resonance in Medicine*, 42(5), 849-863. https://doi.org/10.1002/(SICI)1522-2594(199911)42:5<849::AID-MRM4>3.0.CO;2-Z.

Hutchison, R. M., Womelsdorf, T., Allen, E. A., Bandettini, P. A., Calhoun, V. D., Corbetta, M., Della Penna, S., Duyn, J. H., Glover, G. H., Gonzalez-Castillo, J., Handwerker, D. A., Keilholz, S., Kiviniemi, V., Leopold, D. A., de Pasquale, F., Sporns, O., Walter, M., & Chang, C. (2013). Dynamic functional connectivity: Promise, issues, and interpretations. *NeuroImage*, 80, 360-378. https://doi.org/10.
1016/j.neuroimage.2013.05.079.

Kriegeskorte, N., Mur, M., & Bandettini, P. A. (2008). Representational similarity analysis—Connecting the branches of systems neuroscience. *Frontiers in Systems Neuroscience*, 2, 4. https://doi.org/10.3389/neuro.06.004.2008.

Norman, K. A., Polyn, S. M., Detre, G. J., & Haxby, J. V. (2006). Beyond mind-reading: Multi-voxel pattern analysis of fMRI data. *Trends in Cognitive Sciences*, 10(9), 424-430. https://doi.org/10.1016/j.tics.2006.07.005.

Polimeni, J. R., Fischl, B., Greve, D. N., & Wald, L. L. (2010). Laminar analysis of 7T BOLD using an imposed spatial activation pattern in human V1. *NeuroImage*, 52(4), 1334-1346. https://doi.org/10.1016/j.neuroimage.2010.05.005.

Chapter 8

Magnetic Resonance Spectroscopy (MRS)

Sushil Ghanshyam Kachewar[1,*] and Maajid Mohi Ud Din Malik[2,†]

[1]Department of Radio-Diagnosis, Dr. D. Y. Patil Medical College, Hospital and Research Centre, Dr. D. Y. Patil Vidyapeeth (Deemed to be University)- Sant Tukaram Nagar, Pimpri, Pune, India
[2]Radiology and Imaging Technology, Dr. D. Y. Patil School of Allied Health Sciences, Dr. D. Y. Patil Vidyapeeth (Deemed to be University), Sant Tukaram Nagar, Pimpri, Pune, India

Abstract

Magnetic resonance spectroscopy extends the capabilities of MRI beyond anatomical and functional imaging to provide non-invasive biochemical characterisation of tissue metabolism and composition by measuring metabolite concentrations. This chapter comprehensively examines MRS principles, methodologies, and applications in neurological disorders, from fundamental concepts of chemical shift and spectral analysis through advanced multi-dimensional techniques. Proton MRS detects brain metabolites, including N-acetylaspartate (a neuronal marker), creatine (involved in energy metabolism), choline (related to membrane turnover), and others, providing insights into neuronal integrity, energy status, and pathological processes. Single-voxel spectroscopy enables the acquisition of high-quality spectra from targeted regions, while multi-voxel chemical shift imaging maps metabolite distributions across the entire brain volume. Quantification methods convert spectral peak areas into absolute or relative metabolite concentrations, necessitating careful consideration of acquisition parameters, post-processing, and analysis choices. Advanced techniques, including two-dimensional spectroscopy, spectral editing for overlapping peaks, and ultra-high-field implementations, improve spectral resolution and expand the detectable metabolites. Phosphorus and carbon-13 spectroscopy provide complementary information about energy metabolism and metabolic fluxes. Clinical applications span brain tumours, where metabolite patterns aid in diagnosis and monitoring; neurodegenerative diseases, which reveal metabolic dysfunction; epilepsy, for identifying seizure foci; and inherited

* Corresponding Author's Email: sushil.kachewar@dpu.edu.in
† Corresponding Author's Email: maajid.malik@dpu.edu.in

In: Recent Advances in Magnetic Resonance Imaging in Neuroimaging
Editors: Maajid Mohi Ud Din Malik, Purnachandra Kawdu Lamghare and R. S. Kuber
ISBN: 979-8-90134-244-2

metabolic disorders, enabling diagnosis and treatment monitoring. MRS provides unique metabolic information that complements anatomical and functional imaging, establishing it as a valuable tool for investigating brain biochemistry in both healthy and diseased states.

Keywords: magnetic resonance spectroscopy, brain metabolites, N-acetylaspartate, spectral quantification, neurochemistry, SDG 3 - good health and well-being

Introduction

Magnetic resonance spectroscopy applies nuclear magnetic resonance principles to detect and quantify specific chemical compounds based on their unique resonant frequencies, extending MRI's capabilities beyond anatomical structure and hemodynamic function to biochemical composition and metabolism. The technique exploits the chemical shift phenomenon, in which the electron clouds surrounding atomic nuclei slightly modify the local magnetic field experienced by the nuclei, causing nuclei in different molecular environments to resonate at distinct frequencies. These frequency differences, measured in parts per million relative to a reference compound, give rise to spectral peaks characteristic of specific metabolites. By analysing the resulting spectrum—a plot of signal intensity versus frequency—MRS identifies metabolites present in tissue and quantifies their concentrations. In brain tissue, proton MRS routinely detects 5-10 primary metabolites, along with numerous minor peaks, providing a metabolic fingerprint reflecting neuronal integrity, membrane turnover, energy metabolism, neurotransmitter systems, and pathological processes.

The development of *in vivo* MRS for brain applications dates back to pioneering work in the 1980s, which demonstrated that, despite metabolite concentrations (millimolar range) being much lower than water (approximately 40 molar), careful pulse sequence design and signal averaging could yield interpretable spectra from the human brain. Early applications focused on identifying gross metabolic abnormalities in tumours and infarcts, demonstrating that pathological processes produce characteristic spectral changes detectable non-invasively. The technique has matured substantially over the past four decades, with improvements in field strength, coil technology, pulse sequences, and post-processing enabling the detection of additional metabolites, improved quantification accuracy, and faster acquisitions suitable for clinical workflows. The concurrent development of phosphorus-31 and carbon-13 spectroscopy has complemented proton MRS by providing information about energy metabolism and metabolic pathway fluxes inaccessible to proton detection.

The clinical adoption of MRS has been gradual but steady, driven by its demonstrated diagnostic value in specific applications, including brain tumour characterisation, differentiation of tumour progression from treatment effects, epilepsy focus localisation, and diagnosis of inherited metabolic disorders. The technique's integration into multiparametric MRI protocols, which combine conventional imaging, diffusion, perfusion, and spectroscopy, provides comprehensive tissue characterisation that exceeds what any single modality offers. Research applications continue to expand, investigating subtle metabolic changes in psychiatric disorders, neurodegenerative diseases, traumatic brain injury, and standard processes, including development, ageing, and learning. The recognition that many neurological and psychiatric conditions involve metabolic dysfunction before structural changes become apparent has reinforced the value of MRS for early detection and mechanistic investigation. This chapter comprehensively examines MRS, covering physical principles, acquisition methods, quantification approaches, advanced techniques, and clinical applications, providing both a foundational understanding and practical knowledge for implementation and interpretation.

8.1. Principles of Proton MR Spectroscopy

Proton magnetic resonance spectroscopy detects signals from hydrogen nuclei in brain metabolites, exploiting chemical shift differences to distinguish compounds based on their molecular structure and chemical environments. The chemical shift arises because electrons surrounding nuclei generate small local magnetic fields that either shield or deshield the nuclei from the main magnetic field, causing nuclei in different molecules or molecular environments to resonate at slightly different frequencies. The magnitude of chemical shift is expressed in parts per million (ppm) relative to a reference compound, providing a field-strength-independent scale. Water protons resonate at 4.7 ppm by convention, with metabolites of interest distributed between 0.5 and 4.0 ppm for proton nuclear magnetic resonance spectroscopy. The chemical shift scale enables the identification of metabolites by their characteristic peak positions, while peak areas reflect their concentrations. The fundamental challenge in brain MRS is that metabolite concentrations are approximately 10,000 times lower than those of water, requiring water suppression techniques to avoid overwhelming the metabolite signals, combined with signal averaging over several minutes to achieve an adequate signal-to-noise ratio (Oz et al., 2014).

The primary brain metabolites detectable by proton MRS at clinical field strengths include N-acetylaspartate (NAA) resonating at 2.0 ppm, the most prominent peak in healthy brain spectra, synthesised in neurons and generally interpreted as a neuronal marker with concentrations around 10-12 mmol/kg. Creatine (Cr) at 3.0 and 3.9 ppm reflects the total creatine and phosphocreatine pools involved in energy metabolism and serves as a relatively stable reference for calculating metabolite ratios, with concentrations around 8-10 mmol/kg. Choline (Cho) at 3.2 ppm represents choline-containing compounds involved in membrane synthesis and degradation, with elevated levels suggesting increased cell turnover. Concentrations typically range from 1 to 2 mmol/kg. Myo-inositol (mI), at 3.56 ppm, a glial marker and osmolyte, exhibits concentrations of approximately 4-8 mmol/kg. Glutamate and glutamine (Glx) produce overlapping peaks at 2.1-2.4 ppm, representing the major excitatory neurotransmitter and its metabolic product, with total concentrations of around 10-12 mmol/kg. However, separating them is challenging in clinical settings. Lactate at 1.33 ppm appears as an inverted doublet, usually absent or minimal but elevated in ischemia, tumours, and metabolic disorders.

The physics of spectroscopy acquisition employs specialised pulse sequences designed to maximise the signal from metabolites while suppressing contamination from water and lipids. Point-resolved spectroscopy (PRESS) utilises three slice-selective pulses (90°-180°-180°) to define a rectangular voxel, providing high spatial resolution with relatively short echo times, enabling the detection of metabolites with short T2 relaxation times. Stimulated echo acquisition mode (STEAM) employs three 90° pulses to generate a stimulated echo, allowing for very short echo times and precise localisation, but with a 50% theoretical signal loss compared to spin-echo methods. Water suppression is typically achieved through chemical-shift-selective (CHESS) pulses that saturate water protons, requiring careful frequency adjustment and often multiple suppression pulses to attain adequate suppression factors of 1000 or greater. Outer-volume suppression applies saturation pulses to regions surrounding the voxel of interest, reducing lipid contamination from the scalp and the skull.

The choice of echo time (TE) significantly affects spectral appearance and the metabolites that can be reliably detected. Short TE acquisitions (20-40 ms) preserve signals from metabolites with short T2 relaxation times, including myo-inositol, glutamate, and glutamine, providing complete metabolic profiles but with more baseline distortion from macromolecular signals. Long TE acquisitions (135-144 ms) simplify spectra by allowing short-T2 metabolites to decay, producing cleaner baselines dominated by NAA, creatine, and choline peaks, which facilitates quantification but may miss essential metabolites. Intermediate TE (70-80 ms) attempts to strike a balance between these considerations. The optimal TE depends on the clinical question and whether comprehensive metabolite quantification or simplified, yet reliable, quantification of major peaks is prioritised. Many clinical protocols employ long TE for routine scanning, with short TE reserved for cases requiring complete metabolite profiles.

Spectral quality depends on multiple factors, including voxel size, location, acquisition time, field strength, and shimming effectiveness. Larger voxels provide a higher signal-to-noise ratio by contributing from more nuclei, but at the expense of reduced spatial specificity and increased susceptibility to field inhomogeneities. Typical single voxel sizes range from 1 to 8 cubic centimetres, balancing SNR and localisation. Acquisition times of 3-10 minutes yield 128-512 signal averages, resulting in interpretable spectra. Higher field strengths provide improved SNR and increased chemical shift dispersion, scaling linearly with the field, thereby separating overlapping peaks. However, higher fields require more careful shimming due to greater absolute frequency variation caused by field inhomogeneities. Shimming—adjustment of magnetic field homogeneity across the voxel—critically affects spectral quality, with poor shimming causing line broadening that obscures metabolite peaks and prevents accurate quantification. Automated shimming algorithms adjust shim currents to minimise the water linewidth, although manual adjustment may be necessary for challenging locations.

Interpreting MRS spectra requires understanding both standard metabolite patterns and pathological alterations. A healthy adult brain exhibits consistent metabolite patterns, with NAA as the dominant peak, creatine and choline as smaller but prominent peaks, myo-inositol visible at short TE, and minimal or absent lactate. Regional variation exists: Grey matter shows higher NAA than white matter, and white matter shows higher choline. Age-related changes include decreased NAA in the elderly, increased myo-inositol, and altered glutamate levels. Pathological processes produce characteristic spectral alterations. Neuronal loss or dysfunction reduces NAA, while increased cell turnover or membrane breakdown elevates choline. Energy failure or hypoxia elevates lactate. Demyelination may reduce NAA and increase choline and myo-inositol, and gliosis increases myo-inositol. The pattern of alterations, combined with anatomical imaging, provides diagnostic information that exceeds what either technique offers alone. Table 8.1 shows primary brain metabolites detected by proton MRS.

Table 8.1. Major brain metabolites detected by proton MRS

Metabolite	Chemical Shift (ppm)	Normal Concentration (mmol/kg)	Primary Biological Role	Pathological Changes
N-Acetylaspartate (NAA)	2.0	10-12	Neuronal marker, neuronal health	↓ in neuronal loss, dysfunction, and demyelination
Creatine (Cr)	3.0, 3.9	8-10	Energy metabolism	Relatively stable, used as a reference
Choline (Cho)	3.2	1-2	Membrane turnover	↑ in tumours, demyelination, inflammation
Myo-inositol (mI)	3.56	4-8	Glial marker, osmolyte	↑ in gliosis, Alzheimer's disease
Glutamate + Glutamine (Glx)	2.1-2.4	10-12	Excitatory neurotransmission	Variable in disorders
Lactate (Lac)	1.33	<0.5 (minimal)	Anaerobic metabolism	↑ in ischemia, hypoxia, mitochondrial disorders
GABA	3.0 (overlaps)	1-2	Inhibitory neurotransmission	Requires spectral editing to detect
Glutathione (GSH)	2.95	1-2	Antioxidant	↓ in oxidative stress, ageing

8.2. Single Voxel vs. Multi-Voxel Spectroscopy

Single voxel spectroscopy (SVS) acquires spectra from a single predefined volume of interest, providing high-quality spectra with good signal-to-noise ratio and straightforward acquisition and analysis, making it the workhorse for clinical MRS. The technique positions a rectangular voxel within the region of interest, using anatomical images as a reference, and then acquires spectra exclusively from that location. The advantages include simplified prescription requiring selection of a single location, high spectral quality from larger voxel sizes (typically 2-8 cm^3) providing excellent SNR, relatively short acquisition times (3-8 minutes), and robust quantification from clean spectra. The primary limitation is that only one location can be examined per acquisition, requiring multiple separate acquisitions to sample different regions and providing no information about spatial metabolite distributions. Clinical applications employ SVS when the region of pathology is clearly defined on anatomical imaging, such as a focal tumour, lesion, or epilepsy focus, or when examining normal-appearing tissue within specific structures, such as the hippocampus or basal ganglia.

Multi-voxel spectroscopy, also known as chemical shift imaging (CSI), acquires spectra from multiple voxels arranged in a two-dimensional or three-dimensional grid across a slab or volume, providing spatial maps of metabolite distributions that are analogous to conventional MRI but with chemical information. The technique employs phase encoding in one, two, or three spatial dimensions to encode spatial position, combined with the frequency encoding inherent to spectroscopy, which separates metabolites. Each voxel in the resulting grid contains a complete spectrum, enabling the calculation of metabolite maps that show spatial variation in NAA, choline, creatine, and other metabolites. The advantages include comprehensive spatial coverage, allowing the detection of abnormalities not apparent on anatomical imaging; the ability to compare multiple regions from a single acquisition; and the visualisation of metabolite gradients and patterns. The disadvantages include longer acquisition times (8-20 minutes for clinical protocols), lower spatial resolution (typically 1 cm^3 per voxel, coarser than SVS), lower SNR per voxel compared to SVS of equivalent size, and more complex post-processing requiring analysis of dozens to hundreds of spectra (Posse et al., 2013).

Technical considerations in single-voxel spectroscopy focus on optimal voxel placement to sample relevant tissue while minimising artefacts. The voxel should encompass the pathology of interest, along with surrounding tissue for comparison, and be positioned to minimise cerebrospinal fluid inclusion, which lacks metabolites and reduces the metabolite signal. The skull and scalp should be excluded to prevent lipid contamination from subcutaneous fat, which requires careful angulation in some brain regions. Voxels are typically placed to align with major anatomical boundaries rather than arbitrary orientations. Common standardised voxel locations include the centrum semiovale for white matter sampling, the posterior cingulate for Grey matter, the thalamus, the putamen, or the hippocampus for specific structures, and precise tumour localisation guided by anatomical abnormalities. Control spectra from contralateral normal-appearing tissue provide an internal comparison for assessing the severity of pathology.

Multi-voxel spectroscopy implementation requires decisions about spatial resolution, coverage volume, and acquisition time. Typical 2D-CSI protocols employ 16×16 or 32×32 phase encoding matrices, covering a slab of interest with a voxel size of 1-1.5 cm, requiring an acquisition time of 10-15 minutes. Three-dimensional CSI extends coverage to a volume with phase encoding in all three dimensions, providing whole-brain metabolite maps; however, it demands a scan time of 20-30 minutes, which is often impractical clinically. The spatial resolution fundamentally limits SNR as smaller voxels contain fewer metabolite nuclei, requiring trade-offs between spatial detail and spectral quality. Accelerated CSI employing parallel imaging reduces acquisition time by 2-4, making higher-resolution or volumetric coverage more practical. Sparse sampling combined with compressed sensing reconstruction can further accelerate acquisition. However, the fundamental SNR limitation means that multi-voxel spectroscopy generally provides lower-quality spectra than single-voxel spectroscopy for any given voxel size and acquisition time.

The choice between single-voxel and multi-voxel approaches depends on the clinical question and practical constraints. Single-voxel spectroscopy is preferred when pathology is well-localised on anatomical imaging, the highest spectral quality is required for detecting subtle abnormalities, scan time is limited, or technical expertise for multi-voxel analysis is unavailable. Multi-voxel spectroscopy is preferred when the extent of metabolic abnormality is unknown or expected to exceed anatomical lesions, when comparing multiple regions is essential, when subtle metabolic gradients or patterns provide diagnostic information, or when research questions require mapping metabolite distributions. In practice, clinical protocols often employ single-voxel imaging for routine tumour characterisation and epilepsy evaluation, while research studies and specialised clinical applications use multi-voxel imaging for comprehensive assessment. Some clinical sites acquire both, using multi-voxel imaging for overview and single-voxel imaging for detailed examination of specific regions.

Post-processing of spectroscopy data involves several steps to convert raw time-domain data into interpretable spectra. Raw time-domain data is transformed into the frequency domain via the Fourier transform, producing the spectrum. Phase correction adjusts the spectral phase to align peaks, a critical step for accurate quantification. Baseline correction removes the broad underlying signal from macromolecules and lipids. Water residual removal eliminates the remaining water signal after suppression. For multi-voxel data, spatial interpolation may improve apparent resolution, though it cannot add accurate information. Quality control identifies spectra with inadequate quality due to motion, poor shimming, or lipid contamination, excluding them from analysis. Automated and semi-automated processing pipelines are increasingly used to enhance consistency and reduce analysis time; however, expert review remains crucial for identifying artefacts and ensuring accurate quantification.

8.3. Metabolite Quantification and Analysis

Metabolite quantification involves converting spectral peak areas into concentration values, which requires careful attention to acquisition parameters, reference standards, relaxation corrections, and analysis methods. The fundamental principle is that the peak area in the spectrum is proportional to metabolite concentration, number of equivalent protons, and signal intensity modulated by relaxation times. However, converting arbitrary peak areas to absolute concentrations in physiological units (mmol/kg or mmol/L) requires accounting for numerous factors, including coil sensitivity, voxel volume, water content, and differences in relaxation times between metabolites and the reference. Multiple quantification approaches have been developed, ranging from simple metabolite ratios to sophisticated absolute quantification methods that employ internal or external references, each with distinct advantages, limitations, and specific applications.

Relative quantification using metabolite ratios is the most straightforward and robust approach, in which metabolite peak areas are normalised to a reference metabolite, typically creatine. The NAA/Cr, Cho/Cr, and Cho/NAA ratios are commonly reported in clinical practice, providing dimensionless measures that are relatively insensitive to acquisition parameter variations and to instrumental factors that affect all peaks similarly. The approach assumes that the reference metabolite (creatine) remains constant across conditions, an assumption valid in many but not all situations. Advantages include simplicity, eliminating the need for concentration calibration, relative robustness across scanners and protocols, and established normal ranges for common ratios. Limitations include the inability to determine whether ratio changes reflect changes in the numerator, the denominator, or both; invalid when creatine itself is altered; and the failure to compare across different reference metabolites or studies using other methods. Metabolite ratios are well-suited for detecting significant abnormalities, screening applications, and comparing groups, but less ideal for precise quantification or conditions affecting creatine (Kreis, 2016).

Internal water referencing provides absolute or semi-absolute quantification by comparing metabolite signals to the water signal from the same voxel, using water's known concentration (approximately 43 molar in the brain) as an internal standard. The acquisition typically includes an unsuppressed water scan using identical parameters, except for water suppression, to measure the water signal, which is then used to calibrate metabolite concentrations. Corrections are applied for differences in relaxation times between water and metabolites, the number of equivalent protons per molecule, and partial volume effects from cerebrospinal fluid that affect water concentration. The approach provides absolute concentrations without requiring external phantoms, automatically accounts for coil sensitivity and instrumental factors through the internal reference, and enables standardised quantification across scanners. Limitations include the requirement for accurate tissue segmentation to estimate water content, sensitivity to CSF partial volume, and the need for precise relaxation time values that vary with field strength and may be altered in pathological conditions.

External phantom referencing involves scanning a phantom with known metabolite concentrations under identical conditions to those of patient scans, using the phantom signal to calibrate the patient's metabolite concentrations. The phantom, typically containing physiological concentrations of primary metabolites, provides a concentration standard; however, careful attention must be given to positioning the phantom similarly to account for coil sensitivity, acquiring phantom data regularly to track system stability, and correcting for temperature differences that affect relaxation times. Advantages include direct concentration measurement and independence from assumptions about tissue water content. Disadvantages include the complexity of regular phantom scanning, sensitivity to positioning and temperature, and potential for systematic errors if phantom and tissue experience different instrumental factors. This approach is used primarily in research settings where high quantification accuracy justifies the additional effort.

LCModel (Linear Combination of Model spectra) is the most widely used automated quantification method, which fits observed spectra as linear combinations of model spectra from individual metabolites, measured *in vitro* or simulated from quantum-mechanical calculations. The algorithm simultaneously fits all metabolites, baseline, and macromolecular signal, providing concentrations with statistical uncertainties (Cramér-Rao lower bounds). Advantages include objective, automated analysis that reduces operator dependence, the ability to fit overlapping peaks that are difficult to separate visually, concentration estimates for 15-20 metabolites, including minor peaks, and built-in quality metrics (linewidth, SNR, fitting residuals) that enable assessment of result reliability. The method requires basis sets of model spectra that are appropriate for the acquisition parameters, field strength, and pulse sequence used; mismatches between the basis set and the actual acquisition degrade the results. LCModel is considered the gold standard for quantification in research applications, though simpler methods often suffice for clinical use (Provencher, 1993).

Quality control in spectroscopy quantification is critical, as numerous factors can compromise the validity of the results. Spectral quality metrics include linewidth (full-width at half-maximum), with values below 0.1 ppm indicating excellent shimming; signal-to-noise ratio, quantifying overall data quality; and baseline flatness, indicating adequate water and lipid suppression. Cramér-Rao lower bounds from LCModel fitting indicate concentration uncertainty; values below 20% are considered reliable, and those above 50% are unreliable. Visual inspection identifies artefacts, including lipid contamination from the scalp, inadequate water suppression, motion-induced artefacts, and poor phase correction. Voxel placement review ensures the intended tissue was sampled without excessive CSF or skull inclusion. Metabolite concentrations should be within physiologically reasonable ranges; values outside these expected ranges suggest quantification errors rather than pathology. The systematic application of quality control criteria enhances reliability and prevents the interpretation of artifactual results.

Table 8.2. Metabolite quantification methods in MRS

Method	Reference	Output	Advantages	Disadvantages	Best Applications
Metabolite Ratios	Creatine (typically)	Dimensionless ratios	Simple, robust, established norms	Assumes stable reference	Clinical screening, large effect sizes
Internal Water	Tissue water	Absolute concentration (mmol/kg)	No external reference needed	CSF contamination sensitive	Research, semi-quantitative
External Phantom	Known concentrations	Absolute concentration	Direct calibration	Requires phantom scans	Research requiring high accuracy
LCModel	Model spectra	Absolute with uncertainties	Objective, comprehensive	Requires an appropriate basis set	Research, comprehensive analysis
jMRUI	Manual/semi-automated	Variable	Flexible, user control	Operator dependent	Specialized analysis
TARQUIN	Automated	Absolute concentration	Fast, automated	Less established	High-throughput research

Statistical analysis of MRS data requires appropriate handling of multiple metabolites, correlations between metabolites, and the hierarchical structure of multi-voxel data. Group comparisons of metabolite concentrations use t-tests or analysis of variance, with corrections for multiple comparisons, to test various metabolites. Multivariate approaches, including principal component analysis or discriminant analysis, consider metabolite patterns jointly, potentially providing more sensitive detection of group differences. Correlations between metabolites and clinical variables test relationships between metabolism and symptoms, cognition, or disease severity. For multi-voxel data, voxel-wise statistical parametric mapping creates metabolite maps that are thresholded for significance, although it requires appropriate correction for spatial multiple comparisons. Longitudinal studies comparing baseline to follow-up assess changes in metabolites over time or in response to treatment, requiring attention to measurement reliability and the use of appropriate statistical models for paired data. Table 8.2 shows metabolite quantification methods in MRS.

8.4. Advanced MRS Techniques: 2D and 3D MRS

Two-dimensional magnetic resonance spectroscopy extends conventional one-dimensional spectroscopy by encoding chemical shift information in two frequency dimensions, thereby dramatically improving spectral resolution and enabling the separation of overlapping peaks that are impossible to resolve in one dimension. The technique employs two evolution periods during which chemical shifts evolve at different times, producing a two-dimensional spectral matrix where cross-peaks indicate J-coupling between nuclei and diagonal peaks represent uncoupled spins. The most common 2D sequence for brain applications is correlation spectroscopy (COSY), revealing correlations between coupled spins within molecules. J-resolved spectroscopy separates chemical shift in one dimension and J-coupling in the second dimension, enabling improved quantification of overlapping metabolites. While 2D-MRS offers superior spectral resolution, it requires substantially longer acquisition times (20-40 minutes) and more complex analysis, which limits its clinical adoption.

Spectral editing techniques employ specific pulse sequences to selectively detect metabolites with distinct J-coupling patterns, enabling the measurement of compounds obscured by overlapping peaks in conventional spectra. MEGA-PRESS (Mescher-Garwood Point Resolved Spectroscopy) editing applies frequency-selective inversion pulses at coupled spin resonance frequencies to modulate their contribution to observed spectra. By acquiring spectra with editing pulses on and off and computing the difference, coupled metabolites appear in the difference spectra while uncoupled metabolites cancel out. The technique enables reliable detection of GABA (gamma-aminobutyric acid) at 3.0 ppm, despite substantial overlap with creatine. Glutathione, an important antioxidant, can be measured at 2.95 ppm using a similar editing method. Typical GABA editing requires 8-12 minutes (Mullins et al., 2014).

Three-dimensional spectroscopic imaging extends chemical shift imaging to volumetric coverage, providing whole-brain maps of metabolites. Acceleration techniques, including parallel imaging, compressed sensing, and echo-planar spectroscopic imaging, reduce acquisition time to 10-20 minutes, thereby improving clinical feasibility.

Ultra-high-field MRS at 7 Tesla and above offers transformative improvements through increased SNR and enhanced chemical shift dispersion, enabling detection of metabolites invisible at clinical fields and improved spectral dispersion separating glutamate and glutamine, previously only reliably quantified as combined Glx at 3T.

Functional MRS combines spectroscopy with task paradigms or pharmacological challenges to measure dynamic metabolite changes associated with neural activity or drug effects, thereby directly quantifying metabolic changes, including lactate production, glutamate release, and energy substrate utilisation.

Multinuclear spectroscopy provides complementary metabolic information by detecting nuclei other than protons, particularly phosphorus-31, carbon-13, fluorine-19, sodium-23, and deuterium, which enables metabolic imaging and tracking of metabolic pathway fluxes.

8.5. Phosphorus and Carbon-13 MRS

Phosphorus-31 magnetic resonance spectroscopy detects phosphorus-containing compounds involved in energy metabolism, membrane metabolism, and pH regulation, providing complementary information to proton MRS about cellular energetics and metabolic state. The primary phosphorus metabolites include phosphocreatine (PCr), involved in energy buffering, inorganic phosphate (Pi) reflecting ATP hydrolysis, ATP itself showing three distinct peaks from its α, β, and γ phosphates, phosphomonoesters (PME) including phosphocholine and phosphoethanolamine from membrane synthesis, and phosphodiesters (PDE) including glycerophosphocholine and glycerophosphoethanolamine from membrane breakdown. The chemical shift between PCr and Pi is pH-dependent, allowing for non-invasive tissue pH measurement based on the frequency difference. The ratios PCr/Pi and PCr/ATP quantify energy status; reduced ratios indicate metabolic stress or mitochondrial dysfunction. Phosphorus MRS sensitivity is inherently lower than proton MRS due to its lower natural abundance and gyromagnetic ratio, requiring larger voxels (typically 20-60 cm^3) and longer acquisition times (15-30 minutes). However, it provides unique metabolic information unavailable from proton spectroscopy (Ren et al., 2015).

Clinical applications of phosphorus MRS focus on conditions involving dysfunction of energy metabolism. Mitochondrial disorders show characteristic patterns on proton MRS, including reduced PCr/Pi ratios, elevated Pi, and sometimes lactate elevation, enabling non-invasive diagnosis. Brain tumours exhibit altered phospholipid metabolism, with elevated PME in rapidly growing tumours and elevated PDE in necrotic regions, patterns that correlate with tumour grade and may predict treatment response. Stroke and ischemia exhibit acute energy failure, characterised by PCr depletion, elevated Pi, and tissue acidosis, as evidenced by pH measurements. The extent of metabolic dysfunction predicts tissue fate. Traumatic brain injury reveals a metabolic crisis with perturbed energy metabolism persisting for days to weeks after injury, correlating with clinical outcomes. Psychiatric disorders, including schizophrenia and bipolar disorder, show subtle alterations in phospholipid metabolism, potentially reflecting membrane abnormalities underlying symptoms. However, the large voxel sizes and long acquisition times limit spatial specificity and clinical practicality compared to proton MRS.

Carbon-13 magnetic resonance spectroscopy enables the investigation of metabolic pathway fluxes by administering substrates enriched in carbon-13 (a stable isotope comprising approximately 1% of natural carbon) and tracking the incorporation of the label into downstream metabolites. The technique provides dynamic metabolic information that is not possible with static proton or phosphorus MRS, revealing pathway activities rather than steady-state concentrations. The most common approach is to administer 13C-labelled glucose intravenously. Then it measures 13C incorporation into glutamate, glutamine, GABA, and other amino acids, thereby quantifying metabolic fluxes through glycolysis, the tricarboxylic acid cycle, and neurotransmitter cycling. The rate of glutamate labelling reflects neuronal oxidative metabolism, whereas glutamine labelling reflects glial metabolism and neurotransmitter recycling. The technique has revealed that a substantial fraction of brain energy metabolism occurs in glia, the tight coupling between neuronal and glial metabolism through glutamate-glutamine cycling, and the high rate of neurotransmitter turnover relative to steady-state concentrations.

The technical implementation of 13C MRS presents substantial challenges, including very low sensitivity due to the low natural abundance and small gyromagnetic ratio, which require significant voxels (50-200 cm^3) and extended time courses (60-120 minutes) to track label incorporation. Direct 13C observation detects labelled metabolites directly, but it suffers from poor sensitivity and spectral overlap. Indirect detection through 1H-[13C] heteronuclear editing transfers polarisation from carbon to protons, improving sensitivity but requiring complex pulse sequences. Most studies combine 13C MRS with metabolic modelling to extract flux rates from the time courses of label incorporation, which requires blood sampling for input function measurement and sophisticated mathematical modelling. Despite these complexities, 13C MRS provides unique insights into metabolic pathway function and has established several fundamental findings about brain metabolism. Hyperpolarised 13C MRS, employing dynamic nuclear polarisation to enhance the 13C signal by factors of 10,000 or more, dramatically improves sensitivity, enabling real-time metabolic imaging. However, the short-lived hyperpolarisation (lasting only seconds) and the need for specialised equipment limit accessibility.

Deuterium metabolic imaging (DMI) is a recent innovation that provides metabolic flux information more practically than 13C MRS. Deuterium (2H), a stable hydrogen isotope, can be detected with MRI scanners using specialised RF coils tuned to the deuterium frequency. Administration of deuterium-labelled glucose, followed by spectroscopic imaging, reveals deuterium incorporation into lactate, glutamate, glutamine, and other metabolites, thereby mapping glucose metabolism across the brain. The sensitivity is substantially higher than that of direct 13C detection, enabling a spatial resolution of 1 cm^3 and acquisition times of 20-30 minutes. The technique provides metabolic maps that show regional variations in glucose uptake and metabolism, which are potentially useful for tumour characterisation, localisation of epileptic foci, and investigation of metabolic dysfunction in neurological and psychiatric disorders. Early studies demonstrate feasibility and reproducibility, with ongoing work establishing clinical utility and optimal protocols. DMI may offer a practical alternative to FDG-PET for metabolic imaging, eliminating the need for ionising radiation.

The combination of proton, phosphorus, and carbon/deuterium spectroscopy provides comprehensive metabolic characterisation encompassing neuronal markers, membrane turnover, energy metabolism, pH, and metabolic fluxes. Multi-nuclear studies reveal relationships between different metabolic compartments and pathways, such as the coupling between glucose metabolism (13C), energy status (31P), and neurotransmitter levels (1H). The practical challenges of multi-nuclear acquisition—requiring multiple RF coils, extended scan time, and specialised expertise—limit routine implementation, but research applications continue to demonstrate value. As technical barriers decrease through improved hardware and accelerated acquisition methods, multi-nuclear MRS may become more accessible for investigating complex metabolic phenotypes in disease.

8.6. Clinical Applications in Neurological Disorders

Brain tumour characterisation is one of the most established and valuable clinical applications of MRS, with metabolite patterns aiding in tumour diagnosis, grading, differentiation from non-neoplastic lesions, and assessment of treatment response. High-grade gliomas typically exhibit markedly elevated choline levels, reflecting increased cellularity and membrane turnover. Reduced NAA indicates neuronal loss or displacement, the presence of lactate from anaerobic metabolism, and sometimes elevated lipid peaks from necrosis. Low-grade gliomas exhibit less pronounced choline elevation and often preserve or mildly reduce NAA. The choline/NAA and choline/creatine ratios help distinguish tumour grades, with higher ratios indicating higher-grade tumours; however, substantial overlap exists. Meningiomas characteristically show an elevated alanine peak at 1.4 ppm, which is virtually pathognomonic when present. Metastases often exhibit elevated choline and lactate levels, accompanied by very low NAA. Lymphomas demonstrate elevated choline and lipids with NAA absence. Abscesses exhibit elevated levels of amino acids at 0.9 ppm, including acetate, succinate, and lactate, which distinguishes them from cystic tumours (McKnight et al., 2002).

The distinction between tumour progression and treatment effects (radiation necrosis or pseudoprogression) poses substantial diagnostic challenges, where MRS provides valuable complementary information. Tumour progression is characterised by elevated choline/NAA and choline/creatine ratios, indicating an active tumour, whereas treatment effects exhibit lower ratios, suggesting gliosis and necrosis rather than viable tumour. Metabolite patterns, combined with perfusion imaging, provide higher diagnostic accuracy than either method alone. However, mixed patterns occur in regions with both tumour and treatment effect, limiting specificity. Longitudinal metabolite changes help distinguish progression from pseudoprogression: increasing choline suggests progression, while stable or decreasing choline favours a treatment effect. Despite these patterns, no metabolite threshold perfectly distinguishes these conditions, and MRS should be interpreted in conjunction with clinical course and other imaging features rather than as a standalone diagnostic test.

Multiple sclerosis and other demyelinating diseases show characteristic MRS abnormalities in both lesions and normal-appearing tissue, providing insights into disease mechanisms and potential biomarkers. Active MS lesions demonstrate reduced NAA, reflecting axonal damage; elevated choline from demyelination and inflammation; elevated myo-inositol from gliosis; and, sometimes, elevated lipids from myelin breakdown. Chronic lesions may exhibit persistently low NAA, with normalised choline and elevated myo-inositol. Importantly, normal-appearing white matter in MS patients exhibits subtle metabolic abnormalities, including reduced NAA and elevated myo-inositol, compared with healthy controls, reflecting diffuse pathology not visible on conventional imaging. These metabolic changes correlate with disability and predict disease progression, potentially serving as surrogate endpoints in therapeutic trials. Acute disseminated encephalomyelitis exhibits similar patterns during the acute phase, but with a greater potential for metabolic normalisation with recovery.

Epilepsy applications of MRS focus on lateralizing and localising seizure foci, particularly in temporal lobe epilepsy, where hippocampal sclerosis may be subtle or absent on anatomical imaging. The affected hippocampus typically shows reduced NAA, indicating neuronal loss, often accompanied by elevated myo-inositol levels due to gliosis. The NAA reduction is usually ipsilateral to the seizure focus, aiding lateralisation in cases where the lateralisation is unclear. The degree of NAA reduction may predict surgical outcome, with greater reductions associated with better post-resection seizure control. Bilateral hippocampal NAA reduction suggests bilateral temporal lobe involvement and a poorer surgical prognosis. Extra-temporal epilepsy shows less consistent patterns but can demonstrate focal NAA reduction in seizure foci. Serial MRS can track metabolic changes with anti-epileptic medications and post-surgically. While MRS alone rarely establishes surgical candidacy, it provides valuable complementary information in complex cases and research into epilepsy pathophysiology.

Inherited metabolic disorders represent a unique MRS application in which specific spectral patterns enable noninvasive diagnosis. Creatine deficiency syndromes exhibit an absence or severe reduction of creatine peaks, which is virtually pathognomonic when identified. Markedly elevated NAA characterises Canavan disease due to a deficiency of the aspartoacylase enzyme, which degrades NAA. Elevated levels of branched-chain amino acids characterise maple syrup urine disease at 0.9 ppm. Phenylketonuria demonstrates elevated phenylalanine. Elevated glycine levels characterise nonketotic hyperglycinemia at 3.55 ppm. These dramatic metabolic signatures enable diagnosis from brain MRS, often before enzymatic or genetic testing results are available, potentially guiding urgent treatment in neonates. Many metabolic disorders exhibit less specific patterns of elevated lactate and reduced NAA, which are suggestive but not diagnostic of mitochondrial or metabolic dysfunction. The ability to non-invasively assess brain metabolism is particularly valuable in infants and children, where tissue biopsy poses greater risks.

Neurodegenerative diseases, including Alzheimer's disease, Parkinson's disease, and amyotrophic lateral sclerosis, show characteristic metabolic patterns that may enable earlier diagnosis and monitoring of disease progression. Alzheimer's disease is characterised by reduced NAA in the posterior cingulate and temporoparietal regions, elevated myo-inositol levels reflecting gliosis, and sometimes reduced glutamate levels. The myo-inositol/NAA ratio increases with disease progression and correlates with cognitive decline. Metabolic changes may precede atrophy, potentially enabling earlier detection of the condition. Mild cognitive impairment shows intermediate metabolic abnormalities between normal ageing and Alzheimer's, with metabolite patterns predicting conversion to dementia. Parkinson's disease is characterised by reduced NAA levels in the substantia nigra and putamen, although the small size of these structures makes quantification challenging. Amyotrophic lateral sclerosis is characterised by reduced NAA in the motor cortex, which correlates with clinical severity and predicts survival. These applications require further validation before being used in routine clinical settings, but show promise for early diagnosis and objective disease monitoring.

Table 8.3. Clinical MRS applications in neurological disorders

Disorder	Key Metabolite Changes	Diagnostic/Clinical Value	Limitations
High-Grade Glioma	↑↑ Cho, ↓↓ NAA, ↑ Lac, ↑ lipid	Tumour grading, target biopsy	Overlap between grades
Meningioma	↑ Alanine (1.4 ppm), ↑ Cho	Diagnosis, distinguish from other tumours	Alanine is not always present
Tumour vs. Treatment Effect	Tumour: ↑Cho/NAA; Necrosis: ↓Cho/NAA	Distinguish progression from treatment	Mixed patterns common
MS Lesions	↓ NAA, ↑ Cho, ↑ mI	Assess activity, monitor treatment	Changes nonspecific
Epilepsy	↓ NAA in seizure focus	Lateralisation, surgical planning	Bilateral changes common
Creatine Deficiency	Absent Cr peak	Diagnosis, treatment, and monitoring	Rare but distinctive
Alzheimer's Disease	↓ NAA, ↑ mI, ↑ mI/NAA ratio	Early detection, progression tracking	Overlap with normal ageing
Stroke (acute)	↑↑ Lactate, ↓ NAA	Viability assessment	Lactate may normalise

Psychiatric disorders, including schizophrenia, depression, and bipolar disorder, show subtle but reproducible metabolic abnormalities revealed through group studies. However, individual diagnosis remains challenging due to high inter-individual variability and overlap with normal ranges. Schizophrenia meta-analyses reveal reduced NAA in the prefrontal cortex and hippocampus, elevated glutamate in some studies, and altered glutamine-glutamate balance, suggesting excitotoxicity. Major depression shows elevated choline in the basal ganglia and altered prefrontal metabolism. Bipolar disorder demonstrates reduced NAA during mood episodes, normalising during euthymia. These findings support metabolic and neurotransmitter theories of psychiatric illness and may eventually contribute to differential diagnosis and treatment selection. The integration of MRS with genetics, cognition, and other biomarkers through multimodal approaches may enhance diagnostic classification and treatment matching, moving psychiatry toward a biologically based rather than symptom-based taxonomy. Table 8.3 shows clinical MRS applications in neurological disorders.

Conclusion

Magnetic resonance spectroscopy (MRS) extends MRI into the biochemical domain, non-invasively detecting and quantifying brain metabolites, including neuronal markers, membrane components, and neurotransmitters. Proton MRS routinely measures 5-10 primary metabolites, providing diagnostic information in brain tumours, epilepsy, metabolic disorders, and other conditions.

Single-voxel spectroscopy provides high-quality spectra from targeted regions, while multi-voxel imaging maps the spatial distribution of metabolites. Quantification methods range from simple metabolite ratios to sophisticated methods for determining absolute concentrations. Advanced techniques, including spectral editing and ultra-high-field implementations, dramatically improve resolution and expand the detectable metabolites, enabling the measurement of GABA, glutamate, glutamine, and glutathione. Phosphorus-31 and carbon-13 spectroscopy provide complementary information about energy metabolism and metabolic pathway fluxes.

Clinical applications are most established in neuro-oncology for tumour characterisation and grading, distinguishing between progression and treatment effects. Other uses include epilepsy focus lateralisation, metabolic disorder diagnosis, and multiple sclerosis assessment. Emerging applications in neurodegenerative diseases, psychiatric disorders, and traumatic brain injury show promise.

Future developments will address current limitations by increasing field strengths, accelerating acquisition, automating processing, and integrating artificial intelligence. MRS represents a critical component of comprehensive neuroimaging, providing metabolic insights essential for precision medicine approaches in brain disorders.

Acknowledgments

The authors would like to extend our appreciation to those who offered helpful commentary during the drafting process of this manuscript. We also acknowledge the role the Nova Publishing department played in enabling the work described herein.

References

Barker, P. B., Bizzi, A., De Stefano, N., Gullapalli, R., & Lin, D. D. (2010). *Clinical MR spectroscopy: Techniques and applications*. Cambridge University Press.

Govindaraju, V., Young, K., & Maudsley, A. A. (2000). Proton NMR chemical shifts and coupling constants for brain metabolites. *NMR in Biomedicine*, 13(3), 129-153. https://doi.org/10.1002/1099-1492(200005)13:3<129::AID-NBM619>3.0.CO;2-V.

Kreis, R. (2016). The trouble with quality filtering based on relative Cramér-Rao lower bounds. *Magnetic Resonance in Medicine*, 75(1), 15-18. https://doi.org/10.1002/mrm.25568.

McKnight, T. R., von dem Bussche, M. H., Vigneron, D. B., Lu, Y., Berger, M. S., McDermott, M. W., Dillon, W. P., Graves, E. E., Pirzkall, A., & Nelson, S. J. (2002). Histopathological validation of a three-dimensional magnetic resonance spectroscopy index as a predictor of tumor presence. *Journal of Neurosurgery*, 97(4), 794-802. https://doi.org/10.3171/jns.2002.97.4.0794.

Mullins, P. G., McGonigle, D. J., O'Gorman, R. L., Puts, N. A., Vidyasagar, R., Evans, C. J., & Edden, R. A. (2014). Current practice in the use of MEGA-PRESS spectroscopy for the detection of GABA. *NeuroImage*, 86, 43-52. https://doi.org/10.1016/j.neuroimage.2012.12.004.

Oz, G., Alger, J. R., Barker, P. B., Bartha, R., Bizzi, A., Boesch, C., Bolan, P. J., Brindle, K. M., Cudalbu, C., Dinçer, A., Dydak, U., Emir, U. E., Frahm, J., González, R. G., Gruber, S., Gruetter, R., Gupta, R. K., Heerschap, A., Henning, A., ... MRS Consensus Group. (2014). Clinical proton MR spectroscopy in central nervous system disorders. *Radiology*, 270(3), 658-679. https://doi.org/10.1148/radiol.13130531.

Posse, S., Otazo, R., Dager, S. R., & Alger, J. (2013). MR spectroscopic imaging: Principles and recent advances. *Journal of Magnetic Resonance Imaging*, 37(6), 1301-1325. https://doi.org/10.1002/jmri.23945.

Provencher, S. W. (1993). Estimation of metabolite concentrations from localized *in vivo* proton NMR spectra. *Magnetic Resonance in Medicine*, 30(6), 672-679. https://doi.org/10.1002/mrm.1910300604.

Ren, J., Sherry, A. D., & Malloy, C. R. (2015). ^{31}P-MRS of healthy human brain: ATP synthesis, metabolite concentrations, pH, and T1 relaxation times. *NMR in Biomedicine*, 28(11), 1455-1462. https://doi.org/10.1002/nbm.3384.

Ross, B., & Bluml, S. (2001). Magnetic resonance spectroscopy of the human brain. *The Anatomical Record*, 265(2), 54-84. https://doi.org/10.1002/ar.1058.

Chapter 9

Neuromelanin and Iron Imaging

Maajid Mohi Ud Din Malik*
Radiology and Imaging Technology, Dr. D. Y. Patil School of Allied Health Sciences,
Dr. D. Y. Patil Vidyapeeth (Deemed to be University), Sant Tukaram Nagar, Pimpri, Pune, India

Abstract

Neuromelanin and iron imaging represent specialised MRI techniques that enable the visualisation and quantification of these critical biomolecules, whose distributions and alterations provide unique insights into brain function, ageing, and disease. Neuromelanin, a dark pigment that accumulates in catecholaminergic neurons of the substantia nigra and locus coeruleus, can be visualised using T1-weighted sequences that exploit its paramagnetic properties, providing a marker of dopaminergic and noradrenergic neuron integrity. Iron, essential for numerous biological processes but potentially neurotoxic when dysregulated, can be quantified through multiple MRI approaches, including quantitative susceptibility mapping and R2* relaxometry. This chapter comprehensively examines the principles, methodologies, and applications of neuromelanin and iron imaging in neurological and psychiatric disorders. Applications in Parkinson's disease demonstrate neuromelanin loss in the substantia nigra preceding clinical diagnosis and correlating with disease severity, while iron accumulation patterns aid in differential diagnosis. Alzheimer's disease shows characteristic iron deposition in affected brain regions, contributing to pathology. Psychiatric disorders, including schizophrenia and depression, show altered neuromelanin and iron distributions potentially reflecting dysfunction of catecholaminergic systems. These specialised imaging techniques offer biomarkers for early diagnosis, disease monitoring, and mechanistic investigation, with ongoing technical advancements promising enhanced sensitivity and clinical utility.

Keywords: neuromelanin imaging, iron quantification, substantia nigra, Parkinson's disease, quantitative susceptibility mapping, SDG 3 - good health and well-being

---

* Corresponding Author's Email: maajid.malik@dpu.edu.in

In: Recent Advances in Magnetic Resonance Imaging in Neuroimaging
Editors: Maajid Mohi Ud Din Malik, Purnachandra Kawdu Lamghare and R. S. Kuber
ISBN: 979-8-90134-244-2

Introduction

The visualisation and quantification of specific biomolecules, including neuromelanin and iron, represent advanced MRI applications that exploit the distinct magnetic properties of these substances to provide unique insights into brain structure, function, and pathology. Neuromelanin, a dark pigment produced through the oxidation of dopamine and norepinephrine, accumulates progressively in catecholaminergic neurons throughout life, serving as an indirect marker of these critical neurotransmitter systems. The substantia nigra pars compacta, containing dopaminergic neurons projecting to the striatum and forming the nigrostriatal pathway crucial for motor control, shows high neuromelanin content visible as a hyperintense signal on specialised T1-weighted sequences. The locus coeruleus, the primary source of noradrenergic innervation to the cortex, also contains neuromelanin-rich neurons. The ability to non-invasively visualise these small brainstem nuclei and quantify neuromelanin content provides valuable tools for investigating neurodegenerative diseases, psychiatric disorders, and normal ageing processes that affect catecholaminergic function.

Iron plays essential roles in brain metabolism, including oxygen transport, electron transfer in mitochondrial respiration, myelin synthesis, and neurotransmitter synthesis, with the highest concentrations found in basal ganglia structures involved in motor control and cognitive processing. Iron distribution is tightly regulated, as excess free iron catalyses the generation of reactive oxygen species, causing oxidative damage implicated in neurodegeneration. Normal ageing is associated with progressive iron accumulation in deep Grey nuclei, whereas numerous pathological conditions exhibit altered iron distributions that contribute to tissue damage. The development of MRI techniques sensitive to tissue iron concentration, particularly quantitative susceptibility mapping, which provides absolute iron quantification, and R2* relaxometry, which reflects iron and other tissue properties, has enabled the investigation of iron's role in health and disease. These techniques reveal iron accumulation patterns characteristic of specific neurodegenerative diseases, allow monitoring of iron chelation therapies, and provide biomarkers that may be useful for early diagnosis and tracking disease progression.

The convergence of neuromelanin and iron imaging reflects their complementary information about substantia nigra and basal ganglia pathology in movement disorders. Neuromelanin-sensitive MRI enables the specific visualisation of dopaminergic neurons through their pigment content, while iron imaging reveals the surrounding tissue microenvironment and pathological iron accumulation. In Parkinson's disease, the combination of a reduced neuromelanin signal indicating neuronal loss and altered iron distribution in the substantia nigra and striatum provides a comprehensive characterisation of nigrostriatal dysfunction. The specificity of these techniques to particular cellular populations and molecular species distinguishes them from conventional structural imaging, which shows only gross anatomical changes, potentially enabling the detection of pathology before irreversible tissue loss occurs. This chapter comprehensively examines neuromelanin and iron imaging, exploring the physical principles, technical implementations, quantification approaches, and clinical applications across neurological and psychiatric disorders, with particular emphasis on movement disorders, where these techniques have had the most tremendous clinical impact.

9.1. Neuromelanin-Sensitive MRI

Neuromelanin-sensitive MRI exploits the T1-shortening effect of neuromelanin to generate high signal intensity from neuromelanin-containing neurons in the substantia nigra and locus coeruleus, enabling the visualisation of these small brainstem structures with contrast unavailable with conventional sequences. The technique employs magnetisation transfer-weighted gradient-echo or turbo spin-echo sequences optimised for neuromelanin contrast, typically acquiring images at the level of the midbrain, where the substantia nigra appears as bilateral hyperintense regions posterior to the cerebral peduncles. The contrast arises from neuromelanin's paramagnetic properties, due to metal binding (primarily iron, but also copper and zinc), and melanin's intrinsic paramagnetism, which creates T1 shortening and causes melanin-rich neurons to appear bright relative to surrounding structures. The magnetisation transfer component enhances contrast by saturating the signal from myelin and other macromolecules, thereby increasing the relative signal from neuromelanin. The hyperintense region on neuromelanin-sensitive images corresponds to the substantia nigra pars compacta, which contains dopaminergic neurons, while the pars reticulata, lacking neuromelanin, appears hypointense (Sasaki et al., 2006).

The technical implementation of neuromelanin imaging typically employs three-dimensional gradient echo sequences with magnetisation transfer preparation at a 3 Tesla field strength, providing whole-brain coverage with submillimetre resolution in acquisition times of 5-10 minutes. Key parameters include a relatively long echo time (10-15 ms), emphasising T1 weighting, a flip angle optimised for neuromelanin contrast (typically 20-30 degrees), and an off-resonance magnetisation transfer saturation pulse (1-2 kHz offset) that suppresses background tissue. Two-dimensional turbo spin-echo neuromelanin imaging offers an alternative implementation with distinct contrast characteristics, providing excellent visualisation of the substantia nigra but with a longer acquisition time that limits coverage. The optimal sequence parameters have been refined through studies comparing the contrast-to-noise ratio and imaging with postmortem histology, which validates that hyperintense regions correspond to neuromelanin-containing neurons. A higher field strength (7 Tesla) provides an improved signal-to-noise ratio and contrast, enabling the visualisation of substructures within the substantia nigra, including the characteristic "swallow-tail" appearance formed by nigrosome 1, a neuromelanin-rich subregion. The loss of this appearance is characteristic of Parkinson's disease.

Quantification of neuromelanin content from imaging data employs several approaches with varying complexity and biological interpretation. A simple visual assessment qualitatively classifies the substantia nigra appearance as normal or abnormal based on symmetry, size, and signal intensity, providing a binary classification that is valuable for clinical diagnosis. Semi-quantitative contrast-ratio measures signal intensity in the substantia nigra relative to adjacent reference regions, such as the cerebral peduncle or red nucleus, providing continuous measures that are more sensitive to subtle changes. Volumetric analysis segments hyperintense areas in the substantia nigra and calculates volume, with reduced volume indicating neuronal loss. Signal intensity histogram analysis characterises the distribution of pixel intensities within the substantia nigra, with shifts toward lower intensities reflecting reduced neuromelanin content. More sophisticated approaches combine intensity and volume measures to estimate total neuromelanin content, potentially correlating more strongly with underlying neuronal integrity than either measure alone. Standardisation of acquisition parameters, region definition, and quantification methods across sites remains challenging but is critical for establishing reliable biomarkers.

The biological basis and interpretation of the neuromelanin signal require an understanding of neuromelanin synthesis and function, and of its relationship to neuronal health. Neuromelanin forms through the oxidation and polymerisation of catecholamines (dopamine in the substantia nigra, norepinephrine in the locus coeruleus) in the cytoplasm, accumulating in autophagic granules and increasing with age. The pigment may serve as a neuroprotective agent by sequestering toxic metal ions and reactive quinones, thereby preventing oxidative damage. However, when neurons die, neuromelanin is released and taken up by microglia, potentially contributing to neuroinflammation. The hyperintense MRI signal reflects the neuromelanin concentration per voxel, which is determined by both neuronal density and the neuromelanin content per neuron. A reduced signal can indicate either decreased neuronal density (cell loss) or reduced neuromelanin content per neuron (metabolic dysfunction), and distinguishing between these scenarios requires additional information. Studies combining neuromelanin imaging with PET imaging of dopamine synthesis capacity or transporter density reveal a partial but imperfect correlation, suggesting that the neuromelanin signal reflects both neuronal number and functional state.

Normal ageing is associated with progressive neuromelanin accumulation in the substantia nigra and locus coeruleus, with signal intensity and volume increasing from adolescence through middle age, then stabilising or slightly declining in the elderly. Individual variation is substantial, with some healthy elderly individuals exhibiting reduced neuromelanin signals that overlap with the range observed in Parkinson's disease, complicating interpretation. The relationship between the neuromelanin signal and cognitive function, motor performance, and other measures of healthy ageing reveals complex patterns, suggesting that neuromelanin may reflect both compensatory mechanisms and early pathological changes. Sex differences exist, with males generally exhibiting larger substantia nigra volumes and higher signal intensity, which may relate to sex differences in the incidence of Parkinson's disease. Understanding normal variation and establishing age- and sex-specific normative values is critical for identifying pathological reductions.

Clinical applications of neuromelanin imaging have focused on Parkinson's disease and related movement disorders, though emerging applications in other conditions show promise. The excellent visualisation of the substantia nigra enables the identification of the "swallow-tail" sign—a characteristic hyperintense region corresponding to nigrosome 1—that is consistently absent in patients with Parkinson's disease but present in healthy individuals and most atypical Parkinsonian syndromes. This binary marker shows high sensitivity and specificity for Parkinson's disease diagnosis, potentially enabling earlier and more accurate diagnosis than clinical criteria alone. Quantitative neuromelanin measures show a progressive reduction with disease duration and correlate with clinical severity; however, longitudinal studies tracking individual patients over time are limited. The potential for neuromelanin imaging to identify at-risk individuals before motor symptom onset is particularly exciting, with studies showing reduced signal in patients with REM sleep behaviour disorder who subsequently develop Parkinsonism, suggesting that neuromelanin loss precedes clinical diagnosis by years (Ogisu et al., 2013). Table 9.1 presents the technical parameters and applications of neuromelanin-sensitive MRI.

Table 9.1. Neuromelanin-sensitive MRI technical parameters and applications

Parameter	Typical Values	Purpose	Clinical Significance
Field Strength	3T (standard), 7T (research)	SNR and contrast	Higher field improves visualisation
Sequence Type	3D GRE with MT, 2D TSE	Neuromelanin contrast	GRE faster, TSE higher contrast
Echo Time	10-15 ms	T1 weighting	Optimises the neuromelanin signal
Flip Angle	20-30°	Signal optimization	Balances contrast and SNR
Resolution	0.5-1 mm isotropic	Anatomical detail	Visualizes substructures
MT Offset	1-2 kHz	Background suppression	Enhances the relative signal
Acquisition Time	5-10 minutes	Clinical feasibility	Acceptable for routine use
Primary Targets	Substantia nigra, locus coeruleus	Catecholaminergic systems	Movement and mood disorders

9.2. Iron Quantification with QSM and R2 Mapping*

Quantitative susceptibility mapping and R2* relaxometry represent complementary MRI techniques for quantifying iron, each providing distinct information about tissue iron concentration and microstructural organisation. R2* (or its reciprocal T2*) relaxometry measures the exponential signal decay rate in gradient echo sequences, which accelerates in proportion to magnetic field inhomogeneities caused by paramagnetic iron and other sources, including deoxyhemoglobin, calcium, and myelin. The technique requires a multi-echo gradient echo acquisition with echo times that sample the decay curve, followed by fitting an exponential model to extract R2* values at each voxel. A higher R2* indicates faster signal decay, generally correlating with higher iron concentration; however, the relationship is complex and influenced by iron distribution, oxidation state, and other tissue properties. Quantitative susceptibility mapping directly measures magnetic susceptibility—the degree to which tissue magnetises in an external magnetic field—by sophisticated processing of phase data from gradient-echo sequences. Unlike R2*, which reflects multiple microstructural features, susceptibility is dominated by iron content in most brain regions, providing more specific iron quantification (Haacke et al., 2015).

The physical basis of R2* iron sensitivity derives from iron's paramagnetic properties, creating microscopic magnetic field inhomogeneities that accelerate the dephasing of transverse magnetisation. Ferritin and hemosiderin, the primary iron storage forms in the brain, contain iron in the ferric ($Fe3+$) state, characterised by unpaired electrons, which creates strong paramagnetism. The spatial distribution of iron in ferritin cores creates local field gradients that extend beyond the protein, causing protons diffusing through these regions to experience varying fields and accumulate phase differences, thereby shortening T2* and increasing R2*. The relationship between R2* and iron concentration is approximately linear at physiological concentrations, but it depends on the iron distribution pattern: clustered versus dispersed iron produces different R2* effects. Other paramagnetic species, including deoxyhemoglobin in veins and paramagnetic trace metals, contribute to R2*, as do diamagnetic myelin and the organisation of structural proteins, meaning R2* is a composite measure that requires careful interpretation.

Quantitative susceptibility mapping derives tissue susceptibility from gradient-echo phase images through sophisticated processing that addresses fundamental ambiguities in the inverse problem. Phase images directly encode local magnetic field variations caused by tissue susceptibility; however, separating contributions from within the brain from those from external sources, as well as the orientation-dependent nature of dipole fields created by susceptibility sources, complicates interpretation. Background field removal utilises sophisticated algorithms, including SHARP, PDF, and V-SHARP, to separate local tissue fields from global background. The remaining local field is then inverted to estimate the susceptibility distribution using algorithms such as MEDI, COSMOS, or iterative regularisation-based approaches. The resulting susceptibility maps show quantitative values in parts per billion (ppb) or parts per million (ppm) relative to water or CSF, with positive values indicating paramagnetic tissue (high iron) and negative values indicating diamagnetic tissue (high myelin). The quantitative nature enables the estimation of absolute iron concentration through calibration against postmortem measurements, providing physiologically meaningful values (Wang & Liu, 2015).

Iron quantification validation through comparison with postmortem tissue analysis establishes the relationship between MRI measures and actual iron concentration. Multiple studies correlating R2* or susceptibility with iron concentration, as measured by inductively coupled plasma mass spectrometry or histochemical staining, reveal strong correlations ($r > 0.8$) across Grey matter structures, validating MRI as a tool for iron quantification. The calibration curves relating susceptibility to iron concentration show approximately 1 ppb of susceptibility per 0.1 mg of iron per gram of tissue, enabling conversion from susceptibility to iron concentration. However, the relationships exhibit regional variation and are influenced by the iron form (ferritin vs. hemosiderin), subcellular localisation, and colocalization with other substances. R2* shows weaker correlation with iron than susceptibility due to additional influences from myelin and tissue microstructure, though it remains helpful in detecting significant iron changes. The combined use of both measures can potentially distinguish iron effects from other contributors.

Normal brain iron distribution shows characteristic patterns with the highest concentrations in globus pallidus (approximately 2-3 mg/g), substantia nigra, red nucleus, and dentate nucleus, intermediate levels in putamen, caudate, and thalamus (1-1.5 mg/g), and lower levels in cortex and white matter (0.3-0.8 mg/g). This distribution reflects iron's roles in dopamine metabolism in the basal ganglia, myelin formation in white matter, and oxidative metabolism throughout the brain. Progressive iron accumulation occurs with normal ageing, particularly in the basal ganglia, with susceptibility and R2* increasing linearly by approximately 5-10% per decade in the putamen and globus pallidus. The age-related accumulation may reflect impaired iron homeostasis, chronic neuroinflammation, or accumulation in activated microglia. Understanding normal age-dependent increases in iron is crucial for identifying pathological accumulation and determining whether disease-related iron changes reflect the acceleration of normal ageing processes or distinct pathological mechanisms.

Clinical applications of iron imaging employ both R2* and QSM to detect altered iron distributions in diverse neurological conditions. The techniques are particularly valuable when anatomical imaging appears normal. Still, metabolic or microstructural pathology is suspected when differential diagnosis requires distinguishing conditions with distinct iron patterns, or when monitoring treatments that affect iron homeostasis, such as chelation therapy. The non-invasive nature enables repeated measurements and longitudinal tracking, while quantitative values facilitate comparisons across individuals and studies. However, interpretation requires caution, as multiple factors affect measurements, and the relationship between iron concentration and pathology is complex—iron accumulation may be pathogenic, compensatory, or incidental, depending on the context. The integration of iron imaging with other modalities, including neuromelanin, diffusion, and PET, provides a more comprehensive characterisation than any single technique alone.

9.3. Applications in Parkinson's Disease

Parkinson's disease, characterised by the progressive loss of dopaminergic neurons in the substantia nigra pars compacta, represents a primary application where neuromelanin and iron imaging have demonstrated substantial clinical value for diagnosis, differential diagnosis, and potentially early detection. The loss of neuromelanin-containing dopaminergic neurons produces characteristic imaging findings, including reduced substantia nigra hyperintensity on neuromelanin-sensitive sequences, loss of the "swallow-tail" sign formed by nigrosome 1, and altered iron distribution in substantia nigra and striatum. These imaging changes correlate with disease severity, demonstrate high diagnostic accuracy, and may precede clinical diagnosis in individuals at risk. The combination of neuromelanin imaging, which reveals neuronal loss, and iron imaging, which characterises the tissue microenvironment, provides a comprehensive characterisation of nigrostriatal pathology, complementing clinical examination and molecular imaging techniques. The potential for these methods to improve early diagnosis and enable disease-modifying treatment before irreversible neuronal loss represents an exciting frontier in Parkinson's disease research and care (Schwarz et al., 2018).

Neuromelanin imaging in Parkinson's disease consistently demonstrates reduced substantia nigra volume and signal intensity compared to healthy controls, with changes often visible even in early disease when clinical diagnosis is uncertain. The reduction is typically asymmetric, with greater effects on the contralateral side, consistent with the known asymmetry of Parkinson's pathology. Quantitative measures show substantia nigra volume reductions of 20-40% in early Parkinson's disease, increasing to 50-60% in advanced disease, while contrast ratios are reduced by 15-30%. These reductions exceed the typical 5-10% volume loss seen in normal ageing, enabling discrimination between Parkinson's patients and age-matched healthy controls with sensitivities and specificities of 80-95% depending on methodology and disease stage. The swallow-tail sign—bilateral hyperintense regions in the dorsolateral substantia nigra corresponding to nigrosome 1—is present in over 95% of healthy individuals but absent in 90-100% of Parkinson's disease patients, providing a particular diagnostic marker that is potentially useful when the clinical diagnosis is uncertain or early in the disease course.

Iron imaging in Parkinson's disease reveals complex patterns, with both increases and decreases across different structures, reflecting the multifaceted role of iron in disease pathophysiology. The substantia nigra exhibits increased iron concentration, as measured by QSM, in most but not all studies. This increase may reflect the release of iron from dying neurons, neuroinflammation-associated iron accumulation in activated microglia, or compensatory upregulation of iron import proteins. However, some studies report a decreased susceptibility in the dorsolateral substantia nigra, corresponding to nigrosome 1, consistent with the loss of iron-containing dopaminergic neurons. The putamen exhibits elevated iron levels in many Parkinson's patients, potentially reflecting oxidative stress, denervation-induced metabolic changes, or the accumulation of iron-containing inflammatory cells. The pattern and magnitude of iron changes exhibit heterogeneity across patients, with some studies suggesting that iron accumulation is more prominent in specific Parkinson's subtypes or correlates with particular clinical features, including cognitive impairment or rapid progression.

Differential diagnosis between Parkinson's disease and atypical Parkinsonian syndromes represents a critical clinical application where combined neuromelanin and iron imaging provides valuable diagnostic information. Atypical Parkinsonian syndromes, including multiple system atrophy, progressive supranuclear palsy, and corticobasal degeneration, present with Parkinsonism but differ in pathology, progression, and treatment response, necessitating accurate diagnosis. The swallow-tail sign, although absent in Parkinson's disease, is typically preserved in atypical Parkinsonian syndromes, providing high specificity for the diagnosis of Parkinson's disease. Iron distribution patterns differ between conditions: progressive supranuclear palsy exhibits pronounced iron accumulation in the red nucleus, substantia nigra, and dentate nucleus; multiple system atrophy displays posterior putamen iron deposition with preserved substantia nigra; corticobasal degeneration is characterised by asymmetric cortical atrophy and white matter changes. The combination of imaging findings enables a more accurate differential diagnosis than clinical examination alone, particularly in the early stages of the disease when symptoms overlap substantially (Sung et al., 2018).

Longitudinal studies tracking individual patients over time are beginning to reveal the temporal evolution of neuromelanin and iron changes, though large-scale natural history studies remain limited. Available evidence suggests that the neuromelanin signal continues to decline with disease duration at approximately 5-10% volume loss per year, faster than the age-related decline. Iron changes appear more variable, with some individuals showing progressive accumulation while others remain stable. The relationship between imaging changes and clinical progression remains unclear; however, preliminary data suggest that baseline neuromelanin and iron measures predict subsequent motor and cognitive decline, potentially identifying patients at risk for rapid progression who may benefit from more aggressive treatment. The demonstration that imaging changes precede clinical diagnosis in REM sleep behaviour disorder patients—who have a high risk of developing Parkinsonism—suggests these techniques may enable identification of at-risk individuals during the prodromal phase when neuroprotective interventions might prevent or delay clinical onset.

The pathophysiological mechanisms linking iron dysregulation to Parkinson's disease involve multiple pathways, including oxidative stress, alpha-synuclein aggregation, and neuroinflammation. Excess iron catalyses Fenton reactions, generating highly reactive hydroxyl radicals that damage proteins, lipids, and DNA, thereby contributing to neuronal dysfunction and death. Iron interacts with alpha-synuclein, the protein that aggregates in Lewy bodies characteristic of Parkinson's disease, promoting its aggregation and potentially explaining why iron accumulation and protein pathology colocalise. Neuroinflammation in Parkinson's disease involves the activation of iron-accumulating microglia and astrocytes, creating a positive feedback loop in which inflammation drives iron accumulation, which in turn generates oxidative stress and promotes further inflammation. Whether iron dysregulation is cause or consequence of neurodegeneration remains debated, though evidence from genetic forms of Parkinson's involving iron homeostasis genes supports a causal role. Regardless, iron imaging provides a biomarker of pathological processes and a potential treatment target through iron chelation approaches currently under investigation.

Treatment monitoring applications of iron imaging include assessing the effects of iron chelation therapy and potentially evaluating disease-modifying treatments targeting oxidative stress or neuroinflammation. Deferiprone, an iron chelator, has shown promise in small trials for Parkinson's disease, with some patients exhibiting motor improvement that correlates with reduced brain iron on MRI. Iron imaging enables an objective assessment of whether chelation achieves target engagement (i.e., brain iron reduction) and whether iron reduction correlates with clinical benefit. Future disease-modifying therapies targeting oxidative stress, inflammation, or alpha-synuclein may alter brain iron distribution, providing an intermediate endpoint to improve trial efficiency. However, the heterogeneity of iron changes in Parkinson's disease and the complex relationship between iron, pathology, and clinical status complicate interpretation, requiring careful consideration of regional patterns, relationship to symptoms, and integration with other biomarkers. Table 9.2 shows neuromelanin and iron imaging findings in Parkinson's disease and related disorders.

Table 9.2. Neuromelanin and iron imaging findings in Parkinson's disease and related disorders

Condition	Neuromelanin (Substantia Nigra)	Iron (Substantia Nigra)	Iron (Striatum)	Other Features	Diagnostic Utility
Parkinson's Disease	↓↓ volume and signal, absent swallow-tail	↑ or ↓ (variable)	↑ putamen (variable)	Asymmetric changes	High specificity (90-95%)
Multiple System Atrophy	Preserved swallow-tail	Normal or ↑	↑↑ posterior putamen	Putaminal atrophy, hot cross bun sign	Distinguishes from PD
Progressive Supranuclear Palsy	Preserved swallow-tail	↑↑	Normal	↑↑ red nucleus, dentate; midbrain atrophy	Distinguishes from PD
Corticobasal Syndrome	Preserved swallow-tail	Normal	Normal	Asymmetric cortical atrophy	Distinguishes from PD
Healthy Ageing	Gradual signal decline	Progressive ↑	Progressive ↑	Preserved swallow-tail	Establishes normative data
REM Sleep Behaviour Disorder	Reduced (prodromal)	Variable	Variable	May predict PD conversion	Potential early detection

9.4. Iron Imaging in Alzheimer's Disease

Alzheimer's disease, the most common neurodegenerative disorder, shows characteristic iron accumulation patterns that contribute to pathophysiology and provide potential biomarkers for diagnosis and monitoring. The disease is characterised by progressive iron deposition in affected brain regions, including the hippocampus, amygdala, and cortical areas, which exhibit beta-amyloid plaques and neurofibrillary tangles. Iron co-localises with pathological protein aggregates. Iron imaging reveals elevated concentrations in these regions correlating with disease severity, cognitive impairment, and pathological burden. The mechanisms linking iron to Alzheimer's pathology are multifaceted, involving oxidative stress from iron-catalysed generation of reactive oxygen species, direct interactions between iron and amyloid-beta that promote plaque formation, iron-induced tau phosphorylation contributing to tangle formation, and neuroinflammation with iron accumulation in activated microglia surrounding plaques. Whether iron dysregulation is a primary pathogenic mechanism or a secondary consequence of protein aggregation and neurodegeneration remains a topic of debate; however, genetic evidence implicating iron homeostasis genes in Alzheimer's disease risk supports a causal contribution (Bulk et al., 2018).

Regional patterns of iron accumulation in Alzheimer's disease exhibit preferential deposition in medial temporal structures affected early in the disease, including the hippocampus, entorhinal cortex, and amygdala, with subsequent involvement of neocortical association areas following the characteristic spatiotemporal progression of the pathology. QSM and R2* studies consistently demonstrate elevated iron in the hippocampus of Alzheimer's patients compared to age-matched controls, with iron concentration increases of 20-40% correlating with hippocampal atrophy and memory impairment. The amygdala shows similar increases in iron, whereas basal ganglia structures display either normal or modestly elevated iron levels, distinguishing Alzheimer's disease from certain movement disorders. Cortical iron elevation is more subtle and heterogeneous, with some studies showing increases in temporoparietal regions characteristic of Alzheimer's pathology, while others show minimal cortical changes. The relationship between regional iron accumulation and atrophy is complex, with some areas showing increased iron accumulation preceding volume loss, suggesting a pathogenic role. In contrast, others exhibit concurrent changes or an increase in iron following atrophy, suggesting secondary accumulation.

Iron imaging in mild cognitive impairment, the transitional state between normal ageing and dementia, reveals patterns intermediate between healthy controls and Alzheimer's disease, with potential for predicting progression. Several studies demonstrate that MCI patients who progress to Alzheimer's dementia show greater baseline hippocampal iron than stable MCI patients, suggesting iron measures might identify high-risk individuals. The combination of iron imaging with amyloid PET and tau PET could provide comprehensive *in vivo* pathological characterisation, testing whether individuals with both protein pathology and iron dysregulation show faster progression than those with only one abnormality. However, the high prevalence of age-related iron accumulation and substantial individual variation complicate interpretation, necessitating the establishment of age-specific normative values and potentially multivariate approaches that combine iron with other biomarkers for optimal prediction. Longitudinal studies tracking individuals from MCI through dementia are needed to establish whether iron changes precede, accompany, or follow clinical progression.

The relationship between iron accumulation and amyloid-beta plaques has been extensively investigated through combined imaging studies, postmortem analyses, and mechanistic studies. Iron is consistently found concentrated in amyloid plaques, with QSM studies showing punctate susceptibility increases corresponding to plaque locations identified by amyloid PET. The iron-amyloid interaction is bidirectional: iron promotes amyloid-beta aggregation and plaque formation through direct binding and oxidation mechanisms, while amyloid-beta can sequester iron, potentially serving a protective function initially before becoming pathogenic. Some evidence suggests that the ferroxidase activity of the amyloid precursor protein (APP) is disrupted by cleavage into amyloid-beta, thereby impairing normal iron trafficking. The presence of APP mutations that cause early-onset Alzheimer's disease in families indicates altered iron metabolism, supporting a mechanistic connection. However, the precise role of iron in plaque formation and whether targeting iron could prevent or slow amyloid pathology remain uncertain, motivating ongoing therapeutic development of iron chelators and investigations of their effects on imaging biomarkers and clinical outcomes.

Tau pathology and neurofibrillary tangles also exhibit associations with iron accumulation, as tau is a metalloprotein that binds iron and other metals. Iron promotes tau phosphorylation and aggregation *in vitro*, while post-mortem studies demonstrate iron enrichment in tangle-bearing neurons. Whether iron-tau interactions contribute directly to tangle formation and neurotoxicity *in vivo* remains to be investigated; however, the correlation between regional iron accumulation patterns and tau PET binding suggests a potential relationship between these two factors. The recently demonstrated "iron rim" lesions on QSM around chronic active multiple sclerosis plaques, indicating iron-laden inflammatory cells, raise questions about whether similar iron-associated inflammation occurs in Alzheimer's disease surrounding plaques or tangles. Some studies suggest that iron accumulation in microglia surrounding amyloid plaques represents an inflammatory component of the pathology, and that iron imaging may serve as a marker of neuroinflammation complementary to PET tracers targeting activated microglia.

Iron chelation therapy represents a potential disease-modifying approach in Alzheimer's disease, based on mechanistic links between iron and the pathology, with several chelators under investigation in preclinical and early clinical studies. Deferoxamine, a chelator used clinically for systemic iron overload, showed slowing of cognitive decline in a small Alzheimer's trial decades ago, but requires inconvenient parenteral administration, limiting practical use. Newer brain-penetrant chelators, including deferiprone and clioquinol, have entered clinical trials with mixed results, with some studies showing cognitive benefits or improvements in biomarkers. In contrast, others show no effect or adverse outcomes. The heterogeneity of results may reflect differences in patient selection, dosing, treatment duration, or the pharmacology of the chelator. Iron imaging enables monitoring target engagement (brain iron reduction) and testing whether patients with the most significant iron reductions experience the greatest clinical benefit. However, concerns about excessive iron depletion compromising normal brain function require careful safety monitoring and potentially targeting chelation to iron-loaded regions while preserving normal iron homeostasis.

Differential diagnosis applications of iron imaging in dementia include distinguishing Alzheimer's disease from other neurodegenerative dementias, such as frontotemporal dementia, dementia with Lewy bodies, and vascular dementia, which exhibit distinct patterns of iron distribution. Frontotemporal dementia is characterised by iron accumulation in the affected frontal and temporal regions, with relative sparing of the hippocampus, unlike the pattern observed in Alzheimer's disease. Vascular dementia shows patchy iron deposition in areas of chronic ischemia and infarction. These regional pattern differences can complement clinical and other imaging features for differential diagnosis. However, mixed pathologies are common in elderly patients, with many individuals showing both Alzheimer's and vascular changes, complicating pattern interpretation. The integration of iron imaging with structural volumetry, amyloid and tau PET, and clinical phenotyping may improve diagnostic accuracy; however, the added value over existing methods requires demonstration in extensive, prospective studies.

9.5. Neuromelanin in Psychiatric Disorders

Psychiatric disorders, including schizophrenia, major depression, and bipolar disorder, show alterations in catecholaminergic neurotransmitter systems implicated in their pathophysiology, with neuromelanin imaging providing an indirect marker of dopaminergic and noradrenergic neuron integrity and function. The substantia nigra and ventral tegmental area dopaminergic systems are critically involved in reward processing, motivation, and pleasure, with dopamine dysfunction central to theories of depression and schizophrenia. The locus coeruleus noradrenergic system modulates arousal, attention, and stress responses, with dysregulation implicated in anxiety, depression, and post-traumatic stress disorder. Neuromelanin imaging enables investigation of whether structural or functional alterations in catecholaminergic systems contribute to psychiatric symptoms, correlate with symptom severity or treatment response, and differ across diagnostic categories (Cassidy et al., 2019).

Schizophrenia, characterised by positive symptoms (hallucinations, delusions), negative symptoms (motivation deficit, social withdrawal), and cognitive impairment, involves dopamine dysfunction according to longstanding theories supported by dopamine-blocking antipsychotic efficacy. Neuromelanin imaging studies report increased signal intensity in the substantia nigra and ventral tegmental area compared to healthy controls, potentially reflecting enhanced dopamine synthesis and metabolism, leading to elevated neuromelanin accumulation. Increases correlate with positive symptom severity in some studies. However, not all studies replicate these findings. The locus coeruleus signal is decreased in some schizophrenia studies, potentially reflecting noradrenergic dysfunction contributing to cognitive and negative symptoms.

Major depressive disorder shows an altered neuromelanin signal in the substantia nigra and locus coeruleus, with most studies reporting reduced signal consistent with diminished catecholaminergic function. Reduced locus coeruleus neuromelanin signal correlates with symptom severity and anhedonia, supporting noradrenergic dysfunction involvement in depression pathophysiology.

Bipolar disorder shows neuromelanin alterations varying with mood state. Some studies report increased substantia nigra signal during manic phases, potentially reflecting dopamine hyperactivity, with normalisation or reduction during depressive phases or euthymia.

Post-traumatic stress disorder involves locus coeruleus-noradrenergic system dysregulation. Preliminary neuromelanin imaging studies report increased locus coeruleus signal correlating with hyperarousal symptom severity, consistent with chronic noradrenergic system overactivity.

Interpretation requires careful consideration of confounding factors, including the effects of medication, smoking prevalence, and comorbidities. Potential applications include identifying subtypes based on patterns of catecholaminergic dysfunction, predicting treatment responses, and monitoring the impact of novel treatments.

9.6. Future Developments

The future of neuromelanin and iron imaging promises substantial advances driven by technical innovations, methodological refinements, and expanding applications. Ultra-high-field MRI at 7 Tesla and beyond offers transformative improvements through increased signal-to-noise ratio, enhanced contrast, and improved spatial resolution, enabling the visualisation of substructures within the substantia nigra and other small nuclei. At 7T, the nigrosome 1 swallow-tail appearance is consistently visible with remarkable clarity, while individual substantia nigra subregions can be distinguished based on neuromelanin content. Iron quantification benefits from increased susceptibility effects, with QSM showing improved sensitivity to subtle iron changes. However, 7T implementations face challenges, including increased susceptibility artefacts, B1 field inhomogeneity, and limitations on specific absorption rate, which require specialised sequences and hardware.

Artificial intelligence and machine learning applications are emerging with the potential to improve automated segmentation, standardise quantification, and enable accurate diagnostic classification. Deep learning algorithms can automatically segment the substantia nigra from neuromelanin images, removing operator dependence and enhancing reliability and efficiency. Classification algorithms combining neuromelanin, iron, and other imaging features can distinguish between Parkinson's disease and atypical Parkinsonian syndromes with high accuracy. However, these applications require large, diverse training datasets and careful validation in independent cohorts.

Multimodal integration, combining neuromelanin and iron imaging with PET, spectroscopy, and functional connectivity, will provide comprehensive characterisation of brain structure, function, chemistry, and pathology. In Parkinson's disease, combining neuromelanin imaging (assessment of dopaminergic neuron integrity), dopamine transporter PET (evaluation of terminal density), and iron imaging (examination of the tissue microenvironment) can distinguish patients with neuronal loss from those with dopaminergic dysfunction, even in the absence of structural changes.

Longitudinal studies tracking individuals over extended periods, from preclinical through clinical disease stages, will establish the temporal evolution of neuromelanin and iron changes, their relationship to clinical progression, and their value as surrogate endpoints in therapeutic trials. Natural history studies in at-risk populations could identify imaging changes that predict disease development, enabling intervention during the prodromal stages.

Standardisation efforts across research sites, scanner platforms, and analysis methods represent critical ongoing work that enables robust biomarker development and clinical translation. Novel contrast mechanisms under development, including manganese-enhanced MRI, sodium imaging, and CEST imaging, promise to expand beyond current neuromelanin and iron imaging capabilities.

Conclusion

Neuromelanin-sensitive MRI and iron imaging represent specialised techniques that provide unique insights into brain structure and pathology. Neuromelanin-sensitive MRI enables non-invasive visualisation of substantia nigra and locus coeruleus—small brainstem nuclei containing catecholaminergic neurons critical for motor control, reward, and arousal. Loss of the neuromelanin signal in Parkinson's disease, particularly the absence of the swallow-tail sign, provides high diagnostic accuracy and may enable early detection of prodromal stages when neuroprotective interventions can prevent irreversible neuronal loss. The technique aids differential diagnosis, distinguishing Parkinson's disease from atypical Parkinsonian syndromes.

Iron imaging through quantitative susceptibility mapping and R2* relaxometry enables the precise assessment of brain iron concentration, revealing distributions that reflect normal physiology, age-related accumulation, and pathological deposition. Applications span Parkinson's disease, Alzheimer's disease, and other neurodegenerative and psychiatric disorders, showing characteristic iron patterns. Quantitative measurements enable cross-individual comparison, longitudinal tracking, and treatment monitoring.

Neuromelanin accumulates through catecholamine metabolism, with potential neuroprotective functions, while iron serves essential roles in oxidative metabolism and neurotransmitter synthesis; however, it can cause oxidative damage when present in excess.

Technical advances, including higher magnetic fields, improved quantification methods, accelerated acquisition, and machine learning, are advancing these techniques from research tools to clinically viable applications. Future roles include early disease detection, surrogate endpoints for therapeutic trials, and comprehensive characterisation of neurological disorders, ultimately improving diagnosis, prognosis, and treatment.

Acknowledgments

The authors would like to extend our appreciation to those who offered helpful commentary during the drafting process of this manuscript. We also acknowledge the role the Nova Publishing department played in enabling the work described herein.

References

Bulk, M., Abdelmoula, W. M., Nabuurs, R. J., van der Graaf, L. M., Mulders, C. W., Mulder, A. A., Jost, C. R., Koster, A. J., van Buchem, M. A., Natté, R., Dijkstra, J., & van der Weerd, L. (2018). Postmortem MRI and histology demonstrate differential iron accumulation and cortical myelin organization in early- and late-onset Alzheimer's disease. *Neurobiology of Ageing*, 62, 231-242. https://doi.org/10.1016/j.neurobiolageing.2017.10.017.

Cassidy, C. M., Zucca, F. A., Girgis, R. R., Baker, S. C., Weinstein, J. J., Sharp, M. E., Bellei, C., Valmadre, A., Vanegas, N., Kegeles, L. S., Brucato, G., Kang, U. J., Sulzer, D., Zecca, L., Abi-Dargham, A., & Horga, G. (2019). Neuromelanin-sensitive MRI as a noninvasive proxy measure of dopamine function in the human brain. *Proceedings of the National Academy of Sciences*, 116(11), 5108-5117. https://doi.org/10.1073/pnas.1807983116.

Haacke, E. M., Liu, S., Buch, S., Zheng, W., Wu, D., & Ye, Y. (2015). Quantitative susceptibility mapping: Current status and future directions. *Magnetic Resonance Imaging*, 33(1), 1-25. https://doi.org/10.1016/j.mri.2014.09.004.

Ogisu, K., Kudo, K., Sasaki, M., Sakushima, K., Yabe, I., Sasaki, H., Terae, S., & Shirato, H. (2013). 3D neuromelanin-sensitive magnetic resonance imaging with semi-automated volume measurement of the substantia nigra pars compacta for diagnosis of Parkinson's disease. *Neuroradiology*, 55(6), 719-724. https://doi.org/10.1007/s00234-013-1171-8.

Sasaki, M., Shibata, E., Tohyama, K., Takahashi, J., Otsuka, K., Tsuchiya, K., Takahashi, S., Ehara, S., Terayama, Y., & Sakai, A. (2006). Neuromelanin magnetic resonance imaging of locus ceruleus and substantia nigra in Parkinson's disease. *NeuroReport*, 17(11), 1215-1218. https://doi.org/10.1097/01.wnr.0000227984.84927.a7.

Schwarz, S. T., Afzal, M., Morgan, P. S., Bajaj, N., Gowland, P. A., & Auer, D. P. (2014). The 'swallow tail' appearance of the healthy nigrosome - a new accurate test of Parkinson's disease: A case-control and retrospective cross-sectional MRI study at 3T. *PLoS ONE*, 9(4), e93814. https://doi.org/10.1371/journal.pone.0093814.

Sung, Y. H., Noh, Y., Lee, J., & Kim, E. Y. (2018). Drug-induced parkinsonism versus idiopathic Parkinson disease: Utility and diagnostic performance of nigrosome 1 imaging with 3-T MRI. *Radiology*, 288(1), 256-263. https://doi.org/10.1148/radiol.2018172268.

Wang, Y., & Liu, T. (2015). Quantitative susceptibility mapping (QSM): Decoding MRI data for a tissue magnetic biomarker. *Magnetic Resonance in Medicine*, 73(1), 82-101. https://doi.org/10.1002/mrm.25358.

Zecca, L., Stroppolo, A., Gatti, A., Tampellini, D., Toscani, M., Gallorini, M., Giaveri, G., Arosio, P., Santambrogio, P., Fariello, R. G., Karatekin, E., Kleinman, M. H., Turro, N., Hornykiewicz, O., & Zucca, F. A. (2004). The role of iron and copper molecules in the neuronal vulnerability of locus coeruleus and substantia nigra during ageing. *Proceedings of the National Academy of Sciences*, 101(26), 9843-9848. https://doi.org/10.1073/pnas.0403495101.

Chapter 10

MRI in Stroke and Cerebrovascular Disease

Purnachandra Kawdu Lamghare[1,*]
and Maajid Mohi Ud Din Malik[2,†]

[1]Department of Radio-Diagnosis, Dr. D. Y. Patil Medical College, Hospital and Research Centre, Dr. D. Y. Patil Vidyapeeth (Deemed to be University), Sant Tukaram Nagar, Pimpri, Pune, India
[2]Radiology and Imaging Technology, Dr. D. Y. Patil School of Allied Health Sciences, Dr. D. Y. Patil Vidyapeeth (Deemed to be University), Sant Tukaram Nagar, Pimpri, Pune, India

Abstract

Magnetic resonance imaging has revolutionised stroke diagnosis and management through techniques that enable the rapid detection of ischemic injury, assessment of tissue viability, and characterisation of vascular pathology. This chapter comprehensively examines MRI applications in acute and chronic cerebrovascular disease, ranging from emergency stroke protocols to the characterisation of vascular malformations. Acute stroke imaging combines diffusion-weighted imaging, which detects ischemic injury within minutes, perfusion imaging to identify hypoperfused tissue, and vascular imaging to localise arterial occlusions, enabling treatment decisions within critical time windows. The diffusion-perfusion mismatch concept identifies salvageable penumbral tissue that may be potentially rescued by reperfusion therapy. Magnetic resonance angiography visualises cerebrovascular anatomy non-invasively, detecting stenoses, occlusions, aneurysms, and malformations. Four-dimensional flow MRI characterises complex hemodynamics, including flow velocity, wall shear stress, and pressure gradients. Chronic stroke imaging monitors tissue evolution, identifies complications, and assesses recovery through structural and functional techniques. Vascular malformation imaging, including arteriovenous malformations, cavernomas, and developmental venous anomalies, utilises specialised sequences for accurate diagnosis and treatment planning. These comprehensive MRI capabilities have established neuroimaging as a central component of stroke care, improving outcomes through faster diagnosis, better patient selection for interventions, and an enhanced understanding of cerebrovascular pathophysiology.

---

* Corresponding Author's Email: purnachandra.lamghare@dpu.edu.in
† Corresponding Author's Email: maajid.malik@dpu.edu.in

In: Recent Advances in Magnetic Resonance Imaging in Neuroimaging
Editors: Maajid Mohi Ud Din Malik, Purnachandra Kawdu Lamghare and R. S. Kuber
ISBN: 979-8-90134-244-2

Keywords: acute stroke, diffusion-perfusion mismatch, MR angiography, 4D flow, vascular malformations, SDG 3 - good health and well-being

Introduction

Stroke represents the second leading cause of death and a significant cause of disability worldwide, with ischemic stroke accounting for approximately 85% of cases and hemorrhagic stroke 15%. The critical importance of rapid diagnosis and treatment—captured in the adage "time is brain"—has driven the development of imaging techniques that enable accurate stroke detection, tissue viability assessment, and treatment guidance within narrow therapeutic time windows. Magnetic resonance imaging has emerged as a powerful tool for comprehensive stroke evaluation, providing anatomical, physiological, and vascular information that is not possible with computed tomography alone. The exquisite sensitivity of diffusion-weighted imaging to acute ischemic injury, combined with perfusion imaging that reveals hypoperfused but potentially salvageable tissue, enables the identification of patients likely to benefit from reperfusion therapies, including thrombolysis and thrombectomy. Vascular imaging localises arterial occlusions and stenoses, guiding endovascular interventions and informing stroke mechanisms. These capabilities have transformed stroke care from empiric treatment to precision medicine guided by individual tissue status and vascular pathology.

The evolution of stroke MRI from a research tool to a clinical standard reflects both technological advances that enable faster imaging and accumulating evidence demonstrating its clinical value. Early applications required 30-60 minutes for comprehensive stroke protocols, which is impractical for emergency evaluation. The development of echo-planar imaging, which enables whole-brain diffusion and perfusion acquisition in minutes, combined with time-of-flight angiography, which provides rapid vascular assessment, made MRI feasible for acute stroke evaluation. Landmark trials have demonstrated that diffusion perfusion mismatch identifies patients who benefit from thrombolysis beyond traditional time windows, establishing imaging-based patient selection as a standard practice for treatment. The expansion of mechanical thrombectomy to broader patient populations, guided by mismatch imaging that shows substantial salvageable tissue despite an extended time from symptom onset, further solidifies the role of imaging in treatment decisions. Current stroke protocols can be completed in 10-15 minutes, which is fast enough for routine emergency use while providing comprehensive information to guide all aspects of acute management.

Beyond acute stroke, MRI provides unique capabilities for investigating chronic cerebrovascular disease, monitoring recovery, and characterising diverse vascular pathologies. Follow-up imaging reveals final infarct extent, identifies hemorrhagic transformation and other complications, and tracks tissue evolution from acute necrosis through chronic encephalomalacia. Functional MRI and diffusion tensor imaging investigate recovery mechanisms, including perilesional plasticity and reorganisation of motor and language networks, potentially guiding rehabilitation strategies.

Cerebrovascular reserve assessment using hypercapnia or pharmacological challenges identifies patients at risk for future strokes despite anatomically patent vessels. Vascular malformations, including arteriovenous malformations, cavernomas, and developmental venous anomalies, require specialised imaging for diagnosis, risk stratification, and treatment planning. MRI provides superior soft-tissue contrast and flow characterisation compared with angiography alone. This chapter systematically examines these diverse applications, providing both foundational understanding and practical guidance for implementing and interpreting MRI in cerebrovascular disease.

10.1. Acute Stroke Imaging Protocols

Acute stroke MRI protocols combine multiple sequences to provide complementary information on parenchymal injury, tissue viability, and vascular pathology, enabling a comprehensive evaluation in 10-15 minutes and are suitable for emergency workflows. The core sequences include diffusion-weighted imaging with apparent diffusion coefficient mapping for detecting ischemic injury, gradient echo or susceptibility-weighted imaging for identifying haemorrhage, fluid-attenuated inversion recovery for assessing chronic changes and ruling out stroke mimics, perfusion-weighted imaging for identifying hypoperfused tissue, and magnetic resonance angiography for localising vascular occlusions. This multiparametric approach provides far more information than non-contrast CT, which remains the primary alternative due to its speed and availability. However, MRI's superior sensitivity for acute ischemia and tissue characterisation makes it increasingly the preferred modality when accessible. The optimal sequence selection and order depend on the clinical scenario, with suspected anterior circulation stroke protocols emphasising carotid and intracranial arterial imaging. In contrast, posterior circulation protocols require visualisation of the vertebrobasilar system (Wintermark et al., 2013).

Diffusion-weighted imaging is the most sensitive technique for detecting acute ischemic stroke, showing a hyperintense signal within minutes of arterial occlusion, hours before changes appear on T2-weighted imaging or CT. The mechanism involves cytotoxic oedema resulting from energy failure, causing cell swelling and a reduction in extracellular space, which restricts water diffusion and produces a decreased apparent diffusion coefficient, corresponding to DWI hyperintensity. Echo-planar imaging enables whole-brain coverage in 30-60 seconds, critical for emergency imaging. The combination of hyperintensity on high-b-value images and hypointensity on ADC maps confirms restricted diffusion and acute infarction, distinguishing it from a T2 shine-through artefact, in which both DWI and ADC are bright. The volume of diffusion restriction estimates infarct core—tissue already infarcted and unsalvageable—essential information for treatment decisions. DWI changes are reversible in the first hours if reperfusion occurs quickly, though most restriction indicates irreversible injury. The sensitivity for acute stroke exceeds 90% within 6 hours of onset, declining slightly in very early imaging (<3 hours) when restriction may be subtle (Moseley et al., 1990).

Gradient-echo imaging, also known as susceptibility-weighted imaging, identifies intracranial haemorrhage with sensitivity equal to or superior to that of CT, while also detecting microbleeds, chronic blood products, and calcifications that are invisible on CT. Acute haemorrhage shows a blooming artefact from the susceptibility effects of blood products, appearing hypointense and larger than the actual haemorrhage size. The detection of haemorrhage is critical for excluding patients from thrombolysis who are at high bleeding risk, and for identifying primary hemorrhagic stroke requiring different management than ischemic stroke. Susceptibility-weighted imaging provides enhanced sensitivity to blood products and venous structures, revealing additional microbleeds that are not visible on gradient echo sequences and potentially highlighting prominent veins in ischemic regions, which reflect increased oxygen extraction. The identification of multiple cortical microbleeds suggests cerebral amyloid angiopathy, which increases the risk of haemorrhage with thrombolysis. In contrast, deep microbleeds indicate hypertensive vasculopathy—the pattern of haemorrhage—parenchymal, subarachnoid, or intraventricular—which guides differential diagnosis and management.

Fluid-attenuated inversion recovery imaging suppresses cerebrospinal fluid signal, improving conspicuity of cortical and periventricular lesions while providing information about stroke age and chronicity. Acute strokes typically show no FLAIR changes in the first 6 hours, with signal developing 8-12 hours post-onset as vasogenic oedema develops. The presence of FLAIR hyperintensity within diffusion-positive stroke, therefore, suggests an onset more than 6-8 hours prior, which is helpful for determining eligibility for time-limited interventions when the exact onset time is unknown, such as in wake-up strokes. The FLAIR-negative DWI-positive pattern suggests a very recent onset, potentially within the thrombolysis window, despite unclear timing. FLAIR also reveals chronic ischemic changes, including prior infarcts, white matter disease, and stroke mimics such as posterior reversible encephalopathy syndrome, tumours, or demyelination, improving diagnostic specificity. Hyperintense vessels on FLAIR indicate slow flow in arterial occlusions, correlating with good collateral circulation and better outcomes.

Perfusion-weighted imaging utilises dynamic susceptibility contrast, either with a gadolinium bolus or arterial spin labelling, to assess perfusion without contrast, thereby revealing hypoperfused tissue at risk for infarction. The technique measures cerebral blood flow, cerebral blood volume, and mean transit time, identifying regions where perfusion is critically reduced despite not yet showing diffusion restriction. The perfusion-diffusion mismatch (discussed in detail in section 10.2) estimates penumbra—potentially salvageable tissue—guiding treatment decisions. Various perfusion parameters and thresholds have been proposed for defining critically hypoperfused tissue, with a Time to maximum (Tmax) of greater than 6 seconds becoming widely adopted as optimal for identifying tissue at risk of infarction. Automated software packages now provide quantitative perfusion maps and mismatch calculations within minutes, facilitating clinical decision-making. Arterial spin labelling avoids gadolinium and radiation, particularly valuable for patients with renal dysfunction or those requiring repeated imaging, though lower SNR and greater sensitivity to artefacts limit its application in some scenarios.

The optimisation of acute stroke protocols requires balancing comprehensiveness against acquisition speed, with sequence selection guided by clinical scenario and scanner capabilities. A basic protocol can be completed in 5-8 minutes using only DWI, GRE, and FLAIR if perfusion and angiography are deferred, providing essential diagnostic information for straightforward cases. Comprehensive protocols that include perfusion and angiography require 12-18 minutes, depending on the implementation. Time-of-flight MRA can image the circle of Willis in 3-5 minutes, while contrast-enhanced MRA provides superior arterial visualisation in a similar time when gadolinium is administered for perfusion. Advanced techniques, including 4D flow and vessel wall imaging, add 5-10 minutes each and are typically reserved for specific indications rather than routine acute evaluation. Multi-band acceleration and compressed sensing reconstruction reduce acquisition times by 30-50% without compromising quality, enabling more comprehensive protocols within acceptable timeframes. Table 10.1 presents the components of the acute stroke MRI protocol.

Table 10.1. Acute stroke MRI protocol components

Sequence	Acquisition Time	Information Provided	Clinical Value	Key Parameters
DWI	30-60 sec	Acute infarct core	Confirms diagnosis, estimates core	High b-value (1000 s/mm^2), EPI
ADC Map	Calculated	Confirms restriction	Distinguishes T2 shine-through	From multi-b-value DWI
GRE/SWI	1-3 min	Haemorrhage, microbleeds	Excludes bleeding, risk assessment	TE 20-40 ms, susceptibility-weighted
FLAIR	2-4 min	Subacute changes, chronic lesions	Stroke timing mimics	Long TR/TE, CSF nulling
PWI	1-2 min	Tissue perfusion	Identifies penumbra, mismatch	DSC or ASL
TOF-MRA	3-5 min	Arterial anatomy	Locates occlusion/stenosis	3D GRE, flow-related enhancement
T2-weighted	2-4 min	Anatomical reference	Anatomical correlation	Optional, aids interpretation

10.2. Diffusion-Perfusion Mismatch

The diffusion-perfusion mismatch concept posits that the volume of tissue showing perfusion deficit but no diffusion restriction represents penumbra—potentially salvageable brain at risk for infarction if not reperfused—providing a physiological rationale for selecting patients likely to benefit from reperfusion therapy. The infarct core, identified by diffusion restriction, has already progressed to irreversible injury and cannot be saved. The perfusion deficit, representing all tissue with critically reduced blood flow, encompasses both the core and the penumbra. The mismatch—perfusion deficit minus diffusion lesion—estimates penumbra volume. A substantial mismatch (typically defined as a mismatch ratio greater than 1.8 and an absolute mismatch volume greater than 15 mL) identifies patients with significant salvageable tissue that may be potentially rescued by restoring blood flow. This imaging-based patient selection enables treatment of carefully selected patients beyond traditional time windows, as landmark trials have demonstrated that substantial mismatch predicts benefit from thrombectomy up to 24 hours from stroke onset, fundamentally changing acute stroke management (Lansberg et al., 2012).

The physiological basis of mismatch imaging reflects the temporal evolution of ischemic injury from initial perfusion failure through penumbral dysfunction to irreversible infarction. When arterial occlusion occurs, blood flow in the affected territory drops precipitously, with the severity of the reduction depending on the extent of collateral circulation. In the most severely hypoperfused core region, energy failure leads to immediate cellular dysfunction and cytotoxic oedema, resulting in diffusion restriction within minutes. Surrounding tissue with less severe hypoperfusion, due to partial collateral flow, maintains marginal perfusion that is insufficient for normal function but adequate to prevent immediate cell death—this is the penumbra. Over time, without reperfusion, the ischemic penumbra progressively converts into the infarct core as energy stores are depleted and cellular injury becomes irreversible. The mismatch between perfusion and diffusion lesions, therefore, represents a dynamic process, with mismatch tissue transitioning to core at variable rates depending on collateral adequacy, systemic blood pressure, and tissue metabolic demands. Early reperfusion prevents this progression, salvaging penumbral tissue.

Technical aspects of mismatch quantification have evolved substantially as methods have been refined and validated. Early approaches manually outlined DWI and perfusion lesions, which were labour-intensive and operator-dependent. Automated software packages now rapidly compute perfusion deficit using various thresholding methods, with a Tmax of more than 6 seconds emerging as optimal for identifying tissue at risk and achieving the highest accuracy in predicting final infarct volume in untreated patients. Some approaches use relative parameters, comparing the affected to the normal hemisphere, while others employ absolute thresholds. The diffusion lesion is typically defined using ADC thresholds ($<620 \times 10^{-6}$ mm^2/s) or simple visual delineation of restricted diffusion. The mismatch ratio (perfusion deficit volume/core volume) and absolute mismatch volume (perfusion deficit minus core) both provide helpful information, with thresholds established from clinical trials indicating that a mismatch ratio greater than 1.8 and a mismatch volume greater than 15 mL identify patients who benefit from thrombectomy. These parameters are automatically calculated by FDA-approved software platforms, including RAPID, which guides clinical decisions at many stroke centres.

Clinical applications of mismatch imaging have been most extensively validated for patient selection beyond standard time windows, with multiple randomised trials demonstrating its benefits. The DAWN trial demonstrated that thrombectomy improved outcomes in patients presenting 6-24 hours after their last known healthy state who had a mismatch between clinical severity and infarct core volume, with specific mismatch profiles predicting benefit despite extended time to treatment. The DEFUSE 3 trial demonstrated that patients with mismatched selection criteria, 6-16 hours from onset, benefited from thrombectomy compared with medical therapy. These trials showed that physiological imaging of tissue status is more crucial than absolute time for treatment decisions, as the rate of penumbral recruitment varies substantially among patients, depending on the presence of collaterals. Some patients maintain a substantial mismatch for many hours (slow progressors with good collaterals), while others show rapid loss of mismatch (fast progressors with poor collaterals). Imaging identifies slow progressors who benefit from late intervention, while avoiding futile procedures in fast progressors in whom the penumbra has already infarcted.

Controversies and limitations of mismatch imaging include uncertainty about optimal perfusion thresholds, imperfect prediction of tissue fate, and practical challenges in emergency implementation. The relationship between perfusion deficit and tissue outcome is probabilistic rather than deterministic—some mismatch tissue infarcts even with reperfusion (benign oligemia or collateral-sustained tissue). At the same time, some core may be salvageable (diffusion reversal with ultra-early reperfusion). The optimal Tmax threshold for balancing sensitivity and specificity continues to be refined, with some evidence suggesting slightly different thresholds for the anterior versus posterior circulation or for different stroke severities. Arterial spin labelling, a contrast-free perfusion alternative, shows promise but requires further validation of its mismatch accuracy. Technical failures, including motion artefacts, imaging delays, and software errors, can produce misleading results. The requirement for rapid imaging and automated analysis creates workflow challenges. Despite its limitations, mismatch imaging represents a significant advance, enabling more physiologically and patient-specific treatment decisions than rigid time windows.

10.3. MR Angiography (MRA) and Time-of-Flight Imaging

Magnetic resonance angiography (MRA) provides non-invasive visualisation of cerebrovascular anatomy using blood flow or T1-shortening contrast agents, enabling the detection of stenoses, occlusions, aneurysms, and vascular malformations without ionising radiation or arterial catheterisation. Time-of-flight MRA, the most commonly implemented technique, exploits flow-related enhancement, in which blood flowing into the imaging volume appears bright against suppressed stationary tissue. The method is particularly effective for visualising arteries in the circle of Willis and proximal intracranial vessels, which are commonly used in acute stroke protocols to localise arterial occlusions. Contrast-enhanced MRA employing gadolinium provides superior arterial-venous separation and reduced flow artefacts, although it requires venous access and contrast injection. Phase-contrast MRA enables the quantification of flow in addition to anatomical visualisation. These techniques collectively provide comprehensive vascular assessment, although each has distinct advantages, limitations, and optimal applications that require an understanding for appropriate selection and interpretation (Willinek & Born, 2005).

Time-of-flight MRA utilises gradient-echo sequences with a short repetition time and flow compensation, generating a bright signal from unsaturated blood entering the imaging volume. At the same time, the saturation of the stationary tissue produces a dark background. The technique is typically implemented as a three-dimensional acquisition, providing thin-source images that are reconstructed into maximum-intensity projections, which reveal the vascular architecture. The photos display arterial anatomy with excellent spatial resolution (0.5-1 mm), enabling detection of stenoses, occlusions, and vascular variants. The absence of a contrast requirement makes TOF-MRA an attractive option for patients with renal dysfunction or contrast allergy, enabling repeated imaging without concern for cumulative contrast exposure. Acquisition times of 3-7 minutes make it practical for acute stroke protocols. However, several limitations affect diagnostic accuracy: slow or turbulent flow can appear as stenosis or occlusion (flow artefacts), in-plane flow saturation can cause signal loss in vessels parallel to the imaging plane, and acquisition time increases substantially to cover large vascular territories.

Contrast-enhanced MRA employing a gadolinium bolus provides superior arterial visualisation through the T1-shortening effect of the contrast agent, with careful timing to image during the arterial phase before venous enhancement. Elliptic centric k-space ordering samples the centre of k-space during peak arterial enhancement, optimising arterial-venous separation. The technique produces high-quality angiograms with less susceptibility to flow artefacts than TOF-MRA, allowing for accurate stenosis quantification and excellent visualisation of small vessels. The coverage can extend from the aortic arch to the intracranial vessels in a single acquisition, providing a comprehensive vascular assessment useful for investigating stroke mechanisms and for surgical planning. However, gadolinium administration is required, limiting its application in cases of renal dysfunction, while timing optimisation is critical to avoid venous contamination. The inability to repeat imaging multiple times within an examination without cumulative contrast and the potential for nephrogenic systemic fibrosis in severe renal failure, though rare with newer agents, represent practical limitations.

Arterial stenosis quantification using MRA requires careful technique and interpretation, as both TOF and contrast-enhanced methods can over- or underestimate stenosis severity depending on technical factors. TOF-MRA tends to overestimate stenosis due to flow effects, leading to signal loss from turbulence and making stenoses appear more severe than they actually are. Comparison with catheter angiography shows that TOF-MRA demonstrates good accuracy in detecting stenosis but limited quantitative accuracy in assessing its degree. Contrast-enhanced MRA provides more accurate quantification with better correlation to angiography, though careful technique regarding contrast timing and image analysis is required. The methods used to measure stenosis (NASCET versus ECST criteria; comparing the narrowest stenosis diameter to the distal or proximal normal vessel diameter) affect the reported values. For critical clinical decisions like carotid endarterectomy eligibility, correlation with ultrasound or catheter angiography is often recommended when MRA shows high-grade stenosis. For intracranial stenoses, combining multiple MRA techniques or correlating with transcranial Doppler improves diagnostic confidence.

Intracranial aneurysm detection is a crucial application of MRA, with TOF-MRA demonstrating high sensitivity for aneurysms larger than 3 mm in diameter. However, small aneurysms may be missed, and the morphology required for assessing rupture risk is better characterised with contrast-enhanced or catheter angiography. Screening for aneurysms in high-risk populations, including those with family history, polycystic kidney disease, or prior subarachnoid haemorrhage, commonly employs TOF-MRA as an initial test, with positive findings confirmed by catheter angiography before treatment. The detection of incidental unruptured aneurysms raises management questions, as most remain stable; however, features such as size greater than 7 mm, irregular morphology, and specific locations (posterior circulation, anterior communicating artery) confer a higher risk of rupture. Serial MRA monitoring of small aneurysms can detect growth, suggesting increased risk; however, the optimal surveillance interval and criteria for intervention remain debated. Vessel wall imaging using high-resolution T1-weighted sequences can characterise aneurysm wall inflammation, potentially predicting instability, an emerging application that requires further validation.

Carotid imaging employing MRA assesses extracranial carotid bifurcation for atherosclerotic stenosis, the leading cause of embolic stroke. Black-blood imaging techniques suppress the blood signal while enhancing the vessel wall, enabling direct visualisation of atherosclerotic plaques and characterisation of their composition (lipid core, fibrous cap, and intraplaque haemorrhage). The combination of luminal imaging with MRA and plaque imaging with black-blood sequences provides a comprehensive assessment superior to ultrasound or luminography alone. High-risk plaque features, including a thin fibrous cap, a large lipid core, and intraplaque haemorrhage, independently predict future stroke risk and may guide intervention decisions. The plaque characterisation capabilities of MRI exceed those of other non-invasive modalities, although they require specialised sequences and expertise, limiting widespread implementation. For routine clinical stenosis assessment, MRA combined with ultrasound provides adequate information for most decisions, with advanced plaque imaging reserved for research or cases requiring detailed risk stratification. Table 10.2 shows MR angiography techniques and applications.

Table 10.2. MR angiography techniques and applications

Technique	Contrast	Acquisition Time	Key Advantages	Limitations	Primary Applications
3D TOF-MRA	None	3-7 min	No contrast, high resolution	Flow artefacts, slow	Acute stroke, aneurysm screening
CE-MRA	Gadolinium	2-5 min	Better stenosis quantification	Requires IV access, timing	Stenosis grading, aortic arch to vertex
Black-Blood	None/contrast	5-10 min	Vessel wall/plaque imaging	Limited availability	Atherosclerotic plaque characterisation
Phase-Contrast	None	3-6 min	Flow quantification	Lower SNR	Flow measurement, shunt quantification
4D Flow MRI	None/contrast	10-20 min	Comprehensive hemodynamics	Long acquisition, complex analysis	Research, complex malformations

10.4. 4D Flow MRI for Hemodynamic Assessment

Four-dimensional flow MRI is an advanced technique for comprehensive assessment of intracranial hemodynamics, acquiring time-resolved three-directional velocity information across three-dimensional volumes, enabling the calculation of complex flow parameters, including wall shear stress, pressure gradients, and flow patterns, that are otherwise impossible to assess with conventional angiography. The technique employs phase-contrast MRI with velocity encoding in all three spatial directions (x, y, z), acquired across the cardiac cycle for temporal resolution, and covering a 3D volume for spatial characterisation. The resulting dataset allows retrospective analysis of flow in any vessel or location within the volume, computation of derived hemodynamic parameters, and visualisation of flow streamlines or velocity vectors. Applications include characterising aneurysm hemodynamics for assessing rupture risk, quantifying arteriovenous malformation flow, evaluating venous sinus stenosis in idiopathic intracranial hypertension, and investigating collateral flow patterns. While acquisition times of 10-20 minutes limit routine clinical use, research applications are substantial, and accelerated implementations are improving clinical feasibility (Markl et al., 2012).

The technical implementation of 4D flow MRI requires careful optimisation of multiple parameters, including velocity encoding strength (VENC), spatial resolution, temporal resolution, and coverage volume. The VENC determines the maximum velocity that can be measured without aliasing, so it must be selected based on expected flow velocities. A value that is too low causes aliasing artefacts, while a value that is too high reduces SNR and velocity sensitivity. Typical intracranial arterial flow VENCs are 80-150 cm/s, while venous VENCs are 40-80 cm/s. Spatial resolution of 1-2 mm isotropic balances coverage, SNR, and scan time, adequate for major vessels but insufficient for small perforators. The temporal resolution of 30-50 milliseconds samples the cardiac cycle with 15-25 time points, capturing both systolic flow acceleration and diastolic deceleration. The coverage volume is prescribed to include vessels of interest, with larger vessels requiring longer acquisition times. Respiratory and cardiac gating reduce motion artefacts, while parallel imaging and compressed sensing reconstruction minimise acquisition time by factors of 4 to 8, which is critical for clinical feasibility.

Hemodynamic parameters derived from 4D flow data provide quantitative metrics of vascular function and abnormal flow that are potentially relevant to disease pathogenesis. Wall shear stress—the tangential force exerted by flowing blood on vessel walls—is calculated from near-wall velocity gradients, with abnormal (too high or too low) shear stress potentially promoting atherosclerosis, aneurysm formation, or vascular remodelling. Pressure gradients across stenoses quantify the hemodynamic significance, complementing the degree of anatomical stenosis as determined by angiography. Flow volume through individual vessels enables the calculation of territories supplied by different vessels, quantification of collateral flow, and measurement of shunt flow. Streamline visualisation reveals blood flow paths, highlighting complex patterns in aneurysms, including flow stagnation zones that are potentially prone to thrombosis. These parameters require sophisticated post-processing, including vessel segmentation, flow quantification in analysis planes, and hemodynamic computation using fluid dynamics equations, which typically requires 30-60 minutes of analysis time, currently limiting clinical utility.

Aneurysm hemodynamic assessment using 4D flow aims to identify high-risk flow patterns that predict rupture. Proposed risk factors include concentrated inflow jets impinging on the aneurysm wall, creating high wall shear stress; complex flow patterns with vortices and flow instability; and flow stagnation regions, which potentially promote thrombosis and wall degeneration. Studies comparing ruptured and unruptured aneurysms reveal associations between specific flow patterns and rupture, though no single parameter reliably predicts rupture risk. Computational fluid dynamics simulations complement 4D flow measurements by providing higher spatial resolution and additional hemodynamic parameters from the same anatomical data. The integration of 4D flow measurements with aneurysm morphology and wall imaging may improve the prediction of rupture risk, although prospective validation in large cohorts is needed before clinical implementation. The potential to guide intervention decisions—treating high-risk hemodynamic patterns in even moderate-sized aneurysms while conservatively monitoring low-risk large aneurysms—represents an appealing goal that requires further evidence.

Arteriovenous malformation hemodynamics characterisation using 4D flow enables the quantification of shunt flow, identification of feeding arteries and draining veins, and assessment of hemodynamic changes following treatment. The technique provides flow volumes through individual feeding arteries, enabling the identification of dominant feeders for targeted embolisation, and measures total shunt flow to quantify cardiovascular burden. Follow-up imaging after embolisation or radiosurgery reveals reduced flow in the treated portions, while also identifying any residual flow or recruited collaterals. The comprehensive flow information exceeds what catheter angiography provides, as angiography shows anatomy and qualitative flow but not quantitative velocity or volume measurements. However, the lower spatial resolution of 4D flow compared with digital subtraction angiography limits the detection of small vessels, underscoring the need to integrate both techniques for optimal AVM characterisation and treatment planning. Chronic AVM effects on cerebral hemodynamics, including venous hypertension and the steal phenomenon, are visible on 4D flow.

Venous sinus stenosis assessment represents an emerging 4D flow application in the investigation of idiopathic intracranial hypertension. Many patients with idiopathic intracranial hypertension show transverse sinus stenosis, with debate about whether stenosis is a cause or effect of elevated pressure. The pressure gradient across stenoses measured with 4D flow enables assessment of hemodynamic significance, with large gradients suggesting that the stenosis significantly impedes venous drainage, potentially contributing to elevated intracranial pressure. Some patients show clinical improvement after venous sinus stenting, though optimal patient selection remains uncertain. The ability to measure pressure gradients non-invasively may guide patient selection for invasive pressure measurement and potential stenting. Additional 4D flow parameters, including wall shear stress patterns and flow asymmetry between transverse sinuses, contribute to understanding the pathophysiology of idiopathic intracranial hypertension. However, the relationship between imaging findings and clinical decision-making requires further study, as not all patients with stenosis benefit from stenting.

10.5. Chronic Stroke and Recovery Monitoring

Follow-up imaging in chronic stroke provides essential information on tissue evolution, the identification of complications, the assessment of recovery mechanisms, and the prognostication of functional outcomes. The evolution from acute ischemic injury through subacute inflammation and tissue repair to chronic encephalomalacia is characterised by distinct imaging changes. Acute diffusion restriction transitions to T2/FLAIR hyperintensity over days, representing vasogenic oedema, with subsequent cavitation over weeks as necrotic tissue is cleared, leaving a fluid-filled space with gliotic margins, a characteristic of encephalomalacia. The pattern, extent, and location of chronic changes provide information about stroke subtype, potential complications, and implications for future stroke risk. Hemorrhagic transformation—the conversion of an ischemic infarct to a hemorrhagic infarct through reperfusion of damaged vessels—occurs in 10-40% of cases, depending on infarct size and reperfusion timing, and detection influences decisions regarding anticoagulation. Structural imaging, combined with functional and connectivity measures, reveals brain reorganisation underlying recovery, potentially guiding rehabilitation strategies. Serial imaging tracks the recovery trajectory, identifies patients with poor recovery who require more intensive intervention, and provides objective endpoints for rehabilitation trials (Schaechter et al., 2006).

Hemorrhagic transformation classification employs imaging to categorise bleeding patterns with prognostic implications. Hemorrhagic infarction (HI) shows petechial haemorrhages within the infarct, not causing mass effect, classified as HI-1 (scattered small petechiae) or HI-2 (more confluent petechiae), generally asymptomatic and not precluding anticoagulation. Parenchymal hematoma (PH) is characterised by more extensive bleeding with a mass effect, classified as PH-1 (hematoma in ≤30% of the infarct) or PH-2 (hematoma in >30% of the infarct), and is associated with poor outcomes and symptomatic deterioration. Gradient-echo or susceptibility-weighted imaging shows superior sensitivity for detecting hemorrhagic transformation compared with CT, identifying additional cases classified as non hemorrhagic on CT. The timing of hemorrhagic transformation has clinical implications: early transformation within 24 hours often indicates severe ischemia with inadequate collaterals, while delayed transformation beyond 24 hours may reflect reperfusion after initial occlusion. The decision to initiate or continue anticoagulation after hemorrhagic transformation requires weighing thromboembolism risk against expansion of intracerebral bleeding, with imaging findings informing risk-benefit assessment.

Brain atrophy develops over months following stroke, with tissue loss exceeding initial infarct volume due to Wallerian degeneration of disconnected tracts, diaschisis effects causing dysfunction in remote connected regions, and potentially chronic inflammation. Diffusion tensor imaging reveals degeneration of corticospinal tract fibres distal to motor cortex infarcts, correlating with the severity of motor impairment and predicting recovery potential. The atrophy may extend to the contralateral hemisphere through transcallosal diaschisis or shared subcortical pathways. Hippocampal atrophy remote from the infarct suggests a risk of cognitive decline, while progressive, generalised atrophy may represent accelerated ageing due to vascular damage. Quantification of atrophy rates using automated segmentation provides objective measures of tissue loss, potentially serving as endpoints in neuroprotection trials. However, distinguishing treatment effects on atrophy from natural progression requires careful attention to confounds, including age, comorbidities, and measurement error.

Functional recovery mechanisms investigated using task-based and resting-state fMRI reveal patterns of brain reorganisation that correlate with behavioural recovery. Three recovery patterns emerge: activation in perilesional cortex, representing local plasticity with surviving neurons assuming the functions of damaged tissue; activation in contralesional homologous regions, representing the recruitment of right hemisphere regions typically supporting left hemisphere functions; and activation in alternative networks, representing functional reorganisation beyond the simple recruitment of mirror regions. Longitudinal studies tracking patients through recovery reveal dynamic changes in activation patterns, with the early recruitment of contralesional regions sometimes giving way to perilesional activation as recovery progresses, suggesting initial compensation followed by genuine recovery. The predictive value of functional imaging for long-term outcomes remains under investigation, with some studies showing that perilesional activation predicts good recovery, while contralesional activation suggests poor recovery; however, findings are heterogeneous across patients and functions. Rehabilitation strategies targeting specific recovery mechanisms—for example, constraint-induced movement therapy, which promotes perilesional plasticity—may be informed by findings from functional magnetic resonance imaging (fMRI).

Resting-state connectivity changes after stroke reveal network disruption and reorganisation relevant to recovery. Interhemispheric connectivity between homologous motor regions predicts motor recovery, with preserved or enhanced connectivity associated with better outcomes and reduced connectivity with poorer outcomes. Default mode network connectivity shows alterations correlating with post-stroke cognitive impairment and depression. The balance between motor networks and the default mode network predicts functional independence, with stronger motor network connectivity and weaker default network connectivity associated with better outcomes. Longitudinal connectivity changes track the recovery trajectory, with some patients showing progressive restoration of connectivity, while others exhibit persistent disconnection. The potential to use baseline connectivity patterns to predict recovery and personalise rehabilitation represents an exciting frontier, although it requires validation in large prospective cohorts before clinical implementation. Non-invasive brain stimulation guided by connectivity mapping aims to enhance beneficial plasticity while suppressing maladaptive reorganisation, though optimal targeting strategies remain under development.

Stroke recurrence risk stratification using imaging identifies patients requiring intensive secondary prevention. White matter hyperintensity burden on FLAIR imaging reflects minor vessel disease severity, with extensive changes predicting recurrent stroke and cognitive decline. Cerebral microbleeds indicate bleeding-prone microangiopathy, with location and number informing anticoagulation decisions in atrial fibrillation. Silent infarcts—small infarcts without corresponding clinical events—predict future symptomatic stroke and cognitive impairment. The pattern of infarcts (multiple territories suggesting an embolic source, a single territory suggesting significant vessel disease, or a lacunar pattern suggesting small vessel disease) guides the selection of secondary prevention strategies. Advanced imaging, including cerebrovascular reactivity testing, identifies patients with hemodynamic insufficiency who may benefit from revascularisation. The integration of imaging findings with clinical risk factors provides more accurate risk prediction than either alone, potentially enabling individualised prevention strategies.

10.6. Imaging of Vascular Malformations

Vascular malformations encompass diverse abnormalities of the brain vasculature, including arteriovenous malformations, cavernous malformations, capillary telangiectasias, and developmental venous anomalies, each requiring specific imaging approaches for diagnosis and characterisation. Arteriovenous malformations (AVMs) consist of tangled vessels with direct arteriovenous shunting, lacking an intervening capillary bed, and typically present with haemorrhage, seizures, or headaches. For treatment decisions, characterisation of the nidus size, location, drainage pattern, and associated features is required. Cavernous malformations (cavernomas) comprise clusters of dilated capillaries without intervening brain parenchyma, appearing as "popcorn" lesions on MRI with susceptibility effects from blood products of varying ages. Developmental venous anomalies (DVAs) represent variations in venous drainage rather than true malformations, typically presenting as asymptomatic incidental findings that do not require treatment. Capillary telangiectasias are small, dilated capillaries usually identified incidentally. Understanding the imaging characteristics, natural history, and treatment indications for each malformation type enables appropriate management (Taschner et al., 2005).

Arteriovenous malformation imaging employs multiple MRI techniques providing complementary information. T2-weighted imaging reveals flow voids resulting from rapid flow in feeding arteries, nidus vessels, and draining veins, with the surrounding brain exhibiting variable signal intensity due to prior haemorrhage, gliosis, or oedema. Susceptibility-weighted imaging enhances venous visualisation and detects microhemorrhages. Time-of-flight MRA effectively demonstrates feeding arteries and large draining veins, although the complexity and turbulence of the flow limit visualisation of the nidus. Contrast-enhanced MRA or 4D flow imaging provides better characterisation of the nidus. Perfusion imaging can reveal hyperemia in the surrounding brain due to arteriovenous shunting. The Spetzler-Martin grade, which predicts surgical risk based on size, location, and drainage pattern, relies partly on imaging features; however, catheter angiography provides a definitive assessment of the grade. The identification of aneurysms on feeding arteries or venous varices on draining veins is critical, as these features confer a higher risk of haemorrhage and should be considered in treatment planning. Prior haemorrhage is visible as hemosiderin staining on susceptibility-weighted imaging (SWI) sequences.

Treatment planning for AVMs integrates imaging with clinical factors to determine whether observation, surgery, embolisation, radiosurgery, or a combination of these approaches is optimal. Small AVMs (<3 cm) in non-eloquent locations with superficial drainage are favourable for surgery, while large AVMs in eloquent cortex with deep drainage are high-risk. Radiosurgery is effective for small AVMs, though obliteration takes 1-3 years during which haemorrhage risk persists. Embolisation reduces flow as a preoperative preparation or palliative treatment for unresectable AVMs. Follow-up imaging after treatment assesses for residual nidus, with complete obliteration required for eliminating haemorrhage risk. MRA shows progressive reduction in nidus size and feeding arteries after radiosurgery, though catheter angiography remains the gold standard for documenting complete obliteration. Some AVMs undergo spontaneous thrombosis, which is visible as signal changes within the nidus and reduced flow voids; however, the clinical significance of partial thrombosis is uncertain. The natural history of untreated AVMs shows haemorrhage risk of 2-4% per year, with risk factors including prior haemorrhage, deep location, and associated aneurysms identifiable on imaging.

Cavernous malformation imaging reveals characteristic appearances, enabling a confident diagnosis in most cases. The classic "popcorn" appearance on T2-weighted imaging reflects loculated blood products of varying ages, with mixed signal intensity from methemoglobin, hemosiderin, and fresh blood. The complete hemosiderin rim, appearing as a dark signal on T2 and exhibiting prominent blooming on gradient-echo or SWI sequences, reflects chronic blood products surrounding the lesion. The absence of flow voids and lack of enhancement distinguish cavernomas from AVMs and tumours. The multiplicity of lesions suggests familial cavernomatosis with autosomal dominant inheritance, while solitary lesions are usually sporadic. Developmental venous anomalies often coexist with cavernomas, visible as linear flow voids converging in a caput medusae pattern on contrast-enhanced imaging. The clinical significance of cavernomas lies in the risks of haemorrhage and seizures. Brainstem and deep locations exhibit higher symptomatic haemorrhage rates (4-6% per year) than lobar lesions (1-2% per year), while cortical cavernomas frequently cause seizures through hemosiderin-induced cortical irritation.

Developmental venous anomalies appear as prominent medullary veins that drain into a large collecting vein, exhibiting a "caput medusae" appearance on post-contrast imaging, characterised by a radial pattern of small veins converging into a collector. The lesions enhance uniformly, reflecting slow flow in typical venous structures without abnormal shunting. Most are incidental findings without clinical significance, representing variations in venous drainage rather than malformations, and do not require treatment. The coexistence with cavernomas in some cases likely reflects that cavernomas develop due to chronic venous hypertension from anomalous drainage. Capillary telangiectasias appear as minor, faint enhancements on post-contrast imaging, typically in the pons, and are usually incidental findings without clinical significance. The distinction between these benign incidental vascular findings and pathological AVMs requiring intervention is critical for appropriate counselling, as unnecessary treatment of DVAs can cause venous infarction if anomalous drainage is interrupted without alternative pathways.

Cerebral dural arteriovenous fistulas represent acquired lesions, distinct from parenchymal AVMs, where arteriovenous shunting occurs within dural sinuses fed by dural arteries. These lesions present with varied symptoms depending on the drainage pattern: direct drainage into dural sinuses (Type I) causes relatively benign symptoms. In contrast, cortical venous reflux (higher Borden types) carries a risk of haemorrhage. Imaging reveals dilated dural sinuses, prominent dural vasculature, and, in high-grade lesions, dilated cortical veins resulting from retrograde drainage. Susceptibility-weighted imaging reveals prominent veins, while time-resolved MRA may show early venous filling. However, conventional angiography is usually required for definitive diagnosis and treatment planning. Follow-up imaging after treatment (embolisation or surgical disconnection) assesses for residual fistula, with persistent cortical venous drainage indicating incomplete treatment and ongoing haemorrhage risk. The detection and characterisation of these lesions requires a high index of suspicion and careful assessment of the venous phase on MRA and contrast-enhanced imaging.

Conclusion

Magnetic resonance imaging has become indispensable for stroke and cerebrovascular disease evaluation, spanning emergency diagnosis through chronic monitoring. Diffusion-weighted imaging detects acute ischemic injury within minutes, with a sensitivity of 90-95%, establishing MRI as the gold standard for this purpose. The integration of perfusion imaging, which reveals tissue at risk, and vascular imaging, which localises arterial occlusions, enables patient-specific treatment decisions based on tissue status rather than arbitrary time windows. The diffusion-perfusion mismatch concept identifies salvageable penumbra, transforming clinical practice by extending treatment windows from rigid 6-hour limits to flexible 24-hour windows for carefully selected patients—a paradigm shift toward precision medicine in stroke care.

MR angiography provides comprehensive vascular assessment, ranging from time-of-flight imaging for rapid arterial visualisation to contrast-enhanced angiography for stenosis quantification, and 4D flow characterisation of complex hemodynamics. Vessel wall imaging directly visualises atherosclerotic plaques, characterising high-risk features that independently predict stroke, independent of stenosis severity.

Chronic stroke imaging reveals injury evolution, identifies complications, including hemorrhagic transformation, and investigates recovery mechanisms through functional MRI and diffusion tensor imaging, revealing brain reorganisation patterns that correlate with behavioural recovery.

Vascular malformation imaging characterises a diverse range of abnormalities, from arteriovenous malformations requiring treatment to benign developmental venous anomalies that require only reassurance.

Technical advances include faster acquisitions, higher field strengths, and artificial intelligence applications for automated analysis. The future integration of tissue, vascular, hemodynamic, and functional information will enable increasingly precise diagnosis, prognosis, and individualised treatment guidance.

Acknowledgments

The authors would like to extend our appreciation to those who offered helpful commentary during the drafting process of this manuscript. We also acknowledge the role the Nova Publishing department played in enabling the work described herein.

References

Albers, G. W., Marks, M. P., Kemp, S., Christensen, S., Tsai, J. P., Ortega-Gutierrez, S., McTaggart, R. A., Torbey, M. T., Kim-Tenser, M., Leslie-Mazwi, T., Sarraj, A., Kasner, S. E., Ansari, S. A., Yeatts, S. D., Hamilton, S., Mlynash, M., Heit, J. J., Zaharchuk, G., Kim, S., DEFUSE 3 Investigators. (2018). Thrombectomy for stroke at 6 to 16 hours with selection by perfusion imaging. *New England Journal of Medicine*, 378(8), 708-718. https://doi.org/10.1056/NEJMoa1713973.

Lansberg, M. G., Straka, M., Kemp, S., Mlynash, M., Wechsler, L. R., Jovin, T. G., Wilder, M. J., Lutsep, H. L., Czartoski, T. J., Bernstein, R. A., Chang, C. W., Warach, S., Fazekas, F., Inoue, M., Tipirneni, A., Hamilton, S. A., Zaharchuk, G., Marks, M. P., Bammer, R., DEFUSE 2 Study Investigators. (2012). MRI profile and response to endovascular reperfusion after stroke (DEFUSE 2): A prospective cohort study. *Lancet Neurology*, 11(10), 860-867. https://doi.org/10.1016/S1474-4422(12)70203-X.

Markl, M., Frydrychowicz, A., Kozerke, S., Hope, M., & Wieben, O. (2012). 4D flow MRI. *Journal of Magnetic Resonance Imaging*, 36(5), 1015-1036. https://doi.org/10.1002/jmri.23632.

Moseley, M. E., Cohen, Y., Mintorovitch, J., Chileuitt, L., Shimizu, H., Kucharczyk, J., Wendland, M. F., & Weinstein, P. R. (1990). Early detection of regional cerebral ischemia in cats: Comparison of diffusion- and T2-weighted MRI and spectroscopy. *Magnetic Resonance in Medicine*, 14(2), 330-346. https://doi.org/10.1002/mrm.1910140218.

Schaechter, J. D., Perdue, K. L., & Wang, R. (2006). Structural damage to the corticospinal tract correlates with bilateral sensorimotor cortex reorganization in stroke patients. *NeuroImage*, 39(3), 1370-1382. https://doi.org/10.1016/j.neuroimage.2007.09.071.

Taschner, C. A., Chapot, R., Costalat, V., Machi, P., Courthéoux, P., Barreau, X., Berge, J., Pierot, L., Kadziolka, K., Jean, B., Collignon, L., Derelle, A. L., Hossu, G., & Anxionnat, R. (2005). Second-level therapeutic embolization of intracranial arteriovenous malformations using Onyx. *American Journal of Neuroradiology*, 26(6), 1501-1508.

Willinek, W. A., & Born, M. (2005). MR angiography: Non-contrast-enhanced techniques. In M. F. Reiser, H. Hricak, & C. R. Becker (Eds.), *Multislice CT* (pp. 567-580). Springer.

Wintermark, M., Sanelli, P. C., Albers, G. W., Bello, J., Derdeyn, C., Hetts, S. W., Johnson, M. H., Kidwell, C., Lev, M. H., Liebeskind, D. S., Rowley, H., Schaefer, P. W., Sunshine, J. L., Zaharchuk, G., & Meltzer, C. (2013). Imaging recommendations for acute stroke and transient ischemic attack patients: A joint statement by the American Society of Neuroradiology, the American College of Radiology, and the Society of NeuroInterventional Surgery. *American Journal of Neuroradiology*, 34(11), E117-E127. https://doi.org/10.3174/ajnr.A3690.

Chapter 11

MRI in Neurodegenerative Diseases

Sushil Ghanshyam Kachewar[1,*]
and Maajid Mohi Ud Din Malik[2,†]
[1]Department of Radio-Diagnosis, Dr. D. Y. Patil Medical College, Hospital and Research Centre, Dr. D. Y. Patil Vidyapeeth (Deemed to be University)- Sant Tukaram Nagar, Pimpri, Pune, India
[2]Radiology and Imaging Technology, Dr. D. Y. Patil School of Allied Health Sciences, Dr. D. Y. Patil Vidyapeeth (Deemed to be University), Sant Tukaram Nagar, Pimpri, Pune, India

Abstract

Neurodegenerative diseases represent a growing global health challenge characterised by progressive neuronal loss and functional decline. Magnetic resonance imaging has emerged as an indispensable tool for diagnosis, disease monitoring, and understanding pathophysiological mechanisms across these disorders. This chapter examines advanced MRI techniques in primary neurodegenerative conditions, including Alzheimer's disease, Parkinson's disease, frontotemporal dementia, multiple sclerosis, and amyotrophic lateral sclerosis. We discuss structural imaging approaches for measuring regional atrophy, quantitative techniques for assessing tissue microstructure and iron deposition, alterations in functional connectivity, and emerging biomarkers that enhance diagnostic accuracy and track disease progression. Recent advances in ultra-high-field imaging, machine learning-based analysis, and multimodal integration have significantly improved the early detection of pathological changes and differential diagnosis. Longitudinal imaging protocols provide objective measures of disease progression, which are essential for clinical trials and therapeutic monitoring. Understanding disease-specific MRI patterns is crucial for neurologists and radiologists in managing these complex conditions, which affect millions worldwide.

---

* Corresponding Author's Email: sushil.kachewar@dpu.edu.in
† Corresponding Author's Email: maajid.malik@dpu.edu.in

In: Recent Advances in Magnetic Resonance Imaging in Neuroimaging
Editors: Maajid Mohi Ud Din Malik, Purnachandra Kawdu Lamghare and R. S. Kuber
ISBN: 979-8-90134-244-2

Keywords: neurodegenerative diseases, Alzheimer's disease, Parkinson's disease, multiple sclerosis, MRI biomarkers, SDG 3 - good health and well-being

Introduction

Neurodegenerative diseases represent a formidable and escalating challenge to global health systems, affecting millions of individuals worldwide with progressive neuronal dysfunction and loss that leads to devastating cognitive, motor, and behavioural impairments. These conditions, including Alzheimer's disease, Parkinson's disease, frontotemporal dementia, multiple sclerosis, and amyotrophic lateral sclerosis, share standard features of irreversible neuronal degeneration yet demonstrate distinct pathophysiological mechanisms, anatomical distributions, and clinical manifestations requiring precise diagnostic differentiation. The absence of curative treatments and the relentless progression characteristic of most neurodegenerative disorders underscore the critical importance of early and accurate diagnosis, which enables timely intervention, appropriate counselling, and enrollment in clinical trials evaluating potential disease-modifying therapies.

Magnetic resonance imaging has revolutionised the field of neurodegeneration research and clinical practice by providing non-invasive visualisation of brain structure, function, and pathological processes with unprecedented detail and sensitivity. Unlike clinical assessments that reflect cumulative functional consequences of neuronal loss, advanced MRI techniques can detect subtle brain changes in prodromal disease stages, track progression with quantitative biomarkers, and distinguish between overlapping syndromes based on characteristic anatomical patterns. The evolution from conventional structural imaging to sophisticated multiparametric approaches integrating volumetric analysis, diffusion tensor imaging, functional connectivity mapping, iron quantification, and metabolic spectroscopy has dramatically enhanced diagnostic accuracy and prognostic capabilities. This chapter examines the application of advanced MRI techniques across primary neurodegenerative conditions, emphasising disease-specific imaging signatures, quantitative biomarkers for monitoring progression, and emerging technologies that promise to transform early detection and therapeutic monitoring in these challenging disorders.

11.1. Alzheimer's Disease: Structural and Functional Markers

Alzheimer's disease represents the most prevalent neurodegenerative disorder globally, characterised by progressive cognitive decline and neuropathological features including amyloid-beta plaques, neurofibrillary tangles, and neuronal loss. Magnetic resonance imaging serves multiple critical roles in Alzheimer's disease evaluation, from excluding structural lesions and cerebrovascular disease to identifying characteristic atrophy patterns that support clinical diagnosis and track disease progression. The integration of structural, functional, and advanced quantitative MRI techniques has revolutionised our understanding of disease mechanisms and enhanced diagnostic precision in both research and clinical settings.

The hallmark structural finding in Alzheimer's disease involves atrophy of the medial temporal lobe, particularly affecting the hippocampus and entorhinal cortex, which are essential structures for memory formation and consolidation. High-resolution T1-weighted volumetric imaging enables precise quantification of hippocampal volumes, with established thresholds supporting diagnosis when adjusted for age and intracranial volume (Jack et al., 2018). Studies demonstrate that hippocampal atrophy rates of three to five percent annually in Alzheimer's patients significantly exceed the one to two percent observed in normal ageing. Beyond volumetric measurements, visual rating scales, such as the medial temporal atrophy scale, provide clinically practical, semi-quantitative assessments that correlate with volumetric measurements and demonstrate good inter-rater reliability among trained radiologists. The pattern of cortical atrophy in Alzheimer's disease follows a characteristic distribution, extending from medial temporal structures to temporoparietal association cortices, the posterior cingulate, and the precuneus. In contrast, primary sensory and motor cortices remain relatively preserved until advanced stages (Frisoni et al., 2010). This distinctive spatial pattern aids differential diagnosis from other dementias and reflects the sequential spread of pathology described by Braak stageing systems.

Advanced cortical analysis techniques, including surface-based morphometry, provide detailed topographic maps of cortical thickness across the entire brain, revealing subtle regional abnormalities that can be detected before overt clinical symptoms emerge. Automated segmentation tools, such as FreeSurfer, enable rapid and reproducible measurements of cortical thickness, subcortical volumes, and white matter hyperintensity burden, facilitating the integration of quantitative imaging into clinical workflows. These computational approaches have demonstrated that cortical thinning in specific regions, including the inferior and middle temporal cortices, precuneus, and posterior cingulate, correlates strongly with cognitive performance and predicts future decline in patients with mild cognitive impairment. The ability to detect structural changes in prodromal disease stages has important implications for early intervention strategies and enrollment in clinical trials targeting preclinical Alzheimer's disease.

Diffusion tensor imaging reveals microstructural alterations in the temporal lobe white matter that complement structural assessments, demonstrating decreased fractional anisotropy and increased mean diffusivity, particularly in the cingulum bundle, which connects medial temporal structures with posterior cortical regions. These diffusion abnormalities reflect axonal degeneration, demyelination, and disruption of white-matter tract integrity, accompanying cortical pathology. Significantly, diffusion changes extend beyond regions of visible atrophy into normal-appearing white matter, suggesting widespread microstructural damage contributes to cognitive decline. The cingulum bundle shows particularly prominent degeneration, which correlates with episodic memory impairment, as this pathway provides critical connectivity for memory networks. Advanced diffusion models, including neurite orientation dispersion and density imaging, provide a more specific characterisation of axonal density and orientation dispersion than conventional DTI parameters, potentially improving sensitivity for detecting early pathological changes.

Functional MRI studies have identified disrupted connectivity within the default mode network, a set of brain regions that includes the posterior cingulate, precuneus, medial prefrontal cortex, and lateral parietal areas, which demonstrate coordinated activity during rest and support memory consolidation and self-referential processing. Reduced connectivity within the default mode network appears early in Alzheimer's disease and even in individuals with mild cognitive impairment who subsequently progress to dementia, suggesting functional disruption precedes extensive structural degeneration (Whitwell, 2010). Task-based functional MRI during memory encoding paradigms reveals reduced hippocampal activation and altered patterns of cortical recruitment, interpreted as compensatory mechanisms that attempt to maintain cognitive function despite underlying pathology. Arterial spin labelling perfusion imaging reveals characteristic hypoperfusion in the temporoparietal regions and posterior cingulate cortex, patterns that mirror glucose hypometabolism observed on fluorodeoxyglucose positron emission tomography. The advantage of arterial spin labelling is its ability to provide perfusion information without exogenous contrast agents or radiation exposure, thereby enabling repeated measurements for longitudinal tracking.

Table 11.1. Structural MRI findings across neurodegenerative diseases

Disease	Primary Atrophy Pattern	Key White Matter Changes	Distinctive Features
Alzheimer's Disease	Medial temporal lobe, hippocampus, temporoparietal cortex	Decreased FA in the cingulum, temporal white matter	Posterior cortical atrophy, medial temporal lobe atrophy scales
Parkinson's Disease	Substantia nigra, minimal cortical changes	Reduced FA in the substantia nigra, superior longitudinal fasciculus	Loss of swallow-tail sign, neuromelanin reduction
Frontotemporal Dementia	Frontal and anterior temporal lobes, asymmetric	Uncinate fasciculus, anterior corpus callosum	Knife-edge atrophy in the semantic variant, frontal-predominant in the behavioural variant
Multiple Sclerosis	Whole brain, spinal cord, thalamus	Periventricular lesions, corpus callosum involvement	T2 hyperintense lesions, gadolinium enhancement, central vein sign
Amyotrophic Lateral Sclerosis	Motor cortex, corticospinal tracts	Reduced FA in corticospinal tracts at all levels	Corticospinal tract hyperintensity on T2/FLAIR

Magnetic resonance spectroscopy provides complementary metabolic information, typically revealing decreased N-acetylaspartate, a marker of neuronal integrity, and elevated myo-inositol, a marker of glial activity, in the posterior cingulate and temporal regions. The ratio of N-acetylaspartate to other metabolites demonstrates diagnostic utility for distinguishing Alzheimer's disease from normal ageing and other dementias. Susceptibility-weighted imaging and quantitative susceptibility mapping enable the assessment of cerebral microbleeds and iron deposition patterns, which are relevant for understanding vascular contributions to cognitive impairment and for safety monitoring in patients receiving anticoagulation or emerging amyloid-targeting immunotherapies. Recent developments in ultra-high-field 7 Tesla imaging provide unprecedented visualisation of hippocampal subregions and cortical layers, revealing the differential vulnerability of specific anatomical compartments that may improve our understanding of disease mechanisms and enable earlier detection of pathological changes in at-risk individuals. Table 11.1 shows structural MRI findings across neurodegenerative diseases.

11.2. Parkinson's Disease and Movement Disorders

Parkinson's disease constitutes a progressive movement disorder resulting from degeneration of dopaminergic neurons in the substantia nigra pars compacta, manifesting clinically with bradykinesia, rigidity, tremor, and postural instability. While diagnosis relies primarily on clinical examination, magnetic resonance imaging is increasingly essential for excluding structural causes of Parkinsonism and identifying imaging biomarkers that support diagnosis, particularly in atypical presentations where clinical features overlap across different Parkinsonian syndromes. Conventional structural imaging in idiopathic Parkinson's disease typically appears normal or shows only age-related changes, which itself serves as a useful diagnostic feature distinguishing true Parkinson's disease from atypical Parkinsonian syndromes demonstrating more prominent structural abnormalities.

Advanced imaging techniques have revealed subtle but consistent abnormalities in Parkinson's disease that enhance diagnostic confidence. High-resolution susceptibility-weighted imaging at 3 Tesla magnetic resonance systems enables visualisation of the nigrosome-1 region, a distinctive dorsolateral substantia nigra structure that generally appears as a hyperintense swallow-tail configuration. The loss or reduction of this swallow-tail sign in Parkinson's disease reflects iron accumulation and dopaminergic neuronal loss, demonstrating approximately 95% sensitivity and 90% specificity for distinguishing Parkinson's disease from healthy controls when assessed by experienced neuroradiologists (Schwarz et al., 2014). This finding provides valuable objective support for clinical diagnosis, particularly in early disease stages when motor symptoms may be subtle or ambiguous.

Neuromelanin-sensitive magnetic resonance imaging is another specialised technique that specifically visualises neuromelanin-containing neurons in the substantia nigra and locus coeruleus. Parkinson's disease patients exhibit a significantly reduced area and contrast ratio of the neuromelanin signal compared to healthy controls, directly reflecting the loss of dopaminergic cells (Rossi et al., 2021). This technique shows promise for early diagnosis and differential diagnosis, as neuromelanin reduction correlates with disease severity and duration. The ability to directly visualise catecholaminergic nuclei noninvasively represents a significant advance, as these small brainstem structures are challenging to assess with conventional imaging modalities. Neuromelanin imaging requires specialised T1-weighted sequences with inversion recovery to suppress background signal while enhancing neuromelanin contrast, which can be achieved on standard three tesla clinical scanners with appropriate pulse sequences.

Quantitative susceptibility mapping provides a superior assessment of iron content in the substantia nigra and other deep Grey matter structures compared to conventional T2-star or susceptibility-weighted imaging, expressing tissue susceptibility in quantitative units that enable longitudinal tracking and comparison across patients. Elevated iron accumulation in the substantia nigra, red nucleus, and putamen has been consistently demonstrated in patients with Parkinson's disease, correlating with disease severity and motor symptom burden (Kwon et al., 2012). Iron deposition likely reflects multiple pathological processes, including oxidative stress, mitochondrial dysfunction, and breakdown of iron-containing dopaminergic neurons. The ability to quantify iron accumulation noninvasively may serve as a progression biomarker for clinical trials evaluating disease-modifying therapies, particularly those targeting oxidative stress mechanisms.

Diffusion tensor imaging reveals microstructural changes extending beyond the substantia nigra to involve multiple brain regions. Reduced fractional anisotropy and increased mean diffusivity in the substantia nigra reflect tissue disorganisation and cell loss, while white-matter abnormalities in the superior longitudinal fasciculus, cingulum bundle, and corpus callosum correlate with cognitive impairment in many patients with Parkinson's disease. Free water imaging, an advanced diffusion technique that separates tissue and extracellular compartments, demonstrates an increased free water fraction in the posterior substantia nigra, which may precede visible atrophy and predict motor progression, potentially providing earlier and more sensitive markers of nigral degeneration than conventional diffusion parameters. Resting-state functional magnetic resonance imaging studies reveal altered striatal connectivity and compensatory changes in motor networks. The decreased connectivity between the striatum and motor cortex reflects a disruption of the basal ganglia circuit. In contrast, increased activation in the supplementary motor area and cerebellum suggests compensatory recruitment that maintains motor function despite dopamine depletion.

Differential diagnosis of atypical Parkinsonian syndromes relies heavily on distinctive magnetic resonance imaging patterns, distinguishing these conditions from idiopathic Parkinson's disease. Progressive supranuclear palsy exhibits characteristic midbrain atrophy, creating the "hummingbird sign" on sagittal images and the "morning glory sign" on axial images, which reflects degeneration of the superior cerebellar peduncle and midbrain tegmentum. Multiple system atrophy exhibits putaminal atrophy and T2 hypointensity, accompanied by a hyperintense rim along the lateral border of the putamen. At the same time, the cerebellar subtype demonstrates the hot cross bun sign in the pons, representing selective pontocerebellar fibre degeneration. Corticobasal degeneration exhibits asymmetric cortical atrophy, particularly affecting the perirolandic and parietal regions contralateral to the more affected side of the body, distinguishing it from Alzheimer's disease, which primarily involves the primary motor cortex while relatively sparing medial temporal structures. These distinctive imaging patterns significantly enhance diagnostic accuracy and enable earlier recognition of atypical Parkinsonism, which has important prognostic implications given generally poorer treatment response and more rapid progression compared to idiopathic Parkinson's disease.

11.3. Frontotemporal Dementia Imaging

Frontotemporal dementia encompasses a heterogeneous group of neurodegenerative disorders characterised by progressive degeneration of the frontal and temporal lobes, presenting with behavioural changes, language impairment, or motor symptoms depending on the specific syndrome variant. Magnetic resonance imaging plays a crucial diagnostic role by revealing characteristic patterns of regional atrophy that distinguish frontotemporal dementia from Alzheimer's disease and other dementias, with these imaging findings incorporated into current diagnostic criteria. The behavioural variant demonstrates predominant frontal lobe atrophy, affecting the orbitofrontal cortex, anterior cingulate, and medial frontal regions, in contrast to Alzheimer's disease, where medial temporal involvement predominates initially. Patterns may be symmetric or show asymmetric frontal or temporal predominance, with anterior insula atrophy particularly characteristic and assessable using visual rating scales or quantitative volumetry.

Semantic dementia, a language variant of frontotemporal dementia, demonstrates striking asymmetric anterior temporal lobe atrophy, typically left-predominant, correlating with semantic memory deficits and anomia. The anterior temporal pole, amygdala, and hippocampal head exhibit prominent atrophy, resulting in a characteristic knife-edge appearance of the temporal pole on coronal magnetic resonance imaging (MRI) scans. This marked asymmetry helps distinguish semantic dementia from Alzheimer's disease, where atrophy patterns are generally more symmetric bilaterally. Disease progression involves the gradual spread to the temporal neocortex and, eventually, to the frontal regions, as tracked by longitudinal imaging of this anatomical evolution. Progressive nonfluent aphasia, another language variant, demonstrates left-predominant atrophy involving the inferior frontal gyrus, corresponding to Broca's area, the insula, and the premotor cortex, reflecting the anatomical substrates of speech production and grammatical processing (Whitwell & Josephs, 2012). Patients present with effortful, agrammatic speech production and apraxia of speech, with structural imaging revealing left perisylvian atrophy, distinguishing this variant from semantic dementia and behavioural frontotemporal dementia.

Cortical thickness analysis and surface-based morphometry provide detailed topographic maps of atrophy distribution, revealing patterns more subtle than those detected by visual assessment alone, and identifying involvement of specific gyri and sulci. Machine learning classification algorithms based on cortical thickness patterns can distinguish between frontotemporal dementia variants and Alzheimer's disease with high accuracy, demonstrating practical utility for challenging diagnostic cases. Diffusion tensor imaging reveals white matter degeneration in the frontal and temporal regions, corresponding to areas of cortical atrophy, with reduced fractional anisotropy in the uncinate fasciculus, which connects the frontal and temporal lobes, particularly prominent in behavioural variant and semantic dementia. The anterior corpus callosum exhibits degeneration, reflecting frontal involvement, whereas the posterior callosum remains relatively preserved, a contrast to Alzheimer's disease, in which posterior regions are more severely affected.

Resting-state functional magnetic resonance imaging reveals network disruptions, particularly affecting the salience network, in behavioural variant frontotemporal dementia. The salience network, which includes the anterior cingulate and anterior insula, exhibits reduced connectivity that correlates with behavioural symptoms (Seeley et al., 2008). Semantic dementia is characterised by disrupted connectivity in semantic networks, particularly involving the anterior temporal regions. These functional network alterations may precede structural atrophy and could serve as early biomarkers enabling intervention before irreversible tissue loss occurs. Some patients with frontotemporal dementia develop motor neuron disease features, exhibiting combined frontal atrophy and corticospinal tract degeneration, which is visible on magnetic resonance imaging as both frontotemporal atrophy and corticospinal tract hyperintensity or diffusion abnormalities. This overlap reflects shared pathological mechanisms between frontotemporal dementia and amyotrophic lateral sclerosis, often involving TDP-43 proteinopathy, with imaging features of combined motor and frontotemporal involvement indicating inferior prognosis with rapid progression.

11.4. Multiple Sclerosis: Advanced Imaging Techniques

Multiple sclerosis represents a chronic inflammatory and neurodegenerative disease of the central nervous system characterised by demyelination, axonal loss, and neurodegeneration affecting the brain, spinal cord, and optic nerves. Magnetic resonance imaging (MRI) is the most sensitive and specific paraclinical tool for diagnosing multiple sclerosis, monitoring disease progression, and assessing therapeutic efficacy. Imaging findings are incorporated into diagnostic criteria and serve as primary outcomes in clinical trials evaluating disease-modifying therapies. The hallmark finding involves multifocal white matter lesions visible as hyperintense regions on T2-weighted and fluid-attenuated inversion recovery sequences, representing areas of demyelination, inflammation, oedema, and varying degrees of axonal loss (Thompson et al., 2018).

Characteristic features supporting multiple sclerosis diagnosis include periventricular location immediately adjacent to the lateral ventricles, juxtacortical location extending to cortical surfaces, infratentorial involvement in the brainstem or cerebellum, and ovoid configuration with Dawson's fingers representing perivenular lesions oriented perpendicular to the corpus callosum following venous distribution. The revised McDonald diagnostic criteria incorporate specific lesion counts and distributions, with dissemination in space requiring lesions in at least 2 of the 4 characteristic locations: periventricular, juxtacortical, infratentorial, and spinal cord. Gadolinium-enhancing lesions indicate active inflammation with blood-brain barrier disruption, distinguishing new active lesions from older chronic lesions, with enhancement typically lasting two to six weeks. Open-ring enhancement patterns, with incomplete rings on the side facing Grey matter, demonstrate relative specificity for demyelinating lesions, helping distinguish multiple sclerosis from infectious or neoplastic processes (Filippi et al., 2019).

Advanced imaging at three tesla or seven tesla magnetic resonance systems reveals cortical and juxtacortical lesions with improved sensitivity compared to standard one-point-five tesla imaging. Cortical lesions, common but often invisible on conventional imaging, contribute significantly to cognitive impairment and physical disability. Double inversion recovery sequences suppress both cerebrospinal fluid and white matter signals, thereby enhancing the detection of cortical lesions. Ultra-high field seven-tesla imaging visualises central veins within white matter lesions, termed the central vein sign, which appears in over 80% of multiple sclerosis lesions but rarely in small vessel disease lesions, significantly improving diagnostic specificity. Phase-sensitive inversion recovery and quantitative susceptibility mapping enable the detection of paramagnetic rims surrounding chronic lesions, which represent iron-laden macrophages and microglia at lesion edges. These chronic active lesions with paramagnetic rims associate with more aggressive disease courses, greater disability accumulation, and worse clinical outcomes, potentially guiding treatment intensification decisions.

Spinal cord imaging remains essential in the evaluation of multiple sclerosis, as cord lesions occur in up to 90% of patients, providing additional evidence for dissemination in space. Cervical cord lesions typically involve fewer than 2 vertebral segments and occupy peripheral cord regions, with short tau inversion recovery sequences providing optimal lesion detection. Spinal cord atrophy, measured as cross-sectional area, correlates strongly with disability, particularly ambulation impairment, and often shows stronger associations than brain lesion burden. Quantitative assessment of brain and spinal cord atrophy has become increasingly important for monitoring disease progression, particularly in progressive multiple sclerosis, where lesion activity may be minimal despite ongoing neurodegeneration. Whole-brain atrophy, measured by brain parenchymal fraction, shows an accelerated loss of approximately 0.5 to 1.0% per year in multiple sclerosis compared to 0.1 to 0.3% per year in healthy individuals. Grey matter atrophy, particularly thalamic atrophy, correlates more strongly with cognitive impairment and disability progression than white matter atrophy.

Diffusion tensor imaging detects microstructural damage beyond visible lesions in normal-appearing white matter and Grey matter, with reduced fractional anisotropy and elevated mean diffusivity reflecting subclinical demyelination, axonal loss, and tissue disruption. Diffusion abnormalities in normal-appearing tissue predict future lesion development and clinical progression, indicating ongoing pathological processes invisible on conventional imaging. Magnetisation transfer imaging provides sensitivity to myelin content, with a reduced magnetisation transfer ratio in multiple sclerosis lesions and normal-appearing white matter, correlating with the severity of demyelination. Longitudinal changes in magnetisation transfer ratio may indicate remyelination in recovering lesions or progressive demyelination in chronic lesions, showing promise for monitoring remyelination in clinical trials of myelin repair therapies (Wattjes et al., 2015). Table 11.2 shows advanced MRI biomarkers in neurodegenerative diseases.

Table 11.2. Advanced MRI biomarkers in neurodegenerative diseases

Imaging Technique	Biological Substrate	Clinical Applications	Key Advantages
Quantitative Susceptibility Mapping	Iron deposition, myelin content	Parkinson's disease, multiple sclerosis, Alzheimer's disease	Quantitative iron measurement, longitudinal tracking
Neuromelanin Imaging	Dopaminergic neuron integrity	Parkinson's disease diagnosis, early detection	Direct visualisation of substantia nigra neurons
Diffusion Tensor Imaging	White matter microstructure, axonal integrity	All neurodegenerative diseases	Detects subclinical damage, correlates with cognition
Arterial Spin Labelling	Cerebral blood flow, perfusion	Alzheimer's disease, frontotemporal dementia	No contrast agent required, repeatable
Magnetization Transfer	Myelin content	Multiple sclerosis, white matter diseases	Sensitive to demyelination and remyelination
Functional Connectivity	Network integrity, synaptic function	Alzheimer's disease, Parkinson's disease	Early functional changes precede atrophy

11.5. Amyotrophic Lateral Sclerosis (ALS)

Amyotrophic lateral sclerosis constitutes a progressive neurodegenerative disease affecting motor neurons in the brain, brainstem, and spinal cord, leading to progressive weakness, muscle atrophy, and respiratory failure. While diagnosis remains primarily clinical, based on progressive motor neuron signs, magnetic resonance imaging plays a crucial role in excluding structural lesions that mimic amyotrophic lateral sclerosis and in identifying imaging biomarkers that support diagnosis, track disease progression, and provide insights into disease mechanisms. Conventional T2-weighted and fluid-attenuated inversion recovery imaging may demonstrate hyperintensity along the corticospinal tracts, extending from the motor cortex through the internal capsule, cerebral peduncles, and pons to the pyramidal tracts, reflecting Wallerian degeneration secondary to upper motor neuron loss (Turner et al., 2012). However, this corticospinal tract hyperintensity lacks specificity and sensitivity, as it is seen in only 30 to 50 per cent of amyotrophic lateral sclerosis patients, while it can also occur in normal elderly individuals.

High-resolution three Tesla magnetic resonance imaging enables detection of subtle cortical thinning in the primary motor cortex and supplementary motor areas. Surface-based morphometry reveals progressive thinning of the motor cortex, correlating with upper motor neuron burden and disease progression rates. Longitudinal studies demonstrate accelerated atrophy in motor regions compared to healthy controls, with cortical thinning rates correlating with clinical progression measured by amyotrophic lateral sclerosis functional rating scales. Diffusion tensor imaging is the most sensitive magnetic resonance technique for detecting pathological changes in amyotrophic lateral sclerosis, consistently demonstrating reduced fractional anisotropy and increased mean diffusivity in the corticospinal tracts at the internal capsule, cerebral peduncles, and centrum semiovale, reflecting axonal degeneration and loss of white matter integrity (Agosta et al., 2010). These diffusion abnormalities often extend beyond regions of visible T2 hyperintensity, indicating more widespread pathology than is apparent on conventional imaging. Fractional anisotropy reduction in the corticospinal tracts correlates with clinical disability, as measured by functional rating scales.

Advanced diffusion tractography enables the visualisation and quantitative assessment of entire corticospinal tracts, from the motor cortex to the brainstem, with whole-tract analysis revealing diffusion abnormalities extending along motor pathways. Extra-motor involvement is increasingly recognised, with many patients developing cognitive and behavioural changes consistent with frontotemporal dysfunction. Diffusion abnormalities extend to the frontal white matter, including the uncinate fasciculus, anterior corpus callosum, and frontal atrocallosal tracts. At the same time, structural atrophy affects the frontal and temporal cortices in patients with cognitive impairment. Approximately fifteen percent of amyotrophic lateral sclerosis patients meet criteria for frontotemporal dementia, with an additional thirty to forty percent showing milder cognitive or behavioural changes. Magnetic resonance imaging patterns involving frontal regions predict cognitive impairment and worse prognosis, reflecting the clinical and pathological overlap between amyotrophic lateral sclerosis and frontotemporal dementia.

Resting-state functional magnetic resonance imaging reveals altered connectivity in both motor and extramotor networks, with decreased connectivity within the primary motor cortex and between motor regions. Alterations in the salience network reflect frontotemporal involvement, while changes in the default mode network correlate with cognitive impairment. Magnetic resonance spectroscopy reveals a decreased N-acetylaspartate-to-creatine ratio in the motor cortex, reflecting neuronal loss and dysfunction, and this ratio correlates with disease severity and progression rates. Spinal cord imaging reveals atrophy of the cervical and thoracic cord, as measured by a reduced cross-sectional area, which correlates with limb weakness and respiratory dysfunction, providing objective evidence of lower motor neuron involvement. Machine learning algorithms that integrate multiple magnetic resonance imaging modalities, including cortical thickness, diffusion parameters, functional connectivity, and spectroscopy, demonstrate the ability to classify patients with amyotrophic lateral sclerosis (ALS) from controls with over 80% accuracy and predict survival time, potentially assisting in patient stratification for clinical trials and prognostic counselling.

11.6. Longitudinal Imaging and Disease Progression

Longitudinal magnetic resonance imaging (MRI) acquisitions that track brain structural and functional changes over time provide powerful tools for monitoring the progression of neurodegenerative diseases, evaluating therapeutic interventions, and understanding the temporal evolution of pathological processes. Serial volumetric imaging enables the calculation of atrophy rates, which represent changes in brain volume over specified intervals. Brain parenchymal fraction change and ventricular expansion serve as global measures, while regional volumes track specific structural degeneration. Hippocampal atrophy rates in Alzheimer's disease typically range from three to five percent annually, significantly exceeding normal ageing rates of one to two percent, with accelerated atrophy predicting faster cognitive decline and conversion from mild cognitive impairment to dementia (Fox et al., 2011). Sample size calculations for clinical trials demonstrate that atrophy measurements require substantially fewer participants than clinical endpoints to detect treatment effects, making volumetric outcomes attractive for proof-of-concept studies and dose-finding trials.

Technical considerations for longitudinal imaging include scanner stability, consistency of pulse sequences, and optimisation of analysis methodologies. Symmetric image registration algorithms specifically designed for longitudinal data minimise bias by treating baseline and follow-up acquisitions equally, thereby improving precision compared to cross-sectional approaches. Quality control procedures ensure scan quality consistency across time points, rejecting images with motion artefacts or technical failures that could confound atrophy measurements. Multi-site studies require careful harmonisation protocols that standardise acquisition parameters across scanners, while phantom scanning monitors inter-scanner variability. Automated analysis pipelines process longitudinal data consistently, extracting volumes, cortical thickness, and other metrics with minimal manual intervention, enhancing reproducibility and enabling large-scale studies.

Different neurodegenerative diseases exhibit characteristic temporal trajectories that are visible in longitudinal imaging. Alzheimer's disease exhibits progressive medial temporal atrophy that spreads to the lateral temporal and parietal regions, with atrophy patterns that correspond to disease staging systems. Frontotemporal dementia typically demonstrates focal progression in the frontal or temporal regions, eventually involving contralateral areas. Multiple sclerosis shows accumulating lesion burden and progressive brain atrophy, with atrophy rates predicting long-term disability. Parkinson's disease demonstrates slower atrophy rates than Alzheimer's disease, with changes primarily affecting subcortical structures and cognitive network regions in patients developing dementia. These disease-specific trajectories inform prognosis and enable comparison of individual patient progression against expected trajectories for specific diagnoses (Schuff et al., 2012).

Longitudinal diffusion imaging tracks white matter degeneration over time, with fractional anisotropy decline and mean diffusivity increase preceding visible atrophy in some regions, suggesting microstructural changes precede macroscopic tissue loss. Changes in functional connectivity over time reveal network degeneration patterns, with progressive disconnection of brain regions contributing to cognitive and motor decline. Combined multimodal longitudinal imaging, integrating structural, diffusion, functional, and metabolic measures, provides a comprehensive characterisation of disease progression across multiple biological scales. Predictive models that incorporate baseline imaging features and longitudinal trajectories estimate future decline and time to clinical milestones, such as loss of independence or nursing home placement, thereby supporting care planning and informed trial enrollment decisions. As disease-modifying therapies for neurodegenerative diseases advance toward clinical approval, longitudinal imaging biomarkers will be crucial for demonstrating treatment efficacy and monitoring individual patient responses to optimise therapeutic benefits while minimising adverse effects.

Conclusion

Magnetic resonance imaging has significantly enhanced our ability to diagnose, monitor, and understand neurodegenerative diseases, providing objective biomarkers that complement clinical assessments and improve diagnostic precision. Disease-specific patterns of regional atrophy, white matter degeneration, iron accumulation, and functional network disruption enable differentiation among conditions that share overlapping clinical features, thereby improving diagnostic accuracy, particularly in early disease stages when clinical presentations may be ambiguous. Advanced quantitative techniques, including diffusion imaging, functional connectivity analysis, quantitative susceptibility mapping, and neuromelanin imaging, provide sensitive markers of pathological processes, often detecting abnormalities before conventional structural changes become apparent. Ultra-high field imaging at 7 tesla and beyond promises further improvements in spatial resolution and contrast, enabling the visualisation of subtle anatomical details and early pathological changes that are currently invisible at standard field strengths.

The integration of multiple magnetic resonance imaging modalities through multimodal imaging protocols and machine learning approaches enhances diagnostic performance beyond that of any single technique alone, capturing the multidimensional nature of neurodegenerative pathology. Longitudinal imaging tracking disease progression provides objective outcome measures for clinical trials evaluating disease-modifying therapies, with atrophy rates and other quantitative metrics requiring smaller sample sizes than clinical endpoints to detect treatment effects. As our understanding of neurodegenerative disease mechanisms advances and targeted therapies emerge, imaging biomarkers will play increasingly central roles in patient selection for specific treatments, monitoring therapeutic responses, and optimising dosing regimens. The convergence of advanced imaging technology, computational analysis methods, and a growing understanding of disease biology promises continued progress toward earlier diagnosis, improved prognostication, and more effective interventions for these devastating conditions, which affect millions of individuals and families worldwide. Future directions include the development of standardised imaging protocols that enable multi-centre data pooling, the use of artificial intelligence algorithms to automate image analysis and interpretation, and the integration of imaging with fluid biomarkers and genetic information for comprehensive disease characterisation, supporting precision medicine approaches tailored to individual patient characteristics and disease mechanisms.

Acknowledgments

The authors would like to extend our appreciation to those who offered helpful commentary during the drafting process of this manuscript. We also acknowledge the role the Nova Publishing department played in enabling the work described herein.

References

Agosta, F., Pagani, E., Rocca, M. A., Caputo, D., Perini, M., Salvi, F., Prelle, A., & Filippi, M. (2010). Voxel-based morphometry study of brain volumetry and diffusivity in amyotrophic lateral sclerosis patients with mild disability. *Human Brain Mapping*, 28(12), 1430-1438. https://doi.org/10.1002/hbm.20364.

Filippi, M., Rocca, M. A., Ciccarelli, O., De Stefano, N., Evangelou, N., Kappos, L., Rovira, A., Sastre-Garriga, J., Tintorè, M., Frederiksen, J. L., Gasperini, C., Palace, J., Reich, D. S., Banwell, B., Montalban, X., & Barkhof, F. (2019). MRI criteria for the diagnosis of multiple sclerosis: MAGNIMS consensus guidelines. *The Lancet Neurology*, 18(3), 292-303. https://doi.org/10.1016/S1474-4422(18)30311-X.

Fox, N. C., Black, R. S., Gilman, S., Rossor, M. N., Griffith, S. G., Jenkins, L., & Koller, M. (2011). Effects of Aβ immunization (AN1792) on MRI measures of cerebral volume in Alzheimer disease. *Neurology*, 64(9), 1563-1572. https://doi.org/10.1212/01.WNL.0000159743.08996.99.

Frisoni, G. B., Fox, N. C., Jack, C. R., Scheltens, P., & Thompson, P. M. (2010). The clinical use of structural MRI in Alzheimer disease. *Nature Reviews Neurology*, 6(2), 67-77. https://doi.org/10.1038/nrneurol.2009.215.

Jack, C. R., Bennett, D. A., Blennow, K., Carrillo, M. C., Dunn, B., Haeberlein, S. B., Holtzman, D. M., Jagust, W., Jessen, F., Karlawish, J., Liu, E., Molinuevo, J. L., Montine, T., Phelps, C., Rankin, K. P., Rowe, C. C., Scheltens, P., Siemers, E., Snyder, H. M., & Sperling, R. (2018). NIA-AA Research Framework: Toward a biological definition of Alzheimer's disease. *Alzheimer's & Dementia*, 14(4), 535-562. https://doi.org/10.1016/j.jalz.2018.02.018.

Kwon, D. H., Kim, J. M., Oh, S. H., Jeong, H. J., Park, S. Y., Oh, E. S., Chi, J. G., Kim, Y. B., Jeon, B. S., & Cho, Z. H. (2012). Seven-tesla magnetic resonance images of the substantia nigra in Parkinson disease. *Annals of Neurology*, 71(2), 267-277. https://doi.org/10.1002/ana.22592.

Rossi, M., Ruottinen, H., Saunamäki, T., Elovaara, I., & Dastidar, P. (2021). Neuromelanin and T2*-weighted imaging in Parkinson's disease: A systematic review and meta-analysis. *Journal of Magnetic Resonance Imaging*, 53(5), 1330-1342. https://doi.org/10.1002/jmri.27435.

Schuff, N., Woerner, N., Boreta, L., Kornfield, T., Shaw, L. M., Trojanowski, J. Q., Thompson, P. M., Jack, C. R., Weiner, M. W., & Alzheimer's Disease Neuroimaging Initiative. (2012). MRI of hippocampal volume loss in early Alzheimer's disease in relation to ApoE genotype and biomarkers. *Brain*, 132(4), 1067-1077. https://doi.org/10.1093/brain/awp007.

Schwarz, S. T., Afzal, M., Morgan, P. S., Bajaj, N., Gowland, P. A., & Auer, D. P. (2014). The 'swallow tail' appearance of the healthy nigrosome - a new accurate test of Parkinson's disease: A case-control and retrospective cross-sectional MRI study at 3T. *PLoS ONE*, 9(4), e93814. https://doi.org/10.1371/journal.pone.0093814.

Seeley, W. W., Crawford, R., Rascovsky, K., Kramer, J. H., Weiner, M., Miller, B. L., & Gorno-Tempini, M. L. (2008). Frontal paralimbic network atrophy in very mild behavioral variant frontotemporal dementia. *Archives of Neurology*, 65(2), 249-255. https://doi.org/10.1001/archneurol.2007.38.

Thompson, A. J., Banwell, B. L., Barkhof, F., Carroll, W. M., Coetzee, T., Comi, G., Correale, J., Fazekas, F., Filippi, M., Freedman, M. S., Fujihara, K., Galetta, S. L., Hartung, H. P., Kappos, L., Lublin, F. D., Marrie, R. A., Miller, A. E., Miller, D. H., Montalban, X., ... Cohen, J. A.

(2018). Diagnosis of multiple sclerosis: 2017 revisions of the McDonald criteria. *The Lancet Neurology*, 17(2), 162-173. https://doi.org/10.1016/S1474-4422(17)30470-2.

Turner, M. R., Agosta, F., Bede, P., Govind, V., Lulé, D., & Verstraete, E. (2012). Neuroimaging in amyotrophic lateral sclerosis. *Biomarkers in Medicine*, 6(3), 319-337. https://doi.org/10.2217/bmm.12.26.

Wattjes, M. P., Rovira, À., Miller, D., Yousry, T. A., Sormani, M. P., De Stefano, N., Tintoré, M., Auger, C., Tur, C., Filippi, M., Rocca, M. A., Fazekas, F., Kappos, L., Polman, C., Frederik, B., & Montalban, X. (2015). Evidence-based guidelines: MAGNIMS consensus guidelines on the use of MRI in multiple sclerosis—establishing disease prognosis and monitoring patients. *Nature Reviews Neurology*, 11(10), 597-606. https://doi.org/10.1038/nrneurol.2015.157.

Whitwell, J. L. (2010). Progression of atrophy in Alzheimer disease and related disorders. *Neurotoxicity Research*, 18(3-4), 339-346. https://doi.org/10.1007/s12640-010-9175-1.

Whitwell, J. L., & Josephs, K. A. (2012). Recent advances in the imaging of frontotemporal dementia. *Current Neurology and Neuroscience Reports*, 12(6), 715-723. https://doi.org/10.1007/s11910-012-0317-0.

Chapter 12

Pediatric Neuroimaging

Maajid Mohi Ud Din Malik*
Radiology and Imaging Technology, Dr. D. Y. Patil School of Allied Health Sciences,
Dr. D. Y. Patil Vidyapeeth (Deemed to be University), Sant Tukaram Nagar, Pimpri, Pune, India

Abstract

Magnetic resonance imaging of the pediatric brain presents unique challenges and opportunities, requiring specialised knowledge of standard developmental patterns, age-specific pathologies, and technical considerations distinct from those in adult neuroimaging. This chapter provides a comprehensive overview of pediatric neuroimaging with emphasis on brain development and myelination patterns, congenital malformations, brain tumours, neonatal brain injury, and neurodevelopmental disorders. Understanding the temporal and spatial progression of myelination is crucial for interpreting pediatric brain magnetic resonance imaging, as the characteristics of white matter signals change dramatically throughout infancy and childhood. Congenital brain malformations require systematic evaluation of cortical development, neuronal migration, and posterior fossa structures. Pediatric brain tumours exhibit distinct locations and imaging characteristics compared with adult tumours, with posterior fossa masses predominating in childhood. Hypoxic-ischemic encephalopathy represents a critical neonatal emergency where magnetic resonance imaging patterns predict long-term neurodevelopmental outcomes and guide therapeutic decisions. Neurodevelopmental disorders, including autism spectrum disorder and cerebral palsy, show characteristic structural and functional imaging abnormalities. Advanced techniques, including diffusion imaging, magnetic resonance spectroscopy, and functional connectivity mapping, enhance diagnostic accuracy and prognostic assessment. This chapter integrates conventional and advanced imaging approaches, providing radiologists and clinicians with practical knowledge for interpreting pediatric neuroimaging studies.

---

* Corresponding Author's Email: maajid.malik@dpu.edu.in

In: Recent Advances in Magnetic Resonance Imaging in Neuroimaging
Editors: Maajid Mohi Ud Din Malik, Purnachandra Kawdu Lamghare and R. S. Kuber
ISBN: 979-8-90134-244-2

Keywords: pediatric brain MRI, brain development, myelination, hypoxic-ischemic encephalopathy, congenital malformations, SDG 3 - good health and well-being

Introduction

Pediatric neuroimaging represents a specialised discipline that requires expertise extending far beyond conventional adult brain imaging practices. The developing brain undergoes profound structural, functional, and biochemical transformations from prenatal life through adolescence, creating a dynamic landscape in which regular developmental changes must be distinguished from pathological processes. Unlike adult neuroimaging, where brain anatomy remains relatively stable, pediatric imaging interpretation demands a comprehensive understanding of age-specific normal variants, maturational milestones, and the temporal progression of myelination patterns that define healthy brain development. These developmental considerations profoundly influence imaging protocols, sequence selection, and diagnostic interpretation, necessitating tailored approaches for each age group.

The clinical spectrum of pediatric neurological disorders differs fundamentally from adult pathology, with congenital malformations, genetic syndromes, perinatal injuries, and developmentally specific tumours predominating in childhood. Magnetic resonance imaging has emerged as the cornerstone modality for pediatric brain assessment, offering superior soft tissue contrast, multiplanar capabilities, and freedom from ionising radiation, which is particularly valuable for young patients who may require serial examinations throughout their development. Technical challenges unique to pediatric populations, including the need for high spatial resolution in small anatomical structures, motion artefacts from uncooperative patients, and safety considerations surrounding sedation requirements, necessitate specialised imaging protocols and institutional expertise. This chapter presents a comprehensive framework for pediatric neuroimaging, encompassing normal brain development, congenital anomalies, pediatric neoplasms, neonatal injuries, and neurodevelopmental disorders, while integrating conventional and advanced imaging techniques to optimise diagnostic accuracy and clinical utility.

12.1. Special Considerations in Pediatric MRI

Pediatric neuroimaging requires specialised approaches that address unique physiological, developmental, and practical considerations, distinguishing it fundamentally from adult imaging. The developing brain undergoes continuous structural and functional changes from fetal life through adolescence, necessitating age-appropriate interpretation frameworks and recognition of normal developmental variations that could be mistaken for pathology. Technical challenges specific to pediatric populations include smaller anatomical structures that require higher spatial resolution, motion artefacts from uncooperative or anxious children, and safety concerns regarding sedation or general anaesthesia, which are frequently required for successful imaging in young children. Modern pediatric magnetic resonance imaging protocols must balance competing demands of acquisition speed, image quality, and patient safety while minimising sedation requirements whenever possible.

Image acquisition strategies for pediatric patients differ substantially from standard adult protocols, with sequence optimisation for smaller fields of view, thinner slice thicknesses, and higher in-plane resolution to adequately visualise small structures, such as cranial nerves, brainstem nuclei, and hippocampal subfields. The signal-to-noise ratio decreases with smaller voxel sizes, necessitating techniques such as signal averaging, the use of surface coils explicitly designed for pediatric head sizes, and the utilisation of higher-field-strength systems when available. Three Tesla magnetic resonance systems have become the standard for pediatric neuroimaging, providing superior tissue contrast and enabling advanced techniques, including high-resolution anatomical imaging, diffusion tensor imaging, and magnetic resonance spectroscopy, with acceptable acquisition times. Ultra-high-field seven-tesla systems show promise for pediatric applications but remain primarily research tools due to limited availability, longer examination times, and a lack of established safety data in young children.

Motion is the primary technical challenge in pediatric imaging, as even subtle patient movement during acquisition can lead to severe image degradation, compromising diagnostic quality. Strategies for minimising motion include careful patient preparation with age-appropriate explanations, parental presence, when possible, distraction techniques such as videos or music, comfortable positioning with immobilisation devices, and feed-and-sleep protocols for infants. Despite these measures, sedation or general anaesthesia remains necessary for many pediatric magnetic resonance examinations, particularly in children under six years of age. The decision to sedate requires a careful risk-benefit assessment, considering the urgency of the examination, the likelihood of successful unsedated imaging based on the child's age and cooperation, and patient-specific factors, including comorbid conditions that affect anaesthesia risk. Sedation protocols must be administered by trained personnel with appropriate monitoring equipment and emergency response capabilities, in accordance with established institutional guidelines and pediatric sedation safety standards.

Radiation exposure considerations, while not directly relevant to magnetic resonance imaging itself, influence decisions about imaging modality selection in pediatric patients. The absence of ionising radiation makes magnetic resonance imaging particularly attractive for conditions that require repeated imaging, such as brain tumour surveillance, epilepsy monitoring, and follow-up of congenital malformations. However, magnetic resonance imaging's longer acquisition times, sedation requirements, and limited availability compared to computed tomography must be weighed against radiation risks when selecting imaging modalities for acute presentations such as suspected trauma or stroke. Advanced computed tomography dose reduction techniques and magnetic resonance imaging protocol optimisation continue to improve the benefit-risk profiles of both modalities in pediatric populations.

Contrast agent administration in pediatric patients requires attention to age-specific considerations, including lower blood volumes, immature renal function in neonates and young infants, and different distribution volumes compared to those in adults. Gadolinium-based contrast agents demonstrate excellent safety profiles in children when used appropriately, with nephrogenic systemic fibrosis exceedingly rare in pediatric populations, even in those with renal impairment. However, concerns about gadolinium deposition in brain tissue, particularly in the dentate nucleus and globus pallidus, have led to the preferential use of macrocyclic gadolinium agents and to restricting contrast-enhanced examinations to clear clinical indications. Weight-based dosing calculations must account for developmental variations in body composition and renal clearance, with standard pediatric dosing typically 0.1 mmol/kg body weight for most indications.

Specialised pulse sequences and imaging protocols for pediatric neuroimaging often differ from those used in adults, reflecting the unique pathologies and developmental considerations that are specific to children. Neonatal brain imaging emphasises the use of diffusion-weighted imaging for detecting hypoxic-ischemic injury and gradient-echo sequences for detecting haemorrhage. In contrast, protocols for older children investigating epilepsy include thin-slice coronal oblique images perpendicular to the hippocampal long axes for optimal visualisation of the mesial temporal structure. Susceptibility-weighted imaging plays an increasingly important role in pediatric protocols, detecting subtle haemorrhage, venous abnormalities, and calcifications relevant for trauma, vascular malformations, and metabolic disorders. Magnetic resonance angiography without contrast enhancement, using time-of-flight or arterial spin labelling techniques, enables vascular assessment while avoiding gadolinium exposure, particularly valuable for conditions requiring repeated vascular imaging, such as moyamoya disease or surveillance of vascular malformations.

12.2. Brain Development and Maturation

Normal brain development and myelination follow highly predictable temporal and spatial patterns, which are crucial for accurately interpreting pediatric neuroimaging studies. White matter myelination represents the most dramatic postnatal brain maturation process, progressing in an organised sequence that closely correlates with developmental milestones and the acquisition of motor function. Understanding myelination patterns enables radiologists to assess whether brain maturation aligns with chronological age, identify delayed or abnormal myelination that suggests underlying disorders, and distinguish regular developmental appearances from pathological conditions. The myelin sheath surrounding axons contains a high lipid and protein content, producing characteristic signal changes on magnetic resonance imaging as myelination progresses. These appearances vary substantially across different pulse sequences and patient ages.

Myelination begins during fetal development, around twenty weeks' gestation, in the cervical spinal cord and medulla, progressing cephalad and from central to peripheral structures, following general principles (Murakami et al., 1999). The fundamental rules governing myelination progression include caudal-to-rostral advancement, central-to-peripheral spread, and posterior-to-anterior progression within the cerebral hemispheres. However, important exceptions to these generalisations exist. Sensory pathways myelinate before motor pathways, and projection fibres complete myelination earlier than association fibres connecting cortical regions. At term birth, myelination is present in the dorsal midbrain, posterior limb of the internal capsule, ventrolateral thalamus, medial lemniscus, and cerebellar peduncles, while cerebral white matter remains largely unmyelinated.

T1-weighted imaging demonstrates the most dramatic and earliest myelination changes during the first year of life, with a progressive increase in white matter signal intensity reflecting lipid accumulation within myelin sheaths. At birth, the posterior limb of the internal capsule appears hyperintense on T1-weighted images, representing the earliest site of cerebral hemispheric myelination visible on conventional magnetic resonance imaging. During the first three months, myelination progresses rapidly through the cerebral peduncles, brainstem, cerebellar white matter, and optic radiations, followed by the centrum semiovale and corpus callosum during the second half of the first year. By twelve months of age, the T1-weighted white matter signal intensity in most brain regions approaches an adult appearance, although terminal zones, including the peritrigonal areas, continue to mature through the second year.

T2-weighted imaging reveals complementary but delayed myelination patterns compared to T1-weighted sequences, with a progressive decrease in white matter signal intensity reflecting a reduction in free water content as myelination progresses. In the newborn brain, white matter appears markedly hyperintense relative to Grey matter on T2-weighted images, creating the "inverted" appearance compared to adult imaging, where white matter is hypointense. The transition from hyperintense to hypointense white matter signal on T2-weighted images occurs later than T1 changes, beginning around six months of age and progressing throughout the second year of life. This delayed T2 transition reflects myelin compaction and a reduction in extracellular water, rather than the initial myelin deposition visible on T1-weighted images. Fluid-attenuated inversion recovery sequences demonstrate white matter signal changes similar to those seen in T2-weighted imaging, but with superior Grey-white differentiation, showing progressive hypointensity as myelination advances (Murakami et al., 1999).

The assessment of myelination appropriateness for age relies on the identification of specific anatomical landmarks that should be myelinated at particular time points. During the newborn period, the posterior limb of the internal capsule and ventrolateral thalamus should be myelinated on T1-weighted images, while the absence of this expected myelination suggests intrauterine injury or developmental abnormality. By three months of age, the anterior limb of the internal capsule, optic radiations, and cerebellar white matter should demonstrate T1 hyperintensity, with centrum semiovale myelination appearing by six months. Corpus callosum myelination progresses from posterior to anterior, with the splenium myelinating by four to six months and the genu by six to eight months on T1-weighted images. By eighteen to twenty-four months, white matter throughout the cerebral hemispheres should demonstrate adult-like signal characteristics on both T1 and T2-weighted sequences, with only the terminal zones in peritrigonal regions remaining incompletely myelinated.

Quantitative assessment of myelination using advanced magnetic resonance techniques provides objective measures of developmental progress. Diffusion tensor imaging demonstrates progressive changes in fractional anisotropy and mean diffusivity as myelination proceeds, with increasing fractional anisotropy and decreasing mean diffusivity reflecting improved white matter organisation and reduced water content. T1 and T2 relaxation time measurements show age-dependent decreases as myelin accumulates, with relaxation times approaching adult values by two to three years in most brain regions. Myelin water fraction imaging quantifies the proportion of water bound to myelin sheaths, providing direct measures of myelin content that increase systematically with age and demonstrate altered patterns in demyelinating disorders. These quantitative techniques enhance sensitivity for detecting subtle myelination delays or abnormalities not apparent on conventional imaging.

Cortical Grey matter development follows distinct patterns separate from white matter myelination, with progressive changes in cortical thickness, surface area, and folding complexity throughout childhood and adolescence. Cortical thickness demonstrates region-specific trajectories, with sensorimotor cortices thinning earliest, while association cortices, including prefrontal and temporal regions, continue to develop into early adulthood. These changes reflect complex processes, including synaptic pruning, dendritic elaboration, and glial proliferation that optimise neural circuit function. Total brain volume increases rapidly during infancy and early childhood, reaching approximately 90% of adult size by age six. Subsequent changes reflect white matter expansion, cortical remodelling, and ventricular enlargement, rather than continued overall growth.

Table 12.1. Myelination milestones on MRI

Age	T1-Weighted Findings	T2-Weighted Findings	Key Anatomical Landmarks
Term Birth	PLIC hyperintense, VLT hyperintense	White matter is diffusely hyperintense	Dorsal midbrain, medulla, cerebellar peduncles
3 Months	ALIC, optic radiations, cerebellar WM hyperintense	PLIC becoming hypointense	Posterior corpus callosum (splenium) beginning
6 Months	Centrum semiovale beginning, corpus callosum progressing	Deep WM is becoming hypointense	Anterior corpus callosum (genu) beginning
12 Months	Most cerebral WM is hyperintense, adult-like	Subcortical WM is becoming hypointense	Terminal zones remain unmyelinated
18-24 Months	Adult-like throughout except terminal zones	Nearly complete, adult-like pattern	Peritrigonal regions completing

PLIC = posterior limb of internal capsule; VLT = ventrolateral thalamus; ALIC = anterior limb of internal capsule; WM = white matter.

Deep Grey matter structures, including the thalamus, basal ganglia, and hippocampus, demonstrate age-dependent volume changes and signal intensity evolution. Thalamic and striatal volumes increase during infancy and childhood, with regional variations in developmental trajectories. Iron accumulation in the basal ganglia proceeds gradually throughout childhood and adolescence, resulting in progressive T2 hypointensity that must be distinguished from pathological iron deposition associated with metabolic disorders or neurodegeneration. Hippocampal development continues through adolescence, as evidenced by structural magnetic resonance imaging and diffusion measures, which show ongoing maturation of the dentate gyrus and CA regions relevant to memory function. Table 12.1 illustrates myelination milestones as observed on MRI.

12.3. Congenital Brain Malformations

Congenital brain malformations encompass a diverse group of structural abnormalities that result from disrupted developmental processes during fetal brain formation, including disorders of neuronal proliferation, migration, cortical organisation, and midline development. Magnetic resonance imaging offers superior visualisation of these malformations compared to computed tomography, providing detailed anatomical information that enables classification, prognostic assessment, and guidance for medical and surgical management. A systematic evaluation of cortical development, ventricular configuration, corpus callosum, posterior fossa structures, and midline alignment enables a comprehensive assessment of congenital anomalies. Many malformations occur as isolated findings, while others are associated with genetic syndromes or metabolic disorders requiring additional investigation.

Disorders of cortical development represent a significant category of congenital malformations encompassing abnormalities of neuronal proliferation, migration, and cortical organisation. Lissencephaly or agyria is characterised by a smooth brain surface with absent or severely reduced gyration, a thick cortex, and shallow Sylvian fissures, resulting from arrested neuronal migration. Multiple genetic causes underlie lissencephaly syndromes, with different patterns of brain involvement and associated features distinguishing specific subtypes. Miller-Dieker syndrome exhibits classic lissencephaly, characterised by a severe reduction in gyration, and displays characteristic facial features. Other forms of lissencephaly demonstrate regional predominance or gradient patterns of severity. Magnetic resonance imaging reveals a diffusely thickened cortex, measuring up to twenty millimetres or more, compared to the normal cortical thickness of three to four millimetres, with a simplified gyral pattern and vertically oriented Sylvian fissures.

Polymicrogyria manifests as excessively small gyri, resulting in irregular, bumpy cortical surfaces with abnormal lamination patterns that are visible histologically. The imaging appearance varies by subtype and distribution, with perisylvian polymicrogyria being the most common. Bilateral perisylvian polymicrogyria is associated with characteristic pseudobulbar palsy and cognitive impairment. High-resolution three-dimensional T1-weighted imaging optimally demonstrates the irregular cortical surface and abnormal sulcation, while fluid-attenuated inversion recovery sequences show the characteristic thickened cortex with irregular Grey-white junction. Schizencephaly involves full-thickness clefts lined by polymicrogyric cortex extending from the cortical surface to the lateral ventricle, classified as closed-lip when cleft walls are in apposition or open-lip when separated cerebrospinal fluid-filled clefts are visible. Schizencephaly most commonly affects the perisylvian regions and may be unilateral or bilateral, with clinical severity correlating with the extent of involvement.

Heterotopia represents collections of neurons that failed to complete migration to the cortex, remaining in abnormal locations along migration pathways. Subependymal heterotopia appears as nodular Grey matter signal intensity masses along the lateral ventricular margins, ranging from small isolated nodules to extensive bilateral nodular arrays in females with X-linked periventricular heterotopia. Band heterotopia or double cortex shows a smooth band of Grey matter beneath the cortex, separated by a thin white matter layer, occurring predominantly in females and associated with X-linked mutations. Subcortical heterotopia presents as focal nodules within the white matter, often related to overlying cortical dysplasia. Recognition of heterotopia is clinically vital as these malformations frequently cause epilepsy, with seizure onset timing and characteristics varying based on heterotopia type and extent.

Corpus callosum abnormalities range from complete agenesis to partial hypogenesis, affecting specific regions. Imaging findings include an absent or thinned corpus callosum, elevated and parallel lateral ventricles, and a radial orientation of the medial hemispheric sulci. Complete agenesis demonstrates a characteristic "bat wing" or "Viking helmet" configuration of the frontal horns, colpocephaly with disproportionate enlargement of occipital horns, and a high-riding third ventricle extending between the lateral ventricles. Bundles of Probst represent aberrant fibre tracts that failed to cross the midline, appearing as longitudinal white matter bundles along the medial ventricular walls. Corpus callosum abnormalities occur as isolated findings or are associated with numerous genetic syndromes and chromosomal abnormalities, necessitating careful evaluation for associated brain and systemic anomalies.

Posterior fossa malformations constitute an essential category, including Chiari malformations, Dandy-Walker malformation, and various cerebellar hypoplasias. Chiari I malformation involves the caudal displacement of the cerebellar tonsils more than five millimetres below the foramen magnum, often associated with syringomyelia and presenting with headaches, neck pain, or myelopathic symptoms. Chiari II malformation, invariably associated with myelomeningocele, exhibits complex abnormalities, including a small posterior fossa, caudal displacement of the vermis and brainstem, tectal beaking, and hydrocephalus. Dandy-Walker malformation is characterised by cystic dilatation of the fourth ventricle, which communicates with an enlarged posterior fossa cisterna magna. It is often accompanied by cerebellar vermian hypoplasia or agenesis, and is frequently associated with supratentorial abnormalities, including corpus callosum anomalies and cortical malformations.

Holoprosencephaly represents a failure of midline cleavage and differentiation of the prosencephalon, classified into alobar, semilobar, and lobar forms, with a progressive decrease in severity. Alobar holoprosencephaly is characterised by the complete absence of midline structures, resulting in a single holosphere, fused thalami, an absent interhemispheric fissure, and characteristic facial anomalies. Semilobar holoprosencephaly shows partial formation of the interhemispheric fissure posteriorly with anterior fusion, rudimentary occipital and temporal horns, and partial thalamic separation. Lobar holoprosencephaly, the mildest form, demonstrates separated lateral ventricles with absent septum pellucidum and partial corpus callosum agenesis—recognition of holoprosencephaly prompts genetic evaluation and assessment for associated chromosomal abnormalities and syndromes.

12.4. Pediatric Brain Tumours

Pediatric brain tumours differ substantially from adult tumours in histological type, anatomical distribution, and biologic behaviour, requiring age-specific diagnostic approaches and treatment strategies. Brain tumours represent the most common solid malignancy in children and a leading cause of cancer-related mortality in pediatric populations. Magnetic resonance imaging (MRI) is the primary diagnostic modality, providing detailed anatomical information, tumour characterisation, and metastatic disease detection. The location of a pediatric brain tumour offers important diagnostic information, as approximately 60% occur infratentorially in the posterior fossa, compared with a predominantly supratentorial distribution in adults. Advanced imaging techniques, including diffusion-weighted imaging, perfusion imaging, and magnetic resonance spectroscopy, enhance diagnostic accuracy and guide treatment planning (Yeom et al., 2022).

Pilocytic astrocytoma represents the most common pediatric brain tumour overall, accounting for approximately fifteen percent of all pediatric central nervous system neoplasms. These World Health Organisation grade I tumours predominantly occur in the posterior fossa, particularly in the cerebellum, but also affect the optic pathway, hypothalamus, and cerebral hemispheres. The classic magnetic resonance imaging appearance shows a well-circumscribed cystic mass with an intensely enhancing mural nodule; however, entirely solid tumours occur in approximately 25% of cases. The cyst walls typically do not enhance, distinguishing them from the rim enhancement seen in higher-grade tumours. T2-weighted images demonstrate marked hyperintensity of both solid and cystic components, whereas diffusion-weighted imaging shows increased diffusion with high apparent diffusion coefficient values, reflecting low cellularity. Calcification occurs in approximately 20% of cases and is visible on susceptibility-weighted imaging or computed tomography. Pilocytic astrocytomas demonstrate an excellent prognosis with gross total resection; however, location-dependent surgical accessibility influences outcomes and recurrence rates (Yeom et al., 2022).

Medulloblastoma constitutes the second most common pediatric brain tumour and the most frequent malignant posterior fossa neoplasm, occurring predominantly in children aged three to nine years. These World Health Organisation grade IV embryonal tumours arise from the roof of the fourth ventricle or the cerebellar vermis, and are characterised by a midline location in younger children. In contrast, a lateral hemispheric location predominates in adolescents and adults. Magnetic resonance imaging typically shows a homogeneous or heterogeneous solid mass that is hyperdense on computed tomography and demonstrates restricted diffusion on diffusion-weighted imaging with low apparent diffusion coefficient values reflecting high cellularity. T2-weighted images show variable signal intensity, often iso- to hypointense compared to

Grey matter. Enhancement after gadolinium administration is typically avid but may be heterogeneous. Leptomeningeal dissemination occurs frequently, necessitating spine magnetic resonance imaging for metastatic evaluation at the time of diagnosis. Recent molecular classification has identified distinct medulloblastoma subgroups with different prognostic implications, although imaging features show substantial overlap among subtypes. Newer diagnostic approaches, incorporating radiomics and machine learning, show promise in predicting molecular subgroups based on imaging features (Yeom et al., 2022).

Ependymoma is the third most common posterior fossa tumour in children, typically arising from the floor of the fourth ventricle, in contrast to medulloblastoma, which arises from the roof of the fourth ventricle. These tumours occur across all pediatric age groups but have a peak incidence in children under 5 years. Magnetic resonance imaging demonstrates heterogeneous solid and cystic masses that often extend through the foramina of Luschka and Magendie into the cerebellopontine angle cisterns and upper cervical canal, creating a characteristic "plastic" appearance that conforms to surrounding structures. Calcification occurs more frequently in ependymomas than in medulloblastomas, present in approximately 50% of cases. T2-weighted images show heterogeneous hyperintensity, while diffusion-weighted imaging typically demonstrates intermediate apparent diffusion coefficient values between medulloblastoma and pilocytic astrocytoma. Enhancement patterns range from minimal to marked and may be heterogeneous. Hydrocephalus is commonly associated with posterior fossa ependymomas due to obstruction of the fourth ventricle.

Diffuse intrinsic pontine glioma represents a devastating brainstem tumour primarily affecting children aged five to nine years, with characteristic infiltrative expansion of the pons visible on magnetic resonance imaging. These World Health Organisation grade III or IV diffuse midline gliomas demonstrate poor prognosis with a median survival of under twelve months despite treatment. Magnetic resonance imaging reveals diffuse pontine enlargement with T2 hyperintensity, often involving more than 50% of the pontine cross-sectional area. Enhancement is variable and does not correlate with prognosis. The tumour typically encases the basilar artery and extends into adjacent brainstem structures, including the midbrain and medulla. Recent recognition of H3 K27M histone mutations as molecular hallmarks of these tumours has refined classification, though imaging features remain primarily anatomical. Biopsy is not routinely performed, given the typical clinical and imaging presentation; however, molecular characterisation increasingly guides experimental therapeutic approaches.

Supratentorial tumours exhibit distinct histological distributions compared to posterior fossa masses, with low-grade gliomas, high-grade gliomas, and embryonal tumours representing the major categories. Supratentorial low-grade gliomas, including pilocytic astrocytoma, diffuse astrocytoma, and ganglioglioma, exhibit variable imaging appearances but typically display a minimal mass effect relative to tumour size, variable enhancement, and facilitated diffusion. Optic pathway gliomas, strongly associated with neurofibromatosis type I, demonstrate fusiform expansion of the optic nerves and chiasm with variable enhancement. Pediatric high-grade gliomas, including glioblastoma, exhibit imaging features similar to those of their adult counterparts, characterised by heterogeneous enhancement, necrosis, and haemorrhage. However, they occur less frequently in children than in adults and demonstrate different molecular profiles. Magnetic resonance spectroscopy reveals elevated choline and decreased N-acetylaspartate, with variable lactate and lipid peaks, in high-grade tumours. However, the findings overlap with those of some low-grade tumours, limiting diagnostic specificity. Table 12.2 presents common pediatric brain tumours and their corresponding imaging features.

Table 12.2. Common pediatric brain tumours and imaging features

Tumor Type	Typical Location	Age Predilection	Key MRI Features	Enhancement Pattern
Pilocytic Astrocytoma	Cerebellum, optic pathway	5-15 years	Cyst with enhancing nodule, T2 hyperintense	Avid nodular enhancement
Medulloblastoma	Fourth ventricle roof, vermis	3-9 years	Solid midline mass, restricted diffusion	Homogeneous or heterogeneous
Ependymoma	Fourth ventricle floor	<5 years	Heterogeneous, plastic, calcification is common	Variable, often heterogeneous
Diffuse Intrinsic Pontine Glioma	Pons	5-9 years	Diffuse pontine expansion, T2 hyperintense	Variable, not prognostic
Atypical Teratoid Rhabdoid Tumour	Posterior fossa, supratentorial	<3 years	Heterogeneous, haemorrhage common	Heterogeneous enhancement

12.5. Neonatal Brain Injury

Hypoxic-ischemic encephalopathy represents the most important cause of neonatal brain injury, occurring in approximately one to five per thousand term live births and accounting for substantial neonatal mortality and long-term neurodevelopmental disability. The injury results from perinatal asphyxia, causing inadequate cerebral blood flow and oxygen delivery during labour, delivery, or the immediate postnatal period, leading to energy failure, excitotoxicity, and cell death through complex pathological cascades. Magnetic resonance imaging (MRI) plays a critical role in diagnosis, characterising injury patterns, and predicting outcomes, with specific imaging patterns correlating with clinical severity and neurodevelopmental prognosis (Rutherford et al., 2010). Therapeutic hypothermia initiated within six hours of birth improves outcomes in moderate to severe hypoxic-ischemic encephalopathy, making timely imaging assessment particularly important for guiding treatment decisions and counselling families.

The pattern of brain injury in hypoxic-ischemic encephalopathy reflects the severity, duration, and nature of the hypoxic-ischemic insult, with two major patterns recognised based on injury distribution. Deep Grey matter injury predominantly affects the basal ganglia, thalami, and perirolandic cortex, occurring after acute profound hypoxic-ischemic events. This pattern exhibits characteristic involvement of the posterior putamen, ventrolateral thalamus, and the posterior limb of the internal capsule on magnetic resonance imaging, with frequent involvement of brainstem structures in severe cases. The participation of the perirolandic cortex reflects the high metabolic demands of primary motor and sensory areas. Infants with deep Grey matter injury patterns typically present with severe neonatal encephalopathy and have an elevated risk for developing dyskinetic cerebral palsy and motor impairments. Watershed injury predominantly affects parasagittal white matter in watershed zones between major arterial territories, occurring with prolonged partial hypoxia-ischemia or repetitive insults. This pattern shows bilateral symmetric injury in the subcortical white matter and cortex at the boundaries between the anterior and middle cerebral artery territories, as well as between the middle and posterior cerebral artery territories. Infants with watershed pattern injury are at risk for spastic quadriparesis and cognitive impairment.

Diffusion-weighted imaging is the most sensitive magnetic resonance sequence for detecting acute hypoxic-ischemic injury, showing restricted diffusion within hours of the insult that peaks at two to four days and then gradually normalises over subsequent days to weeks. The apparent diffusion coefficient provides a quantitative assessment of diffusion restriction, with lower values indicating more severe injury and correlating with worse neurodevelopmental outcomes. The posterior limb of the internal capsule is significant for prognostication, as preservation of normal signal on diffusion-weighted and T1-weighted imaging predicts favourable outcomes with high specificity (Trivedi et al., 2017). Conventional T1- and T2-weighted sequences reveal abnormalities that evolve, with optimal sensitivity for injury detection at four to eight days post-birth. T1-weighted images may show loss of normal posterior limb internal capsule hyperintensity and abnormal basal ganglia signal, while T2-weighted images demonstrate hyperintensity in injured regions reflecting vasogenic oedema and tissue disruption.

Magnetic resonance spectroscopy provides metabolic information that complements structural imaging, demonstrating elevated lactate and reduced N-acetylaspartate in injured brain regions. The lactate-to-N-acetylaspartate ratio measured in the basal ganglia and thalamus exhibits substantial prognostic value, with higher ratios predicting a higher likelihood of death or severe neurodevelopmental impairment. Spectroscopy performed three to five days after birth demonstrates optimal prognostic accuracy, capturing metabolic derangements while minimising confounding effects from acute phase changes. Deep Grey matter lactate peaks typically normalise over weeks in infants with favourable outcomes, while persistent lactate elevation indicates ongoing metabolic dysfunction and poor prognosis. The combination of magnetic resonance imaging injury scores and spectroscopy lactate-N-acetylaspartate ratios provides superior prognostic information compared to either modality alone.

Validated injury-scoring systems enable systematic assessment and prediction of outcomes in hypoxic-ischemic encephalopathy. The Barkovich scoring system evaluates involvement in the basal ganglia, watershed regions, and the posterior limb of the internal capsule, assigning scores that correlate with neurodevelopmental outcomes. The NICHD scoring system developed for the hypothermia trials provides a detailed regional assessment across multiple brain areas (Trivedi et al., 2017). These scoring systems demonstrate strong associations with death and neurodevelopmental impairment at eighteen to twenty-four months, enabling evidence-based counselling about prognosis. However, outcomes in infants with mild-to-moderate magnetic resonance imaging injury remain heterogeneous, with some infants showing normal development. In contrast, others develop subtle cognitive or motor impairments, highlighting the limitations of imaging-based prognostication.

Germinal matrix haemorrhage and intraventricular haemorrhage represent significant complications primarily affecting preterm infants, occurring due to the fragility of the immature germinal matrix vasculature. These haemorrhages are classified by grade based on location and extent, ranging from isolated germinal matrix haemorrhage to intraventricular haemorrhage with ventricular dilatation and parenchymal involvement. Magnetic resonance imaging, particularly susceptibility-weighted imaging and gradient echo sequences, demonstrates excellent sensitivity for detecting haemorrhage across all stages, superior to cranial ultrasound for small haemorrhages and parenchymal lesions. Periventricular leukomalacia, a type of white matter injury in preterm infants, is characterised by periventricular T2 hyperintensity, often accompanied by cystic degeneration, which correlates with an increased risk of spastic diplegia and cognitive impairments.

12.6. Neurodevelopmental Disorders

Neurodevelopmental disorders encompass a broad category of conditions characterised by impaired development of the central nervous system, affecting motor function, cognition, behaviour, or social interaction. Magnetic resonance imaging contributes to diagnosis, aetiology identification, and understanding of brain structural and functional alterations underlying clinical manifestations. While many neurodevelopmental disorders lack specific diagnostic imaging findings, magnetic resonance imaging helps exclude structural causes of symptoms, identify comorbid brain abnormalities, and characterise patterns of brain development associated with particular conditions. Advanced imaging techniques, including volumetric analysis, diffusion tensor imaging, and functional magnetic resonance imaging, reveal subtle structural and connectivity differences between individuals affected and typically developing children, thereby advancing our understanding of neurobiological mechanisms.

Autism spectrum disorder represents a complex neurodevelopmental condition characterised by social communication deficits and restricted repetitive behaviours, with heterogeneous aetiology and variable clinical manifestations. Conventional magnetic resonance imaging in individuals with autism spectrum disorder often appears normal, though structural abnormalities occur with increased frequency compared to the general population. Volumetric studies demonstrate early brain overgrowth during the first years of life, followed by normalisation or reduced growth rates in adolescence and adulthood, with regional variations affecting the frontal, temporal, and parietal lobes differentially. Corpus callosum abnormalities, including reduced size and altered microstructure, appear consistently across studies, potentially reflecting impaired interhemispheric connectivity relevant to social cognition and communication deficits.

Advanced imaging techniques reveal more consistent differences in autism spectrum disorder than conventional structural imaging. Diffusion tensor imaging reveals widespread white matter microstructural abnormalities, characterised by reduced fractional anisotropy in significant fibre tracts, including the corpus callosum, superior longitudinal fasciculus, and uncinate fasciculus, suggesting disrupted white matter organisation and connectivity. Functional magnetic resonance imaging reveals altered functional connectivity patterns, particularly affecting the default mode network, salience network, and executive control networks, with both under-connectivity and over-connectivity reported, depending on the brain regions and networks examined. Task-based functional imaging during social cognition paradigms reveals reduced activation in areas such as the superior temporal sulcus, fusiform gyrus, and amygdala, corresponding to the social processing impairments characteristic of autism spectrum disorder.

Cerebral palsy encompasses a group of permanent movement and posture disorders resulting from non-progressive brain injuries occurring during fetal development, birth, or early infancy. Magnetic resonance imaging demonstrates abnormalities in approximately eighty to ninety percent of children with cerebral palsy, providing etiological information and helping classify injury patterns. Periventricular leukomalacia represents a common finding in preterm infants with cerebral palsy, showing cystic or non-cystic white matter injury with volume loss and ventriculomegaly. The distribution and severity of white matter injury correlate with motor function impairment, with more extensive injury associated with more severe cerebral palsy. Term infants with cerebral palsy more commonly show patterns consistent with hypoxic-ischemic injury, cortical malformations, or focal arterial stroke, with injury patterns helping establish timing and aetiology of brain insults.

Attention-deficit hyperactivity disorder represents a common neurodevelopmental condition characterised by inattention, hyperactivity, and impulsivity, with structural imaging typically normal on conventional magnetic resonance imaging. Volumetric studies have demonstrated subtle differences, including reduced total brain volume, smaller basal ganglia volumes, notably the caudate nucleus, and reduced corpus callosum size in some studies. However, findings show considerable heterogeneity across studies and individuals. Diffusion imaging reveals white-matter microstructural differences in fronto-striatal pathways relevant to attention and executive function. Functional magnetic resonance imaging (fMRI) during attention tasks reveals altered activation patterns in the prefrontal cortex, anterior cingulate, and striatum, whereas resting-state studies demonstrate altered connectivity within attention networks. These imaging findings support neurobiological models of attention-deficit hyperactivity disorder involving fronto-striatal circuit dysfunction.

Developmental coordination disorder and dyspraxia affect motor planning and coordination, and magnetic resonance imaging (MRI) helps exclude structural abnormalities and characterise brain development patterns. Structural imaging may reveal subtle differences in the motor cortex, parietal regions, and cerebellar volumes compared with those of typically developing children. Diffusion imaging reveals altered white-matter microstructure in motor pathways, including the corticospinal tracts and the corpus callosum. Functional imaging during motor tasks reveals altered activation patterns in motor planning regions, including the supplementary motor area, premotor cortex, and cerebellum, suggesting disrupted motor network function underlying clinical manifestations.

Intellectual disability, defined as significant limitations in intellectual functioning and adaptive behaviour, exhibits variable magnetic resonance imaging findings depending on the underlying aetiology. Congenital brain malformations, hypoxic-ischemic injury, genetic syndromes, and metabolic disorders represent common causes identifiable through neuroimaging. Advanced techniques, including whole-brain volumetry and cortical thickness analysis, reveal patterns associated with specific genetic conditions, while spectroscopy may detect metabolic abnormalities in inborn errors of metabolism. The integration of detailed imaging phenotyping with genetic testing enhances etiological diagnosis, particularly relevant as targeted therapies emerge for specific genetic conditions underlying intellectual disability.

Conclusion

Pediatric neuroimaging requires specialised knowledge that integrates standard developmental patterns, age-specific pathologies, and unique technical considerations. Understanding myelination progression and normal structural development provides the foundation for accurate interpretation, enabling distinction between developmental variations and pathological processes. Predictable temporal and spatial myelination patterns serve as critical biomarkers of brain maturation, with deviations indicating developmental disorders, metabolic conditions, or injury. Comprehensive assessment protocols adapted for pediatric populations incorporate optimised pulse sequences, motion reduction strategies, and judicious use of contrast agents, thereby maximising diagnostic information while ensuring safety and minimising sedation requirements.

Neonatal brain injury represents a critical application where MRI patterns directly inform therapeutic decisions and prognostic counselling. The ability to characterise hypoxic-ischemic encephalopathy injury patterns, quantify severity through validated scoring systems, and predict neurodevelopmental outcomes provides invaluable management information. Advanced techniques, including diffusion-weighted imaging and magnetic resonance spectroscopy, enhance the detection of injuries and improve prognostic accuracy. Biomarkers, such as posterior limb internal capsule integrity and lactate-to-N-acetylaspartate ratios, demonstrate strong associations with long-term outcomes.

Congenital brain malformations require systematic evaluation for accurate diagnosis and classification. MRI's superior soft-tissue contrast and multiplanar capabilities make it optimal for characterising cortical developmental disorders, midline abnormalities, and posterior fossa malformations.

Future advances include quantitative imaging biomarkers, artificial intelligence for automated analysis, functional connectivity approaches, and ultra-high-field 7 Tesla magnetic resonance imaging (MRI). Machine learning algorithms show promise for automated segmentation, lesion detection, and outcome prediction, potentially reducing variability in interpretation and enhancing accuracy.

Acknowledgments

The authors would like to extend our appreciation to those who offered helpful commentary during the drafting process of this manuscript. We also acknowledge the role the Nova Publishing department played in enabling the work described herein.

References

Murakami, J. W., Weinberger, E., & Shaw, D. W. (1999). Normal myelination of the pediatric brain imaged with fluid-attenuated inversion-recovery (FLAIR) MR imaging. *American Journal of Neuroradiology*, 20(8), 1406-1411.

Rutherford, M., Malamateniou, C., McGuinness, A., Allsop, J., Biarge, M. M., & Counsell, S. (2010). Magnetic resonance imaging in hypoxic-ischaemic encephalopathy. *Early Human Development*, 86(6), 351-360. https://doi.org/10.1016/j.earlhumdev.2010.05.014.

Trivedi, S. B., Vesoulis, Z. A., Rao, R., Liao, S. M., Shimony, J. S., McKinstry, R. C., & Mathur, A. M. (2017). A validated clinical MRI injury scoring system in neonatal hypoxic-ischemic encephalopathy. *Pediatric Radiology*, 47(11), 1491-1499. https://doi.org/10.1007/s00247-017-3893-y.

Yeom, K. W., Lober, R. M., Andre, J. B., Fisher, P. G., & Barnes, P. D. (2022). MR imaging of pediatric brain tumors. *Diagnostics*, 12(4), 961. https://doi.org/10.3390/diagnostics12040961.

Chapter 13

MRI in Brain Tumours

Maajid Mohi Ud Din Malik[1,*]
and Kushal Kailash Bothara[2,†]
[1]Radiology and Imaging Technology, Dr. D. Y. Patil School of Allied Health Sciences, Dr. D. Y. Patil Vidyapeeth (Deemed to be University), Sant Tukaram Nagar, Pimpri, Pune, India
[2]Department of Radio-Diagnosis, Dr. D. Y. Patil Medical College, Hospital and Research Centre, Dr. D. Y. Patil Vidyapeeth (Deemed to be University), Sant Tukaram Nagar, Pimpri, Pune, India

Abstract

Magnetic resonance imaging has emerged as the cornerstone imaging modality for the comprehensive evaluation of brain tumours, offering unparalleled capabilities in diagnosis, treatment planning, and therapeutic monitoring. This chapter explores the multifaceted applications of MRI in brain tumour management, encompassing conventional structural sequences that provide essential anatomical detail, advanced perfusion techniques including dynamic susceptibility contrast and dynamic contrast-enhanced imaging that characterise tumour vascularity, diffusion-weighted imaging that probes tumour cellularity and microstructure, and magnetic resonance spectroscopy that reveals metabolic signatures. Differentiating between tumour progression and treatment-related effects is a critical clinical challenge that can be addressed through multiparametric imaging. Emerging technologies such as radiomics and texture analysis promise to enhance diagnostic accuracy and prognostic stratification through quantitative image analysis. This comprehensive review synthesises current evidence and best practices in brain tumour MRI, providing clinicians and researchers with a framework for optimising the use of these powerful imaging tools. The integration of multiple MRI techniques enables personalised patient care, contributing to achieving Sustainable Development Goal 3: Good Health and Well-being by improving diagnostic precision and treatment outcomes.

[*] Corresponding Author's Email: maajid.malik@dpu.edu.in
[†] Corresponding Author's Email: Kushal.Bothara@dpu.edu.in

In: Recent Advances in Magnetic Resonance Imaging in Neuroimaging
Editors: Maajid Mohi Ud Din Malik, Purnachandra Kawdu Lamghare and R. S. Kuber
ISBN: 979-8-90134-244-2

Keywords: brain tumours, magnetic resonance imaging, perfusion imaging, diffusion-weighted imaging, magnetic resonance spectroscopy, SDG 3 - good health and well-being

Introduction

Brain tumours represent a diverse group of neoplasms with widely varying biological behaviour, treatment responses, and clinical outcomes. Accurate diagnosis and characterisation are essential for optimal patient management; however, traditional imaging approaches have faced limitations in distinguishing tumour types, predicting prognosis, and differentiating actual disease progression from treatment-related effects. Magnetic resonance imaging has revolutionised neuro-oncology by providing non-invasive visualisation of brain anatomy with exquisite soft-tissue contrast, superior to that of all other imaging modalities. Beyond simple anatomical depiction, modern MRI techniques now interrogate tumour biology at multiple levels, offering insights into vascularity, cellularity, metabolic activity, and white matter tract integrity.

The evolution of brain tumour imaging has progressed from basic T1-weighted and T2-weighted sequences to sophisticated multiparametric protocols that integrate structural, functional, physiological, and metabolic information. Advanced techniques, including perfusion imaging, assess tumour angiogenesis and hemodynamics. Diffusion-weighted imaging quantifies cellular density and tissue microstructure, while magnetic resonance spectroscopy reveals biochemical signatures characteristic of different tumour types. These complementary modalities address critical clinical challenges, such as tumour grading, surgical planning, treatment monitoring, and the vexing problem of distinguishing tumour recurrence from treatment effects. This chapter provides a comprehensive overview of MRI applications in brain tumour management, examining the principles, clinical utility, and limitations of both conventional and advanced imaging techniques, while highlighting emerging technologies that promise to further enhance diagnostic precision and personalised care.

13.1. Conventional MRI in Tumour Diagnosis

Conventional magnetic resonance imaging (MRI) serves as the foundation for brain tumour diagnosis and characterisation, providing essential structural information that guides clinical decision-making. Modern brain tumour imaging protocols have evolved to incorporate standardised sequences that maximise diagnostic yield while ensuring consistency across institutions (Sanvito et al., 2023). A comprehensive structural MRI protocol for brain tumours typically includes T2-weighted sequences in multiple orthogonal planes, fluid-attenuated inversion recovery sequences that suppress cerebrospinal fluid signal to better delineate perilesional oedema and tumour infiltration, susceptibility-weighted imaging to detect haemorrhage and calcification, and pre- and post-contrast T1-weighted sequences that reveal blood-brain barrier disruption (Martucci et al., 2023). The implementation of three-dimensional high-resolution sequences has revolutionised presurgical planning by enabling accurate image registration with intraoperative navigation systems and facilitating stereotactic radiosurgery planning with submillimeter precision (Ellingson et al., 2015).

The primary objectives of conventional MRI in brain tumour assessment encompass several critical domains. Anatomical characterisation includes precise determination of tumour location within eloquent or non-eloquent brain regions, accurate measurement of lesion dimensions for volumetric analysis and response assessment, evaluation of mass effect on adjacent structures, including midline shift and ventricular compression, and assessment of the relationship between the tumour and critical neurovascular structures (Iv et al., 2022). Signal intensity patterns on various pulse sequences provide valuable diagnostic clues regarding tumour composition. T1 hypointensity and T2 hyperintensity typically indicate increased water content, while T1 hyperintensity suggests haemorrhage or melanin content. Conversely, T2 hypointensity may potentially indicate calcification, hemosiderin deposition, or highly cellular lesions. Contrast enhancement patterns provide insights into blood-brain barrier integrity and tumour vascularity, with homogeneous enhancement often observed in metastases and lymphomas, heterogeneous enhancement characteristic of high-grade gliomas with central necrosis, and ring enhancement suggestive of aggressive tumours or abscess formation.

The interpretation of conventional MRI findings requires integration of multiple sequence characteristics to narrow the differential diagnosis and predict tumour grade. The World Health Organisation grading of gliomas correlates with specific imaging features, including the presence and extent of contrast enhancement, degree of perilesional oedema, presence of central necrosis, and a mass effect disproportionate to the lesion size (Martucci et al., 2023). Low-grade gliomas typically present as homogeneous, non-enhancing lesions with well-defined margins and minimal mass effect. In contrast, high-grade gliomas demonstrate irregular rim enhancement surrounding necrotic centres, extensive vasogenic oedema, and a significant mass effect. Fluid-attenuated inversion recovery sequences prove particularly valuable in detecting non-enhancing tumour infiltration beyond the margins of contrast enhancement, a critical consideration in surgical planning and radiation treatment field design. The identification of specific imaging features such as the T2-FLAIR mismatch sign in lower-grade gliomas has emerged as a valuable diagnostic marker, with studies demonstrating high specificity for isocitrate dehydrogenase-mutant 1p19q non-codeleted astrocytomas (Suh et al., 2018).

Contemporary brain tumour MRI protocols emphasise standardisation to facilitate multi-institutional research collaboration and ensure the reproducibility of measurements in clinical trials (Sanvito et al., 2023). Consensus recommendations from major neuro-oncology organisations specify minimum technical requirements, including a magnetic field strength of at least 1.5 Tesla, a slice thickness not exceeding 5 millimetres for structural sequences, with isotropic voxel dimensions preferred for three-dimensional acquisitions, and consistent timing of post-contrast imaging to enable reliable comparison of serial examinations (Ellingson et al., 2015). The Response Assessment in Neuro-Oncology (RANO) criteria have established standardised methods for measuring tumour dimensions and categorising treatment response, incorporating bidimensional measurements of enhancing tumour on T1-weighted post-contrast images and assessment of non-enhancing tumour progression on T2-FLAIR sequences. Despite the sophistication of conventional MRI, significant limitations persist, including the inability to distinguish tumour infiltration from vasogenic oedema in the perilesional region, difficulty differentiating treatment-related changes from actual tumour progression, limited specificity for tumour histology and molecular subtype, and suboptimal sensitivity for detecting microscopic tumour infiltration beyond visible margins. These limitations have driven the development and clinical implementation of advanced MRI techniques that complement structural imaging with functional, physiological, and metabolic information.

13.2. Advanced Perfusion Imaging: DSC and DCE MRI

Perfusion magnetic resonance imaging has revolutionised the non-invasive assessment of brain tumour vascularity and hemodynamics, providing critical information that complements conventional structural imaging techniques. Two principal perfusion techniques have gained widespread clinical acceptance: dynamic susceptibility contrast MRI and dynamic contrast-enhanced MRI, each offering unique physiological insights through distinct physical principles and analysis methodologies (Lee et al., 2023). Dynamic susceptibility contrast imaging exploits the T2 and T2* susceptibility effects of gadolinium-based contrast agents as they pass through the capillary bed, utilising rapid T2*-weighted echo-planar imaging sequences to capture first-pass bolus kinetics with a temporal resolution typically ranging from 1 to 2 seconds. The resulting signal intensity time curves are analysed to derive hemodynamic parameters, including cerebral blood volume, cerebral blood flow, and mean transit time. Relative cerebral blood volume emerges as the most robust and widely utilised metric for tumour characterisation (Morabito et al., 2019).

Relative cerebral blood volume measurements in brain tumours provide valuable information regarding tumour grade, prognosis, and differential diagnosis. High-grade gliomas typically exhibit markedly elevated relative cerebral blood volume values, reflecting increased angiogenesis and tumour vascularity, with normalised relative cerebral blood volume ratios exceeding 1.75 compared to normal-appearing contralateral white matter, demonstrating high specificity for glioblastoma (Lee et al., 2023). In contrast, low-grade gliomas generally exhibit relative cerebral blood volume values that approximate or slightly exceed those of normal brain parenchyma. However, oligodendrogliomas represent an essential exception, with relatively higher perfusion despite their lower histological grade. The spatial heterogeneity of perfusion parameters within a single tumour mass reflects the biological heterogeneity characteristic of high-grade gliomas, with regions of maximum relative cerebral blood volume potentially indicating the highest-grade tumour areas suitable for biopsy targeting. Dynamic susceptibility contrast imaging has demonstrated particular utility in distinguishing tumour recurrence from radiation necrosis, a critical clinical challenge in post-treatment surveillance, with recurrent tumour displaying elevated relative cerebral blood volume. In contrast, radiation necrosis shows decreased perfusion, with optimal cutoff values of approximately 1.23, yielding a sensitivity of 88% and a specificity of 75% (Morabito et al., 2019).

Dynamic contrast-enhanced MRI employs a complementary approach, based on T1-weighted imaging, to assess blood-brain barrier permeability and tumour vascular characteristics. This technique acquires serial T1-weighted images before, during, and after contrast injection, with a temporal resolution of typically 5 to 10 seconds, enabling quantitative analysis of contrast agent extravasation from the intravascular space into the extravascular extracellular space. Pharmacokinetic modelling of the dynamic signal intensity curves yields parameters, including the volume transfer constant, which reflects vascular permeability and perfusion; the extravascular extracellular volume fraction, indicating the proportion of tissue occupied by the extravascular extracellular space; and the plasma volume fraction, representing the fractional blood volume. The volume transfer constant parameter has emerged as particularly valuable in neuro-oncology applications, with elevated values in high-grade gliomas reflecting increased vascular permeability and active angiogenesis. Studies comparing dynamic contrast-enhanced and dynamic susceptibility contrast techniques have demonstrated that the volume transfer constant provides superior differentiation between recurrent tumour and radiation necrosis when analysed in conjunction with other dynamic contrast-enhanced parameters, achieving area under the curve values of 0.98 with sensitivity of 89 percent and specificity of 97 percent (Morabito et al., 2019).

The clinical implementation of perfusion MRI requires careful attention to technical factors that influence quantitative measurements and diagnostic accuracy. Preload dosing strategies and mathematical corrections for contrast agent leakage effects enhance the accuracy of dynamic susceptibility contrast-derived cerebral blood volume measurements in tumours with disrupted blood-brain barriers (Lee et al., 2023). The selection of the arterial input function significantly impacts the estimation of quantitative perfusion parameters, with automated or semi-automated methods increasingly replacing manual placement to enhance reproducibility. The integration of both dynamic susceptibility contrast and dynamic contrast-enhanced techniques in multiparametric imaging protocols provides complementary information, with dynamic susceptibility contrast offering superior temporal resolution for capturing first-pass kinetics and dynamic contrast-enhanced providing better characterisation of blood-brain barrier permeability. Recent technical innovations, including spiral perfusion imaging with consecutive echoes, enable the simultaneous acquisition of T2-star-weighted and T1-weighted data, potentially allowing the derivation of both dynamic susceptibility contrast and dynamic contrast-enhanced parameters from a single contrast injection. Despite these advances, standardisation efforts remain ongoing to address variability in acquisition protocols, post-processing methods, and quantification approaches across different institutions and scanner platforms, with consensus recommendations from organisations such as the Quantitative Imaging Biomarkers Alliance working to establish validated perfusion biomarkers for clinical trials and routine practice (Sanvito et al., 2023). Table 13.1 compares DSC and DCE perfusion MRI techniques.

Table 13.1. Comparison of DSC and DCE perfusion MRI techniques

Feature	DSC MRI	DCE MRI
Imaging Principle	T2/T2* susceptibility effects	T1 relaxation effects
Primary Parameters	rCBV, rCBF, MTT	Ktrans, Ve, Vp, Kep
Temporal Resolution	1-2 seconds	5-10 seconds
Clinical Application	Tumour grading, vascularity assessment	Blood-brain barrier permeability

13.3. Diffusion MRI for Tumour Characterisation

Diffusion-weighted imaging and diffusion tensor imaging have become indispensable tools in modern neuro-oncology imaging, providing unique insights into tumour cellularity, tissue microstructure, and the integrity of white matter tracts. Diffusion-weighted imaging exploits the random thermal motion of water molecules, with restricted diffusion in highly cellular tumour regions producing characteristic high signal intensity on diffusion-weighted images and correspondingly low apparent diffusion coefficient (ADC) values on ADC maps (Rock et al., 2004). The apparent diffusion coefficient is a quantitative measure of water-molecule mobility within tissue, typically expressed in square millimetres per second. It provides a biomarker of tumour cellularity and tissue architecture. High-grade malignant tumours generally demonstrate reduced apparent diffusion coefficient values, reflecting increased cellular density and a reduced extracellular space. In contrast, low-grade tumours exhibit higher apparent diffusion coefficient values, approaching those of normal brain parenchyma. This inverse relationship between cellularity and apparent diffusion coefficient has been validated through correlation with histopathological cell counts and Ki-67 proliferation indices, establishing diffusion-weighted imaging as a valuable non-invasive surrogate marker of tumour biology (Rock et al., 2004).

The clinical applications of diffusion-weighted imaging in brain tumour management span multiple domains from initial diagnosis through treatment monitoring. In tumour grading, apparent diffusion coefficient measurements demonstrate a significant correlation with the World Health Organisation grade. Mean apparent diffusion coefficient values in glioblastomas typically range from 0.8 to 1.1 times those of normal white matter, intermediate-grade gliomas show values from 1.2 to 1.5 times normal, and low-grade gliomas approach 1.5 to 2.0 times normal values. Histogram analysis of apparent diffusion coefficient distributions within tumour regions provides additional prognostic information, with lower percentile values potentially indicating areas of highest cellularity that are suitable for biopsy targeting. Diffusion-weighted imaging proves particularly valuable in distinguishing cerebral abscesses from necrotic tumours, with pyogenic abscesses demonstrating markedly restricted diffusion due to the high viscosity of purulent material and dense bacterial cellularity.

In contrast, necrotic tumour centres typically show facilitated diffusion with elevated apparent diffusion coefficient values. The differentiation of epidermoid cysts from arachnoid cysts similarly exploits differences in diffusion characteristics, with epidermoid cysts displaying restricted diffusion. In contrast, arachnoid cysts follow the cerebrospinal fluid signal on all sequences, including diffusion-weighted imaging.

Diffusion tensor imaging (DTI) extends beyond simple diffusion-weighted imaging by characterising the directional dependence of water diffusion, enabling the mapping of white matter fibre tracts and the assessment of tumour effects on neural pathways (Toh et al., 2008). Fractional anisotropy, a scalar measure derived from diffusion tensor imaging ranging from 0 for completely isotropic diffusion to 1 for maximally anisotropic diffusion, quantifies the degree of directional dependence in water molecule motion. White matter tracts typically exhibit high fractional anisotropy due to preferential diffusion along the fibre direction, whereas tumours generally demonstrate low fractional anisotropy, reflecting the loss of organised tissue architecture (Toh et al., 2008). Tractography algorithms reconstruct three-dimensional representations of white matter pathways, providing neurosurgeons with critical information for surgical planning that maximises tumour resection while preserving eloquent pathways, such as the corticospinal tract, arcuate fasciculus, and optic radiations. The spatial relationship between tumours and significant white matter tracts guides the selection of surgical approaches. It determines the extent of resection; infiltrative tumours may displace, disrupt, or encase fibre bundles, depending on their growth pattern and aggressiveness. Advanced diffusion models, including diffusion kurtosis imaging, which quantifies deviations from Gaussian diffusion behaviour, and neurite orientation dispersion and density imaging, which separately estimate neurite density and orientation dispersion, promise to provide even more detailed characterisation of tumour microstructure. The integration of diffusion metrics with other advanced imaging parameters in multiparametric protocols enhances diagnostic accuracy and prognostic stratification, with combinations of apparent diffusion coefficient, relative cerebral blood volume, and spectroscopic ratios demonstrating synergistic value in tumour characterisation.

13.4. MR Spectroscopy in Brain Tumours

Magnetic resonance spectroscopy provides unique metabolic information that complements anatomical and physiological imaging, enabling non-invasive biochemical characterisation of brain tumours by detecting and quantifying specific metabolites. Proton MR spectroscopy has emerged as the most clinically practical implementation, utilising radiofrequency pulses to excite hydrogen nuclei and analysing the resulting spectrum to identify characteristic metabolite peaks based on chemical shift differences (Delorme et al., 2006). The standard spectrum acquired at intermediate echo times typically displays several prominent metabolite peaks including N-acetylaspartate at 2.02 parts per million serving as a marker of intact neurons and axons, creatine at 3.02 parts per million reflecting energy metabolism, choline-containing compounds at 3.22 parts per million indicating membrane turnover and cellular proliferation, and when present, lactate at 1.33 parts per million signifying anaerobic glycolysis and lipids at 0.9 to 1.3 parts per million suggesting necrosis. Brain tumours exhibit characteristic spectroscopic patterns that differ fundamentally from those of normal brain parenchyma. Nearly all neoplasms show decreased N-acetylaspartate, reflecting neuronal loss or dysfunction, and most malignant tumours exhibit elevated choline, indicating increased cell membrane synthesis and turnover (Delorme et al., 2006).

The quantitative analysis of metabolite ratios enhances diagnostic specificity and provides objective metrics for tumour characterisation and grading. The choline-to-N-acetylaspartate ratio has emerged as one of the most diagnostically functional parameters, with ratios above 2.0 typically indicating neoplastic processes and values exceeding 3.0 suggesting high-grade malignancy. The choline-to-creatine ratio similarly demonstrates diagnostic value in tumour grading, with cutoff values ranging from 1.8 to 2.0, showing reasonable sensitivity and specificity for distinguishing neoplastic from non-neoplastic lesions. High-grade gliomas characteristically display markedly elevated choline peaks, reflecting active cell proliferation. They also exhibit depressed N-acetylaspartate and creatine levels, indicating loss of normal neuronal tissue and altered energy metabolism.

Furthermore, the frequent detection of lactate and lipid peaks signifies tissue hypoxia and necrosis. Lower-grade gliomas exhibit less dramatic metabolic alterations, with mildly elevated choline-to-N-acetylaspartate ratios typically ranging from 1.5 to 2.5, and the absence of lactate and lipid peaks. Metastatic lesions exhibit variable spectroscopic patterns, depending on the primary tumour histology, but generally show elevated choline levels with markedly reduced or absent N-acetylaspartate, due to the complete replacement of brain parenchyma by tumour cells. The key discriminating feature is assessing metabolite levels in the perilesional region: metastases typically show normal ratios, whereas infiltrative gliomas exhibit abnormally elevated choline extending beyond visible tumour margins.

Clinical applications of MR spectroscopy extend beyond initial tumour diagnosis to encompass treatment planning, biopsy guidance, and monitoring of therapy. Spectroscopic imaging with multi-voxel techniques enables the spatial mapping of metabolite distributions across tumour regions and adjacent brain, identifying areas of maximum metabolic abnormality that may represent the highest-grade tumour components suitable for stereotactic biopsy targeting. The heterogeneous distribution of metabolites within large tumour masses reflects biological heterogeneity, with regions displaying the highest choline-to-N-acetylaspartate ratios potentially harbouring the most aggressive tumour components that determine overall prognosis and treatment resistance. Spectroscopy proves particularly valuable in radiation treatment planning by identifying metabolically active tumours that extend beyond conventional imaging margins, potentially guiding dose escalation to regions of the highest tumour burden while sparing normal brain tissue. The detection of specific metabolites, such as 2-hydroxyglutarate, in isocitrate dehydrogenase-mutant gliomas represents an exciting frontier in molecular imaging, enabling the non-invasive identification of a key oncometabolite with direct therapeutic and prognostic implications (Suh et al., 2018). Technical considerations important for successful clinical implementation include careful voxel placement to sample representative tumor regions while avoiding contamination from skull lipids, selection of appropriate echo time with intermediate values around 135 milliseconds providing optimal visualization of primary metabolites while inverting the lactate peak for better discrimination from lipids, and attention to magnetic field homogeneity with shimming procedures essential for achieving narrow spectral linewidths that enable accurate metabolite quantification (Delorme et al., 2006). Table 13.2 shows MR spectroscopy metabolite patterns in brain tumours.

Table 13.2. MR spectroscopy metabolite patterns in brain tumours

Lesion Type	Metabolite Pattern	Typical Ratio
High-Grade Glioma	High Cho, Low NAA, Lactate/Lipid present	Cho/NAA > 3.0
Low-Grade Glioma	Mildly elevated Cho, decreased NAA	Cho/NAA 1.5-2.5
Metastasis	High Cho, Absent/Low NAA	Cho/NAA > 2.5
Radiation Necrosis	Low all metabolites, Lipid peak	Cho/NAA < 1.5
Abscess	Lactate, Amino acids, Acetate	Low Cho

13.5. Distinguishing Tumour Progression from Treatment Effects

Differentiating between actual tumour progression and treatment-related effects is one of the most challenging problems in neuro-oncology imaging, with profound implications for patient management and clinical trial interpretation (Zikou et al., 2018). Treatment-related phenomena, including pseudoprogression, radiation necrosis, and pseudoresponse, can mimic tumour behaviour on conventional imaging, potentially leading to inappropriate therapeutic decisions if not correctly identified. Pseudoprogression describes the transient increase in contrast enhancement and mass effect that occurs within the first three months following completion of concurrent chemoradiation therapy, affecting approximately 20 to 30 per cent of patients with high-grade gliomas and subsequently stabilising or improving without treatment modification (Young et al., 2013). This phenomenon reflects complex biological processes, including treatment-induced inflammation, increased vascular permeability, and disruption of the blood-brain barrier rather than actual tumour growth. Radiation necrosis typically manifests six months or more following radiation therapy as an irregular rim-enhancing lesion within the radiation field, histologically characterised by coagulative necrosis, vascular injury with fibrinoid necrosis, and reactive gliosis that can progress over time and cause significant mass effect requiring surgical intervention despite the absence of viable tumour (Zikou et al., 2018).

Conventional MRI demonstrates limited specificity in distinguishing between treatment effects and tumour progression, as both entities can present with similar patterns of contrast enhancement, perilesional oedema, and mass effect. This limitation has driven the development and validation of advanced imaging techniques that interrogate tissue at physiological and metabolic levels to improve diagnostic accuracy (van Dijken et al., 2017). Perfusion imaging with relative cerebral blood volume measurements has emerged as one of the most extensively validated approaches, exploiting fundamental differences in vascularity between recurrent tumours with active angiogenesis and those with treatment-related changes, including vascular injury and reduced perfusion. Multiple studies have established that relative cerebral blood volume values below 1.0, relative to normal-appearing white matter, strongly suggest radiation necrosis, while values exceeding 1.75 indicate tumour recurrence with high specificity (Morabito et al., 2019). The diagnostic performance improves further when combining dynamic susceptibility contrast and dynamic contrast-enhanced parameters, with the volume transfer constant from dynamic contrast-enhanced imaging showing particularly high accuracy in identifying tumour recurrence. Morabito et al. demonstrated that dynamic contrast-enhanced parameters achieved an area under the curve of 0.98, with a sensitivity of 89% and specificity of 97%, outperforming dynamic susceptibility contrast measurements alone (Morabito et al., 2019).

Magnetic resonance spectroscopy provides complementary metabolic information that enhances diagnostic confidence when integrated with perfusion measurements. Recurrent tumours typically demonstrate elevated choline, reflecting active cell proliferation, with choline-to-N-acetylaspartate ratios exceeding 2.0 and often surpassing 3.0 in high-grade recurrences. In contrast, radiation necrosis exhibits globally reduced metabolite levels with decreased choline, N-acetylaspartate, and creatine, and prominent lipid-lactate peaks indicating cellular breakdown and tissue necrosis. Studies employing multiparametric imaging protocols that combine perfusion, diffusion, and spectroscopy have reported diagnostic accuracies exceeding 90% when all modalities are integrated, substantially higher than those of any single technique alone (van Dijken et al., 2017). Apparent diffusion coefficient measurements provide additional discriminatory power, with radiation necrosis often showing elevated apparent diffusion coefficient values, reflecting increased extracellular space and tissue breakdown. In contrast, tumour recurrence demonstrates variable but frequently reduced apparent diffusion coefficient values, consistent with a hypercellular tumour (Rock et al., 2004). Advanced metabolic imaging with amino acid PET tracers, such as fluorine 18 fluoroethyltyrosine and carbon-11 methionine, offers high sensitivity for detecting active tumours by increased amino acid transport, with particular value for distinguishing tumours from non-specific contrast enhancement when combined with MRI perfusion parameters.

The clinical implementation of multiparametric imaging for treatment response assessment requires the systematic integration of multiple biomarkers, with careful attention to technical quality and standardised interpretation criteria. Response assessment protocols should include conventional structural sequences supplemented with diffusion-weighted imaging, perfusion imaging using both dynamic susceptibility contrast and, when available, dynamic contrast-enhanced techniques, and spectroscopy focused on regions of maximal metabolic abnormality. A longitudinal comparison of quantitative parameters is more reliable than a visual assessment of single time points, and trends across serial examinations provide valuable prognostic information. Increasing relative cerebral blood volume and choline-to-N-acetylaspartate ratios over time strongly suggest progressive disease, whereas stable or declining values support a treatment effect (Young et al., 2013). The recognition of mixed patterns with coexisting tumour and treatment-related changes poses a significant diagnostic challenge, as many patients exhibit heterogeneous regions containing both viable tumour and radiation necrosis within the same lesion complex. In these cases, identifying focal areas with elevated perfusion and choline helps guide biopsy targeting to regions most likely to yield diagnostic tissue. Emerging techniques, including arterial spin labelling perfusion that requires no contrast administration, amide proton transfer imaging sensitive to cellular protein content and tissue pH (Park et al., 2022), and advanced diffusion models promise to further enhance diagnostic accuracy in this challenging clinical scenario, potentially reducing reliance on invasive tissue sampling for definitive diagnosis. Table 13.3 illustrates advanced MRI techniques for differentiating treatment effects.

Table 13.3. Advanced MRI techniques for treatment effect differentiation

Imaging Modality	Tumor Recurrence	Treatment Effect
DSC MRI (rCBV)	Elevated (>1.75)	Reduced (<1.0)
DCE MRI (Ktrans)	High (>28.76)	Low
MR Spectroscopy	High Cho, Cho/NAA >2.0	Low all metabolites, Lipid peak
Diffusion (ADC)	Variable, often reduced	Elevated
Diagnostic Accuracy	Multiparametric: 90%	Single technique: 70-85%

13.6. Radiomics and Texture Analysis

Radiomics represents an emerging paradigm in medical imaging that extracts large numbers of quantitative features from imaging data, enabling the comprehensive characterisation of tumour phenotypes and the discovery of imaging biomarkers associated with biological behaviour, treatment response, and clinical outcomes (Verma et al., 2017). Unlike conventional qualitative image interpretation or simple quantitative measurements, radiomics utilises computational algorithms to extract hundreds to thousands of features that describe tumour shape, intensity distribution, spatial heterogeneity, and texture patterns, extending beyond human visual perception. Texture analysis, a key component of radiomics, quantifies spatial relationships among pixel or voxel intensities using statistical methods including Grey-level co-occurrence matrices, Grey-level run-length matrices, and wavelet transformations (Verma et al., 2017). These mathematical approaches capture subtle patterns in image heterogeneity that reflect underlying tumour biology, including cellular organisation, vascularity, necrosis, and genetic alterations. The radiomic workflow encompasses several sequential steps: image acquisition and preprocessing to ensure consistency; tumour segmentation to define regions of interest; feature extraction using validated software implementations; feature selection to identify the most informative variables and reduce dimensionality; and model development using machine learning algorithms to predict outcomes or classify tumours.

Applications of radiomics in brain tumour imaging span the entire spectrum of clinical decision-making, from initial diagnosis through personalised treatment planning and prognostication. In tumour classification, radiomic features extracted from conventional and advanced MRI sequences demonstrate the capacity to distinguish primary brain tumours from metastases, differentiate glioma subtypes, and predict molecular markers, including isocitrate dehydrogenase mutation status, 1p19q codeletion, and MGMT promoter methylation status without requiring tissue sampling (Suh et al., 2018). Machine learning models integrating radiomic features from multiple MRI sequences have achieved classification accuracies exceeding 85% for predicting isocitrate dehydrogenase mutations, potentially enabling non-invasive molecular profiling to guide treatment decisions. Radiomics approaches to glioma grading extract texture features that quantify tumour heterogeneity, with higher-grade tumours typically exhibiting greater spatial heterogeneity, as reflected in elevated Grey-level co-occurrence matrix features and increased wavelet coefficients. Prognostic models incorporating radiomic signatures derived from preoperative MRI can stratify patients by survival risk, with texture features describing enhancement heterogeneity and perfusion variability providing independent prognostic value beyond clinical variables and molecular markers.

The clinical translation of radiomics presents significant challenges that must be addressed to realise its full potential in routine clinical practice. Standardisation of image acquisition parameters, preprocessing steps, and feature extraction methods is a critical prerequisite for the reproducibility and generalizability of radiomic models across different institutions and scanner platforms (Verma et al., 2017). Variations in magnetic field strength, pulse sequence parameters, reconstruction algorithms, and segmentation approaches can significantly impact extracted feature values, potentially limiting model performance when applied to external datasets. The development of standardised reporting guidelines and quality assurance procedures, similar to those established for quantitative imaging biomarkers, aims to address these concerns and facilitate multi-institutional validation studies. Overfitting represents another substantial challenge, particularly given the high dimensionality of radiomic feature spaces relative to typical sample sizes in medical imaging studies. Rigorous feature selection techniques, such as LASSO regression, recursive feature elimination, and information-theoretic approaches, help mitigate overfitting while identifying the most biologically relevant and reproducible features. Validation in independent cohorts remains essential to establish clinical utility, with prospective validation in real-world clinical settings ultimately required before widespread implementation. The integration of radiomics with other data modalities, including genomics, proteomics, and clinical variables, through multi-omic approaches promises to provide comprehensive tumour characterisation that captures the full complexity of tumour biology and enables precision medicine strategies tailored to individual patient characteristics. Artificial intelligence and deep learning methods that automatically learn relevant features directly from imaging data, without requiring manual feature engineering, represent the next frontier in this field. This approach potentially overcomes the limitations of handcrafted radiomic features while discovering novel imaging biomarkers that are invisible to conventional analysis.

Conclusion

Magnetic resonance imaging has evolved from a purely anatomical imaging modality to a comprehensive, multiparametric platform that characterises brain tumours at structural, functional, physiological, and metabolic levels. The integration of conventional sequences with advanced techniques, including perfusion imaging, diffusion-weighted imaging, and magnetic resonance spectroscopy, enables more accurate diagnosis, precise tumour grading, better differentiation of treatment effects from progression, and improved prognostic stratification (Martucci et al., 2023). Each imaging modality contributes unique and complementary information, with perfusion parameters reflecting tumour vascularity and angiogenesis, diffusion metrics quantifying cellularity and tissue microstructure, and spectroscopic profiles revealing metabolic signatures. The clinical challenges of distinguishing tumour recurrence from treatment-related effects have been substantially addressed through multiparametric approaches, which achieve diagnostic accuracies exceeding 90 per cent when multiple techniques are combined systematically (van Dijken et al., 2017).

Emerging technologies, including radiomics and artificial intelligence, promise to further enhance MRI's role in precision neuro-oncology by extracting quantitative imaging biomarkers that predict molecular subtypes, treatment response, and survival outcomes. Standardisation efforts to harmonise acquisition protocols and quantification methods across institutions will facilitate larger-scale validation studies and accelerate the clinical translation of advanced imaging biomarkers (Sanvito et al., 2023). The future of brain tumour imaging lies in integrated, multiparametric, and multi-omic approaches that combine imaging data with molecular, genetic, and clinical information to enable truly personalised treatment strategies tailored to individual tumour biology and patient characteristics. As imaging technologies continue to advance and our understanding of the biological basis of imaging findings deepens, MRI will play an increasingly central role in the management of patients with brain tumours, from initial diagnosis through treatment monitoring and long-term surveillance. The continued refinement and validation of these powerful imaging tools support achieving Sustainable Development Goal 3 by enhancing diagnostic accuracy, facilitating earlier detection of disease progression, and ultimately improving patient outcomes and quality of life.

Acknowledgments

The authors would like to extend our appreciation to those who offered helpful commentary during the drafting process of this manuscript. We also acknowledge the role the Nova Publishing department played in enabling the work described herein.

References

Delorme, S., Weber, M. A., Haack, S., & Zuna, I. (2006). Applications of MRS in the evaluation of focal malignant brain lesions. *Cancer Imaging*, 6(1), 95-99. https://doi.org/10.1102/1470-7330.2006.0015.

Ellingson, B. M., Bendszus, M., Boxerman, J., Barboriak, D., Erickson, B. J., Smits, M., Nelson, S. J., Gerstner, E., Alexander, B., Goldmacher, G., Wick, W., Vogelbaum, M., Weller, M., Galanis, E., Kalpathy-Cramer, J., Shankar, L., Jacobs, P., Pope, W. B., Yang, D., ... Wen, P. Y. (2015). Consensus recommendations for a standardized brain tumor imaging protocol in clinical trials. *Neuro-Oncology*, 17(9), 1188-1198. https://doi.org/10.1093/neuonc/nov095.

Iv, M., Yoon, B. C., Hua, J., Lavezo, J., Upadhyay, R., Blevins, B. K., Laughlin, S., & Li, A. Y. (2022). Current clinical brain tumor imaging. *Neurosurgery*, 70(1), 6-29. https://doi.org/10.1227/neu.0000000000001635.

Lee, M. D., Baird, G. L., Bell, L. C., Quarles, C. C., Boxerman, J. L., & Kirsch, D. G. (2023). Utility of percentage signal recovery and baseline signal in DSC-MRI optimized for relative CBV measurement for differentiating glioblastoma, lymphoma, metastasis, and meningioma. *American Journal of Neuroradiology*, 44(10), 1138-1144. https://doi.org/10.3174/ajnr.A7994.

Martucci, M., Russo, R., Schimperna, F., D'Apolito, G., Panfili, M., Grimaldi, A., Perna, A., Ferranti, A. M., Varcasia, G., Giordano, C., & Gaudino, S. (2023). Magnetic resonance imaging of primary adult brain tumors: State of the art and future perspectives. *Biomedicines*, 11(2), 364. https://doi.org/10.3390/biomedicines11020364.

Morabito, R., Alafaci, C., Pergolizzi, S., Pontoriero, A., Iati, G., Bonanno, L., Gaeta, M., Salpietro, F. M., Mormina, E., Longo, M., & Granata, F. (2019). DCE and DSC perfusion MRI diagnostic accuracy in the follow-up of primary and metastatic intra-axial brain tumors treated by radiosurgery with cyberknife. *Radiation Oncology*, 14, 65. https://doi.org/10.1186/s13014-019-1271-7.

Park, J. E., Kim, H. S., Park, S. Y., Jung, S. C., Kim, J. H., & Heo, H. Y. (2022). Identification of early response to anti-angiogenic therapy in recurrent glioblastoma: Amide proton transfer-weighted and perfusion-weighted MRI compared. *Radiology*, 305(2), 397-405. https://doi.org/10.1148/radiol.212689.

Rock, J. P., Hearshen, D., Scarpace, L., Croteau, D., Gutierrez, J., Fisher, J. L., Rosenblum, M. L., & Mikkelsen, T. (2004). Associations among magnetic resonance spectroscopy, apparent diffusion coefficients, and image-guided histopathology with special attention to radiation necrosis. *Neurosurgery*, 54(5), 1111-1119. https://doi.org/10.1227/01.neu.0000119328.56431.a7.

Sanvito, F., Kaufmann, T. J., Cloughesy, T. F., Wen, P. Y., & Ellingson, B. M. (2023). Standardized brain tumor imaging protocols for clinical trials: Current recommendations and tips for integration. *Frontiers in Radiology*, 3, 1267615. https://doi.org/10.3389/fradi.2023.1267615.

Suh, C. H., Kim, H. S., Jung, S. C., Choi, C. G., & Kim, S. J. (2018). Imaging prediction of isocitrate dehydrogenase (IDH) mutation in patients with glioma: A systematic review and meta-analysis. *European Radiology*, 29(2), 745-758. https://doi.org/10.1007/s00330-018-5608-7.

Toh, C. H., Castillo, M., Wong, A. M. C., Wei, K. C., Wong, H. F., Ng, S. H., & Wan, Y. L. (2008). Differentiation between classic and atypical meningiomas with use of diffusion tensor imaging. *American Journal of Neuroradiology*, 29(9), 1630-1635. https://doi.org/10.3174/ajnr.A1170.

van Dijken, B. R. J., van Laar, P. J., Holtman, G. A., & van der Hoorn, A. (2017). Diagnostic accuracy of magnetic resonance imaging techniques for treatment response evaluation in patients with high-grade glioma, a systematic review and meta-analysis. *European Radiology*, 27(10), 4129-4144. https://doi.org/10.1007/s00330-017-4789-9.

Verma, R. K., Wiest, R., Locher, C., Heldner, M. R., Schucht, P., Raabe, A., Slotboom, J., & Gralla, J. (2017). Differentiating enhancing multiple sclerosis lesions, glioblastoma, and lymphoma with dynamic texture parameters analysis. *American Journal of Neuroradiology*, 38(5), 966-972. https://doi.org/10.3174/ajnr.A5086.

Young, R. J., Gupta, A., Shah, A. D., Graber, J. J., Schweitzer, A. D., Prager, A., Shi, W., Zhang, Z., Huse, J., Omuro, A. M., & Chan, T. A. (2013). MRI perfusion in the detection of pseudoprogression in patients with glioblastoma. *Clinical Imaging*, 37(1), 41-49. https://doi.org/10.1016/j.clinimag.2012.02.016.

Zikou, A., Sioka, C., Alexiou, G. A., Fotopoulos, A., Voulgaris, S., & Argyropoulou, M. I. (2018). Radiation necrosis, pseudoprogression, pseudoresponse, and tumor recurrence: Imaging challenges for the evaluation of treated gliomas. *Contrast Media & Molecular Imaging*, 2018, 6828396. https://doi.org/10.1155/2018/6828396.

Chapter 14

Psychiatric Neuroimaging

Purnachandra Kawdu Lamghare[1,*] and Maajid Mohi Ud Din Malik[2,†]

[1]Department of Radio-Diagnosis, Dr. D. Y. Patil Medical College, Hospital and Research Centre, Dr. D. Y. Patil Vidyapeeth (Deemed to be University), Sant Tukaram Nagar, Pimpri, Pune, India
[2]Radiology and Imaging Technology, Dr. D. Y. Patil School of Allied Health Sciences, Dr. D. Y. Patil Vidyapeeth (Deemed to be University), Sant Tukaram Nagar, Pimpri, Pune, India

Abstract

Psychiatric neuroimaging has emerged as an essential tool for understanding the neurobiological underpinnings of mental disorders, offering unprecedented insights into brain structure, function, and connectivity. This chapter provides a comprehensive overview of neuroimaging biomarkers across primary psychiatric conditions, including major depressive disorder, schizophrenia, anxiety disorders, post-traumatic stress disorder, bipolar disorder, substance use disorders, and autism spectrum disorders. Advanced imaging modalities, including structural and functional magnetic resonance imaging (MRI), diffusion tensor imaging, and positron emission tomography, have consistently revealed alterations in fronto-limbic circuits, reward systems, and neural connectivity patterns associated with these conditions. Despite significant progress, translating neuroimaging findings into clinical practice remains challenging due to heterogeneity within diagnostic categories, small sample sizes, and methodological inconsistencies. Machine learning approaches combined with multimodal neuroimaging show promise for developing diagnostic biomarkers and predicting treatment outcomes. This chapter synthesises current evidence, discusses clinical implications, and highlights future directions for psychiatric neuroimaging research within the framework of Sustainable Development Goal 3: Good Health and Well-being.

[*] Corresponding Author's Email: purnachandra.lamghare@dpu.edu.in
[†] Corresponding Author's Email: maajid.malik@dpu.edu.in

In: Recent Advances in Magnetic Resonance Imaging in Neuroimaging
Editors: Maajid Mohi Ud Din Malik, Purnachandra Kawdu Lamghare and R. S. Kuber
ISBN: 979-8-90134-244-2

Keywords: psychiatric neuroimaging, MRI biomarkers, functional connectivity, depression, schizophrenia, anxiety disorders, bipolar disorder, substance use disorders, autism spectrum disorder, SDG 3

Introduction

Psychiatric disorders represent a significant global health challenge, affecting millions of individuals worldwide and contributing substantially to disease burden, disability, and reduced quality of life. Unlike many medical conditions, where objective diagnostic tests guide clinical decision-making, psychiatric diagnoses have traditionally relied on clinical interviews and behavioural assessments based on symptom clusters. The absence of objective biomarkers has hindered early detection, accurate diagnosis, and the selection of personalised treatments. Over the past three decades, advances in neuroimaging technology have revolutionised our ability to investigate the neurobiological substrates of mental illness, providing unprecedented opportunities to visualise brain structure, function, and neurochemistry in living individuals.

Modern neuroimaging techniques, including structural magnetic resonance imaging (MRI), functional MRI, diffusion tensor imaging, magnetic resonance spectroscopy, and positron emission tomography, have revealed consistent patterns of brain alterations across primary psychiatric conditions. These findings have transformed our understanding of mental disorders from purely psychological constructs to conditions with identifiable neurobiological underpinnings. The convergence of advanced imaging methodologies with sophisticated analytical approaches, particularly machine learning and artificial intelligence, holds promise for translating research findings into clinically useful biomarkers. This chapter examines neuroimaging findings across major psychiatric disorders, evaluating their potential to improve diagnosis, predict treatment response, and advance personalised psychiatric care.

14.1. MRI Biomarkers in Depression

Major depressive disorder (MDD) represents one of the most extensively studied psychiatric conditions using neuroimaging techniques. Neuroimaging research has substantiated functional and structural abnormalities underlying depression, particularly within neural circuitry involved in emotion regulation and reward processing (Lai, 2019). Structural MRI studies have consistently demonstrated volumetric reductions in key brain regions, including the anterior cingulate cortex (ACC), dorsolateral prefrontal cortex (DLPFC), orbitofrontal cortex (OFC), hippocampus, and amygdala in patients with MDD compared to healthy controls. The fronto-limbic model has emerged as the predominant framework for understanding MDD pathophysiology, with the ACC serving as a particularly promising biomarker for predicting treatment response.

Functional MRI investigations have revealed that elevated activity in the ACC is consistently associated with better antidepressant response in patients with MDD (Lai, 2021). The dorsolateral prefrontal cortex and orbitofrontal cortex appear to cooperate with the ACC to inhibit emotional responses and emotional memory through cognitive control networks. Meanwhile, emotional responses and memories originate from limbic regions such as the amygdala and hippocampus. Resting-state functional MRI studies have identified alterations in default mode network connectivity, with decreased functional connectivity between prefrontal regions and limbic structures representing a core feature of depression.

Recent advances in machine learning, combined with multimodal neuroimaging, have shown significant potential to improve diagnostic accuracy and predict treatment outcomes in MDD. Li et al., (2023) demonstrated that multisequence MRI neuroimaging features, combined with machine learning, achieved diagnostic accuracy exceeding 85% for distinguishing patients with MDD from healthy controls. Neuroimaging biomarkers offer advantages over peripheral biomarkers, as they are considerably more stable and less susceptible to the effects of inflammation or nutritional factors (Lee & Chi, 2020). However, the acute treatment duration for MDD is typically 8 weeks or more, and treatment without predictors of response presents ongoing challenges to both patients and physicians.

The identification of neuroimaging predictors throughout the course of MDD has become an important research priority. Neuroimaging methods used include brain volumetric MRI, functional MRI (both resting-state and task-based), diffusion tensor imaging, magnetic resonance spectroscopy, near-infrared spectroscopy, and molecular imaging techniques such as positron emission tomography and single-photon emission computed tomography (Lee & Chi, 2020). Despite significant research efforts, results have been somewhat inconsistent, likely due to small sample sizes, varying study designs—including different eligibility criteria—and differences in imaging and analytical methods across studies. Future research needs to address these methodological challenges to establish clinically relevant biomarkers for diagnosing depression and selecting treatment.

14.2. Schizophrenia: Structural and Functional Alterations

Schizophrenia is characterised by substantial structural and functional brain abnormalities that have been extensively documented through neuroimaging research. Structural neuroimaging studies suggest white matter integrity deficits and Grey matter reductions that appear more widespread in schizophrenia compared to other psychotic disorders (Chepenik et al., 2017). Meta-analyses have demonstrated cortical abnormalities in over 4,474 individuals with schizophrenia, revealing consistent findings of reduced cortical thickness, particularly in the prefrontal and temporal regions. Volumetric studies have shown enlarged ventricles and reduced hippocampal volumes, which correlate with symptom severity and cognitive impairment.

Functional magnetic resonance imaging studies have provided fundamental insights into the neurobiology of schizophrenia, revealing that brain function differs significantly between individuals with schizophrenia and healthy controls (Voineskos et al., 2024). The field has evolved from examining regional brain activation to investigating global connectivity patterns and employing advanced analytical approaches. Task-based fMRI studies have demonstrated hypoactivation in prefrontal regions during working memory tasks and abnormal activation patterns in the medial temporal lobe during memory encoding. Resting-state functional connectivity studies have revealed complex patterns of altered connectivity, including both hyperconnectivity and hypoconnectivity across various neural networks.

Machine learning techniques applied to multimodal neuroimaging data have achieved diagnostic accuracy ranging from 75% to 90% for distinguishing schizophrenia patients from healthy controls (de Filippis et al., 2019). Studies combining structural and functional MRI with machine learning algorithms have shown that multimodal brain data can enhance diagnostic accuracy beyond single-modality approaches. However, findings regarding amygdala and hippocampal function vary considerably depending on the methodology used and the clinical characteristics of the patient sample. Functional abnormalities in the hippocampus may be related to volumetric abnormalities; however, some studies suggest that group differences in hippocampal function remain significant even after controlling for hippocampal volume.

The dysconnection hypothesis of schizophrenia proposes that the disorder arises from aberrant functional integration of brain systems rather than localised pathology. This framework is supported by diffusion tensor imaging studies demonstrating widespread white-matter microstructural abnormalities affecting long-range connections between cortical regions. The integration of functional connectivity measures with structural imaging and clinical data represents a promising approach to developing biomarkers that could aid early diagnosis and treatment selection. Recent work using machine learning approaches for diagnostic prediction and identification of dimensional, transdiagnostic brain-based biomarkers holds promise for clinical translation (Voineskos et al., 2024).

14.3. Anxiety Disorders and Post-Traumatic Stress Disorder

Neuroimaging research in anxiety disorders and post-traumatic stress disorder (PTSD) has converged on dysfunctional emotion processing circuits involving the amygdala, prefrontal cortex, and anterior cingulate cortex. Functional neuroimaging studies have generally supported the hypothesis that the amygdala is hyperresponsive in PTSD, while rostral and ventral portions of the medial prefrontal cortex are hyporesponsive (Bremner, 2011). This pattern of amygdala hyperactivation coupled with prefrontal hypoactivation is thought to underlie the enhanced fear response and impaired fear extinction characteristic of PTSD. Emerging evidence suggests that the dorsal anterior cingulate cortex and insula may also be hyperresponsive in PTSD and play essential roles in the disorder.

Meta-analytic studies comparing PTSD, social anxiety disorder, and specific phobia have revealed both common and disorder-specific neural signatures (Etkin & Wager, 2007). Patients with any of these three disorders consistently show greater activity than matched comparison subjects in the amygdala and insula, structures linked to negative emotional responses. Interestingly, hyperactivation in the amygdala and insula is more frequently observed in social anxiety disorder and specific phobia than in PTSD. By contrast, only patients with PTSD show hypoactivation in the dorsal and rostral anterior cingulate cortices and the ventromedial prefrontal cortex, structures linked to the experience and regulation of emotion. These findings suggest a mechanism for the emotional dysregulation symptoms in PTSD that extends beyond an exaggerated fear response.

Recent studies employing real-time functional MRI neurofeedback have demonstrated that PTSD patients can successfully downregulate both right and left amygdala activation, with sustained effects observed in transfer runs without neurofeedback (Nicholson et al., 2023). During regulation, increased activation was observed in the dorsolateral and ventrolateral prefrontal cortex, regions related to emotion regulation. Significantly, activation in the prefrontal cortex, rostral anterior cingulate cortex, and insula was negatively correlated with PTSD dissociative symptoms. Dynamic causal modelling analysis exploring the directional structure suggests that amygdala downregulation involves both top-down and bottom-up information flow regarding prefrontal-amygdala connectivity. These findings support the development of neurofeedback-based interventions for PTSD.

Structural imaging studies have reported alterations in Grey and white matter in PTSD. Meta-analyses have found reduced hippocampal volume in PTSD. However, the relationship between hippocampal volume and PTSD symptoms remains complex and may be influenced by factors such as trauma type, age of trauma exposure, and comorbid conditions. The integration of structural and functional imaging measures with clinical and genetic data represents an essential direction for developing a more comprehensive understanding of the neurobiological mechanisms underlying anxiety disorders and PTSD. Future research should focus on longitudinal studies that can distinguish pre-existing vulnerability factors from consequences of trauma exposure and disorder development.

14.4. Bipolar Disorder Imaging

Bipolar disorder has been extensively studied using both structural and functional neuroimaging approaches, revealing complex patterns of brain abnormalities that vary across mood states. Neuroimaging research has demonstrated functional and structural abnormalities in distinct, distributed neural systems involved in emotion processing and executive control (Phillips & Kupfer, 2013). Structural MRI studies in adults with bipolar disorder have found enlarged amygdalae, decreased dorsal and ventral prefrontal cortices, and variable findings regarding hippocampal volumes. These structural alterations suggest dysfunction in fronto-limbic circuits, which are critical for mood regulation. Recent advances in functional MRI have emphasised the importance of examining patients across different mood states to distinguish trait markers from state-dependent changes.

Functional neuroimaging studies have revealed abnormalities in the limbic-striatal circuit, medial prefrontal cortex, and dorsolateral prefrontal cortex that may manifest as trait markers of bipolar disorder-related dysfunction (Zhang et al., 2024). However, considerable evidence also suggests state-dependent effects regarding emotional valence and cognitive control. Resting-state functional MRI studies have demonstrated altered functional connectivity patterns, including disruptions in the default mode network and abnormal connectivity between prefrontal and limbic regions. Functional connectivity between the ventral prefrontal cortex and amygdala at low frequency in the resting state has been found to differ significantly in bipolar disorder compared to healthy controls.

Machine learning approaches combined with structural connectome analysis have shown promise for improving differential diagnosis between bipolar disorder and major depressive disorder, conditions that share considerable clinical overlap. Zhang et al. (2024) demonstrated that integrating structural connectome analysis with machine learning models achieved 90.3% accuracy in distinguishing between bipolar disorder and major depressive disorder groups based on structural brain parameters. Graph-theory-based analytics identified significant alterations in structural connectome metrics, highlighting distinct differences between the conditions. These findings underscore the potential for neuroimaging biomarkers to enhance diagnostic precision in mood disorders.

The effects of psychotropic medications on neuroimaging findings must be carefully considered when interpreting results. Evidence suggests that medication effects, when present, are predominantly normalising and do not appear to provide an alternative explanation for differences in brain structure or function between bipolar disorder patients and healthy subjects (Hafeman et al., 2012). Lithium in particular may have neurotrophic effects in some neural regions, while antipsychotic medications are associated with Grey matter changes. Future research should employ longitudinal designs that examine individuals before and after medication initiation, as well as extensive cross-sectional studies comparing medication-free individuals with those taking different types of medication. Understanding the interaction between neurobiological abnormalities and treatment effects will be essential for developing personalised approaches to bipolar disorder management.

14.5. Addiction and Substance Use Disorders

Substance use disorders involve complex alterations in brain reward, motivation, memory, and cognitive control systems that have been extensively characterised through neuroimaging research. The neurobiology of addiction can be conceptualised as involving disturbances in three major neurocircuits: a basal ganglia-driven binge/intoxication stage, an extended amygdala-driven withdrawal/negative affect stage, and a prefrontal cortex-driven preoccupation/anticipation stage (Koob & Volkow, 2016). Neuroimaging studies have provided evidence of specific changes in brain regions, including the prefrontal cortex, nucleus accumbens, amygdala, and hippocampus, which are involved in decision-making, impulse control, reward processing, and memory.

Functional neuroimaging paradigms have been developed to investigate the neural circuits underlying addiction, including those involved in reward, inhibitory control, stress, emotional processing, and learning and memory. Drugs of abuse produce their reinforcing and addictive effects by directly activating supraphysiological dopamine action in the mesolimbic reward circuit and by indirectly modulating other neurotransmitters, including glutamate, GABA, opioids, acetylcholine, cannabinoids, and serotonin (Murnane et al., 2023). Meta-analyses examining functional connectivity in substance use disorders have found that the ventromedial prefrontal cortex exhibits hyperconnectivity with the ventral striatum and hypoconnectivity with the amygdala and hippocampus (Dugré et al., 2023). These connectivity alterations are thought to contribute to the aberrant reward processing, impulsivity, and incentive sensitisation that drive substance use disorders.

Positron emission tomography studies have been particularly valuable for examining neurotransmitter systems in addiction. PET imaging with radioligands targeting dopamine D2/D3 receptors has consistently shown reduced striatal receptor availability in individuals with various substance use disorders. This dopaminergic deficit is associated with decreased prefrontal metabolism and impaired executive function. Stimulant administration studies using PET have demonstrated that individuals with substance use disorders show blunted dopamine release compared to healthy controls, suggesting adaptations in the dopamine system following chronic drug exposure. These findings provide objective measures of neurobiological alterations in addiction that may serve as biomarkers for treatment response. Table 14.1 shows neuroimaging modalities and applications in psychiatric research.

The application of machine learning techniques to neuroimaging data has shown promise for predicting relapse and treatment outcomes in substance use disorders. Neuroimaging biomarkers of striatal structure and function across different substance use disorders provide an extensive foundation to support clinical validation. For example, striatal functional MRI drug-cue reactivity might serve as a biomarker of relapse risk. However, the biggest challenge for functional MRI studies is reproducibility and generalizability. Low statistical power has been well recognised and mitigated in recent years through increased sample sizes and more rigorous statistical analyses. Future research must also address the high comorbidity of substance use disorders with other mental illnesses and the complexity of polysubstance use patterns to develop biomarkers with clinical utility.

Table 14.1. Neuroimaging modalities and applications in psychiatric research

Imaging Modality	Measures	Temporal Resolution	Spatial Resolution	Primary Applications	Advantages	Limitations
Structural MRI (sMRI)	Brain anatomy, volume, cortical thickness	N/A (static)	1-2 mm	Volumetric analysis, morphometry, structural abnormalities	Non-invasive, widely available, excellent spatial resolution	Cannot assess function; Limited in understanding dynamic processes
Functional MRI (fMRI)	Blood oxygen level-dependent (BOLD) signal	1-3 seconds	2-4 mm	Neural activation patterns, functional connectivity, task-related changes	Non-invasive, good spatial resolution, no radiation	Indirect measure of neural activity; Sensitive to motion artefacts
Diffusion Tensor Imaging (DTI)	White matter integrity, fibre tracking	N/A (static)	2-3 mm	Connectivity analysis, white matter microstructure	Quantifies white matter pathways, tract-specific analysis	Complex analysis and interpretation challenges with crossing fibres
Magnetic Resonance Spectroscopy (MRS)	Neurochemical concentrations (NAA, glutamate, GABA)	Minutes	1-8 cm^3	Neurotransmitter levels, metabolic changes	Direct measurement of brain chemistry	Lower spatial resolution, technically demanding
Positron Emission Tomography (PET)	Receptor binding, metabolism, neurotransmitter release	Minutes to hours	4-6 mm	Neurotransmitter systems, receptor availability, metabolic activity	Direct measure of neurochemical function	Radiation exposure is expensive and has limited availability
Single Photon Emission Computed Tomography (SPECT)	Regional cerebral blood flow, receptor binding	Minutes to hours	8-10 mm	Cerebral perfusion, dopamine transporter imaging	Lower cost than PET, clinical availability	Lower resolution than PET, radiation exposure

Table 14.2. Summary of key neuroimaging findings across psychiatric disorders

Disorder	Structural Findings	Functional Findings	Connectivity Alterations	Key Biomarkers
Major Depressive Disorder	Reduced volume in ACC, DLPFC, hippocampus, amygdala	Decreased activation in prefrontal regions; Increased amygdala reactivity to negative stimuli	Decreased fronto-limbic connectivity; DMN abnormalities	ACC activity predicts treatment response
Schizophrenia	Enlarged ventricles; Reduced cortical thickness; White matter abnormalities	Prefrontal hypoactivation during working memory; Altered temporal lobe activity	Widespread dysconnectivity; Reduced fronto-temporal connectivity	Striatal dopamine dysfunction; Prefrontal-hippocampal disconnection
PTSD	Reduced hippocampal volume; Grey matter reductions in mPFC	Amygdala hyperactivation; mPFC hypoactivation during fear processing	Decreased amygdala-prefrontal connectivity	Amygdala-mPFC balance during fear extinction
Bipolar Disorder	Enlarged amygdala; Decreased prefrontal cortex volume	Altered limbic-striatal activation; State-dependent prefrontal changes	Abnormal ventral PFC-amygdala connectivity at rest	Structural connectome patterns distinguish MDD
Substance Use Disorders	Reduced Grey matter in prefrontal regions; Striatal atrophy	Decreased striatal response to reward; Increased cue reactivity	Hyperconnectivity of vmPFC-ventral striatum; Hypoconnectivity with amygdala	Reduced D2 receptor availability; Blunted dopamine release
Autism Spectrum Disorder	Enlarged brain volume (early); Reduced cortical thickness (later); Amygdala abnormalities	Decreased DMN connectivity; Altered social processing network activity	Over- and under-connectivity in different networks; White matter disruptions	Early brain overgrowth; Atypical connectivity patterns in infancy

Table 14.3. Machine learning applications in psychiatric neuroimaging

Psychiatric Disorder	ML Technique	Neuroimaging Modality	Sample Size	Accuracy	Key Features	Reference
Major Depressive Disorder	Support Vector Machine	Multisequence MRI	102 participants	85.3%	Hippocampal volume, cortical thickness, and functional connectivity	Li et al., 2023
Bipolar Disorder vs MDD	Machine Learning + Graph Theory	Structural MRI	167 participants	90.3%	Structural connectome metrics, nodal centralities	Zhang et al., 2024
Schizophrenia	Multiple ML algorithms	sMRI + fMRI	Meta-analysis (35 studies)	75-90%	Grey matter volume, functional connectivity patterns	de Filippis et al., 2019
Autism Spectrum Disorder	Hybrid CNN-RNN	sMRI + rs-fMRI	1,112 participants	87.6%	Structural and functional connectivity features	Koc et al., 2023
Substance Use Disorders	Meta-analytic approach	Resting-state fMRI	5,757 participants	Variable	vmPFC-striatum connectivity, reward circuit function	Dugré et al., 2023
PTSD	Multivariate pattern analysis	Task-based fMRI	Meta-analysis	70-85%	Amygdala-prefrontal connectivity during fear processing	Etkin & Wager, 2007

14.6. Autism Spectrum Disorders

Autism spectrum disorder (ASD) is characterised by persistent difficulties in social communication, repetitive behaviours, and restricted interests, with considerable heterogeneity in symptom presentation and severity. Neuroimaging research has revealed atypical brain morphometry, altered functional connectivity, and disruptions in white matter integrity within neural networks supporting social cognition and communication. Structural MRI studies have demonstrated volumetric abnormalities in key brain regions, including an enlarged total brain volume in early childhood, followed by a reduction in cortical thickness in adolescence and adulthood. The amygdala and superior temporal sulcus, critical areas for social processing, show consistent alterations in individuals with ASD.

Functional MRI studies have revealed abnormalities in the default mode network that impair the ability to integrate and process information about oneself in relation to others, as well as to adapt and attend to social stimuli (Kana et al., 2024). Resting-state functional connectivity studies have revealed complex patterns of altered connectivity, with evidence of both overconnectivity and underconnectivity across short- and long-range networks. Task-based functional MRI studies examining social processing have demonstrated atypical regional brain activity in the fusiform face area, the superior temporal sulcus, and the medial prefrontal cortex during face processing and theory-of-mind tasks. These functional abnormalities correlate with the severity of social communication deficits characteristic of ASD.

Diffusion tensor imaging has highlighted disruptions in white matter connectivity, with most studies reporting increased fractional anisotropy and decreased radial diffusivity in various tracts, including the corpus callosum, uncinate fasciculus, and superior longitudinal fasciculus in young children with autism (Lau & Leung, 2024). These white matter alterations suggest that atypical neural connections may underlie the core symptoms of ASD. Longitudinal neuroimaging studies in infants at elevated familial risk for ASD have shown that changes in Grey matter growth and white matter connectivity across the first 6-24 months can robustly predict later ASD diagnosis. Increased extra-axial fluid volume in babies and toddlers who are later diagnosed with ASD has also been reported, suggesting early developmental markers.

Machine learning approaches combined with multimodal neuroimaging have achieved promising results for ASD classification. Koc et al., (2023) demonstrated that hybrid convolutional recurrent neural networks analysing both structural and functional MRI data achieved superior performance compared to single-modality approaches for distinguishing ASD patients from healthy controls. The integration of neuroimaging with genetic and phenotypic data represents an essential direction for understanding the relationship between heterogeneous neuropathological phenotypes and clinical manifestations of ASD. However, the heterogeneity of ASD poses significant challenges for identifying consistent neuroimaging-based biomarkers. Future research must account for individual differences, comorbidities, and developmental trajectories to develop neuroimaging biomarkers with clinical utility for early diagnosis and personalised intervention planning.

14.7. Clinical Implications and Future Directions

The accumulation of neuroimaging findings across psychiatric disorders has substantially advanced our understanding of the neurobiological basis of mental illness. However, translating these findings into clinical practice remains limited. Several key challenges must be addressed to realise the clinical potential of psychiatric neuroimaging. First, the heterogeneity within diagnostic categories poses significant obstacles, as current psychiatric diagnoses are based on symptom clusters rather than underlying neural mechanisms. This heterogeneity contributes to inconsistent findings across studies and limits the specificity of identified biomarkers. Second, small sample sizes in many neuroimaging studies limit statistical power and reduce the replicability of findings. Large-scale collaborative initiatives and data-sharing efforts are essential for overcoming these limitations. Table 14.2 summarises key neuroimaging findings across psychiatric disorders.

The integration of multimodal neuroimaging approaches represents a promising direction for developing more robust and clinically useful biomarkers. Combining structural, functional, and neurochemical imaging with machine learning techniques has demonstrated superior performance compared to single-modality approaches for diagnostic classification and outcome prediction. The development of standardised imaging protocols and analytical pipelines across research sites will be critical for ensuring reproducibility and facilitating meta-analyses. Additionally, longitudinal studies examining individuals from pre-illness stages through disease progression and treatment are needed to distinguish cause from consequence and to identify predictive biomarkers for early intervention. Table 14. 3 shows machine learning applications in psychiatric neuroimaging.

The application of advanced analytical techniques, including machine learning, deep learning, and network-based approaches, holds particular promise for extracting clinically relevant information from complex neuroimaging data. These methods can identify subtle patterns and relationships that may not be apparent through traditional analytical approaches. However, concerns regarding interpretability, generalizability, and clinical implementation must be carefully addressed. The development of explainable artificial intelligence methods that can provide clinically meaningful insights into the features driving classification decisions will be essential for clinical acceptance. Furthermore, prospective validation studies demonstrating the clinical utility and cost-effectiveness of neuroimaging biomarkers are necessary before widespread clinical adoption.

Emerging technologies, including ultra-high-field MRI, advanced diffusion imaging techniques, and novel PET radioligands, continue to expand our ability to characterise brain structure and function with increasing precision. The integration of neuroimaging with other data modalities, including genetics, transcriptomics, proteomics, and digital phenotyping, creates opportunities for developing comprehensive models of psychiatric disorders that span from molecular mechanisms to symptoms and behaviour. Such integrative approaches align with Research Domain Criteria (RDoC) frameworks, which emphasise dimensional constructs that cut across traditional diagnostic boundaries. The ultimate goal is to develop neurobiologically-informed classification systems that can guide personalised treatment selection and improve outcomes for individuals with psychiatric disorders.

The ethical considerations surrounding the clinical use of neuroimaging biomarkers must also be carefully considered. Issues such as privacy, consent, potential misuse of neuroimaging data, and the implications of probabilistic predictions for individuals necessitate thoughtful discussion among researchers, clinicians, ethicists, and patient advocacy groups. As neuroimaging biomarkers move closer to clinical implementation, establishing appropriate guidelines for their responsible use will be essential. The development of psychiatric neuroimaging biomarkers represents a critical step toward achieving Sustainable Development Goal 3 (Good Health and Well-being) by enabling more accurate diagnosis, personalised treatment approaches, and improved outcomes for the millions of individuals affected by mental illness worldwide.

Conclusion

Psychiatric neuroimaging has evolved from a purely research endeavour to an increasingly clinically relevant discipline that enhances our understanding of mental illness and holds promise for transforming diagnostic and therapeutic approaches. The convergence of advanced imaging techniques with computational methods has revealed consistent neurobiological alterations across major psychiatric disorders, fundamentally reshaping conceptualisations of mental illness from purely psychological constructs to conditions with identifiable brain-based substrates. Structural abnormalities in fronto-limbic circuits, disruptions in functional connectivity networks, alterations in neurotransmitter systems, and abnormal patterns of brain development represent core findings that transcend traditional diagnostic boundaries, suggesting shared neurobiological mechanisms underlying diverse clinical presentations.

Despite substantial progress, significant challenges remain in translating neuroimaging discoveries into routine clinical practice. The heterogeneity within diagnostic categories, modest effect sizes of many findings, the limited specificity of biomarkers, and substantial individual variability all constrain the immediate clinical utility. However, integrating multimodal neuroimaging with machine learning approaches demonstrates encouraging diagnostic classification and treatment response prediction accuracy, suggesting feasible pathways toward clinical implementation. Large-scale collaborative initiatives, standardised protocols, and prospective validation studies are essential for establishing neuroimaging biomarkers that meet clinical standards for sensitivity, specificity, and generalizability.

The future of psychiatric neuroimaging lies in personalised medicine approaches that combine neurobiological, genetic, and clinical data to inform individualised treatment selection and predict outcomes. As neuroimaging technologies continue to advance and analytical methods become more sophisticated, the field moves closer to achieving the goal of objective biomarkers that enhance diagnosis, optimise treatment matching, and monitor therapeutic response. These advances directly support Sustainable Development Goal 3 by enabling earlier intervention, reducing treatment-related morbidity, and ultimately improving outcomes for millions affected by psychiatric disorders worldwide.

Acknowledgments

The authors would like to extend our appreciation to those who offered helpful commentary during the drafting process of this manuscript. We also acknowledge the role the Nova Publishing department played in enabling the work described herein.

References

Bremner, J. D. (2011). Functional neuroimaging studies of post-traumatic stress disorder. *Expert Review of Neurotherapeutics, 11*(2), 275-285. https://doi.org/10.1586/ern.10.198.

Chepenik, L. G., Raffo, M., Hampson, M., Lacadie, C., Wang, F., & Jones, M. M. (2017). Brain structure, function, and neurochemistry in schizophrenia and bipolar disorder: A systematic review of the magnetic resonance neuroimaging literature. *npj Schizophrenia, 3*(1), 15. https://doi.org/10.1038/s41537-017-0013-9.

de Filippis, R., Carbone, E. A., Gaetano, R., Bruni, A., Pugliese, V., Segura-Garcia, C., & De Fazio, P. (2019). Machine learning techniques in a structural and functional MRI diagnostic approach in schizophrenia: A systematic review. *Neuropsychiatric Disease and Treatment, 15*, 1605-1627. https://doi.org/10.2147/NDT.S202418.

Dugré, J. R., Orban, P., & Potvin, S. (2023). Disrupted functional connectivity of the brain reward system in substance use problems: A meta-analysis of functional neuroimaging studies. *Addiction Biology, 28*(1), e13257. https://doi.org/10.1111/adb.13257.

Etkin, A., & Wager, T. D. (2007). Functional neuroimaging of anxiety: A meta-analysis of emotional processing in PTSD, social anxiety disorder, and specific phobia. *American Journal of Psychiatry, 164*(10), 1476-1488. https://doi.org/10.1176/appi.ajp.2007.07030504.

Hafeman, D. M., Chang, K. D., Garrett, A. S., Sanders, E. M., & Phillips, M. L. (2012). Effects of medication on neuroimaging findings in bipolar disorder: An updated review. *Bipolar Disorders, 14*(4), 375-410. https://doi.org/10.1111/j.1399-5618.2012.01023.x.

Kana, R. K., Uddin, L. Q., Kenet, T., Chugani, D., & Müller, R. A. (2024). Neuroimaging insights into autism spectrum disorder: Structural and functional brain. *Health Psychology Research, 12*, 123439. https://doi.org/10.52965/001c.123439.

Koc, A., Yildirim, M., & Baygin, M. (2023). Autism spectrum disorder detection by hybrid convolutional recurrent neural networks from structural and resting state functional MRI images. *Autism Research and Treatment, 2023*, 4136087. https://doi.org/10.1155/2023/4136087.

Koob, G. F., & Volkow, N. D. (2016). Neurobiology of addiction: A neurocircuitry analysis. *The Lancet Psychiatry, 3*(8), 760-773. https://doi.org/10.1016/S2215-0366(16)00104-8.

Lai, C. H. (2019). Promising neuroimaging biomarkers in depression. *Psychiatry Investigation, 16*(9), 662-670. https://doi.org/10.30773/pi.2019.07.25.2.

Lai, C. H. (2021). Development of neuroimaging-based biomarkers in major depression. *Advances in Experimental Medicine and Biology, 1305*, 19-33. https://doi.org/10.1007/978-981-33-6044-0_2.

Lau, W. K. W., & Leung, M. K. (2024). Early diagnosis of autism spectrum disorder using structural connectivity biomarker. *Psychoradiology, 4*, kkae004. https://doi.org/10.1093/psyrad/kkae004.

Lee, J., & Chi, S. (2020). Neuroimaging biomarkers for predicting treatment response and recurrence of major depressive disorder. *International Journal of Molecular Sciences, 21*(6), 2148. https://doi.org/10.3390/ijms21062148.

Li, Q., Dong, F., Gai, Q., Che, K., Ma, H., Zhao, F., Chu, T., Mao, N., & Wang, P. (2023). Diagnosis of major depressive disorder using machine learning based on multisequence MRI neuroimaging features. *Journal of Magnetic Resonance Imaging, 58*(5), 1420-1430. https://doi.org/10.1002/jmri.28650.

Murnane, K. S., Edinoff, A. N., Cornett, E. M., & Kaye, A. D. (2023). Updated perspectives on the neurobiology of substance use disorders using neuroimaging. *Substance Abuse and Rehabilitation, 14*, 99-116. https://doi.org/10.2147/SAR.S381832.

Nicholson, A. A., Friston, K. J., Zeidman, P., Harricharan, S., McKinnon, M. C., Densmore, M., Neufeld, R. W., Théberge, J., Corrigan, F., Jetly, R., & Lanius, R. A. (2023). Amygdala downregulation training using fMRI neurofeedback in post-traumatic stress disorder: A randomized, double-blind trial. *Translational Psychiatry, 13*(1), 38. https://doi.org/10.1038/s41398-023-02467-6.

Phillips, M. L., & Kupfer, D. J. (2013). Bipolar disorder diagnosis: Challenges and future directions. *The Lancet, 381*(9878), 1663-1671. https://doi.org/10.1016/S0140-6736(13)60989-7.

Voineskos, A. N., Hawco, C., Neufeld, N. H., Turner, J. A., Ameis, S. H., Anticevic, A., Buchanan, R. W., Cadenhead, K., Dazzan, P., Dickie, E. W., Gallucci, J., Lahti, A. C., Malhotra, A. K., Öngür, D., Lencz, T., Sarpal, D. K., & Oliver, L. D. (2024). Functional magnetic resonance imaging in schizophrenia: Current evidence, methodological advances, limitations and future directions. *World Psychiatry, 23*(1), 26-51. https://doi.org/10.1002/wps.21159.

Zhang, G., Liang, Q., Li, S., Liao, H., & Zhao, J. (2024). Innovative neuroimaging biomarker distinction of major depressive disorder and bipolar disorder through structural connectome analysis and machine learning models. *Biomedicines, 12*(2), 391. https://doi.org/10.3390/biomedicines12020391.

Chapter 15

Artificial Intelligence and Machine Learning in MRI

Kushal Kailash Bothara[1,*]
and Maajid Mohi Ud Din Malik[2,†]

[1]Department of Radio-Diagnosis, Dr. D. Y. Patil Medical College, Hospital and Research Centre, Dr. D. Y. Patil Vidyapeeth (Deemed to be University), Sant Tukaram Nagar, Pimpri, Pune, India
[2]Radiology and Imaging Technology, Dr. D. Y. Patil School of Allied Health Sciences, Dr. D. Y. Patil Vidyapeeth (Deemed to be University), Sant Tukaram Nagar, Pimpri, Pune, India

Abstract

Artificial intelligence (AI) and machine learning (ML) are revolutionising magnetic resonance imaging (MRI) by enhancing image quality, accelerating acquisition times, and improving diagnostic accuracy. This chapter explores the integration of deep learning techniques in MRI image reconstruction, automated segmentation, and diagnostic classification. We examine how convolutional neural networks (CNNs) and other AI architectures are transforming clinical workflows through automated analysis, predictive modelling, and quality control mechanisms. The application of AI in MRI addresses critical challenges, including reducing scan time, detecting artefacts, and addressing inter-observer variability, while raising ethical considerations regarding data privacy, algorithmic bias, and clinical validation. This chapter provides a comprehensive overview of current AI applications in MRI, discusses implementation challenges, and outlines future directions for this rapidly evolving field. The integration of AI technologies aligns with Sustainable Development Goal 3 (Good Health and Well-being) by improving access to accurate diagnostic imaging and enhancing the efficiency of healthcare delivery.

Keywords: artificial intelligence, machine learning, deep learning, mri reconstruction, image segmentation, diagnostic classification, convolutional neural networks, SDG 3 - good health and well-being

---

* Corresponding Author's Email: Kushal.Bothara@dpu.edu.in
† Corresponding Author's Email: maajid.malik@dpu.edu.in

In: Recent Advances in Magnetic Resonance Imaging in Neuroimaging
Editors: Maajid Mohi Ud Din Malik, Purnachandra Kawdu Lamghare and R. S. Kuber
ISBN: 979-8-90134-244-2

Introduction

The convergence of artificial intelligence and magnetic resonance imaging represents one of the most significant technological advances in modern medical imaging, fundamentally transforming how we acquire, analyse, and interpret diagnostic images. Over the past decade, machine learning algorithms, intensive learning neural networks, have demonstrated unprecedented capabilities in addressing longstanding challenges in MRI, including lengthy scan times, image artefacts, variability in subjective interpretation, and labour-intensive quantitative analysis. These AI-powered solutions are transitioning from research laboratories into clinical practice, with several systems already receiving regulatory approval and many more in various stages of clinical validation (Lundervold & Lundervold, 2019).

The application of AI in MRI encompasses the entire imaging pipeline, from initial data acquisition through final clinical decision-making. Deep learning networks can reconstruct high-quality images from undersampled data, enabling dramatic reductions in scan time without compromising diagnostic quality. Automated segmentation algorithms can delineate anatomical structures and pathological tissues with human-level accuracy in minutes, rather than hours, facilitating the extraction of quantitative biomarkers and longitudinal disease monitoring. Diagnostic classification systems can detect and characterise diseases with performance approaching or exceeding that of expert radiologists in specific tasks, potentially improving diagnostic accuracy and consistency, particularly in settings with limited subspecialty expertise (Akkus et al., 2017).

Beyond these established applications, AI is enabling entirely new capabilities, such as predictive modelling of disease progression and treatment response, automated quality control to ensure consistent image quality, and the integration of multimodal data sources to support precision medicine approaches. However, the clinical implementation of AI in MRI also raises essential considerations regarding algorithmic bias, data privacy, clinical validation, and equitable access that must be thoughtfully addressed to ensure these powerful technologies benefit all patients (Char et al., 2020). This chapter provides a comprehensive examination of current AI applications in MRI, their clinical impact, implementation challenges, and future directions for this rapidly evolving field.

15.1. Deep Learning for Image Reconstruction

The application of deep learning to MRI image reconstruction represents one of the most transformative advances in medical imaging technology. Traditional MRI reconstruction methods rely on mathematical algorithms, such as Fourier transforms and iterative optimisation techniques, that are effective but often require lengthy computation times and produce images with inherent limitations in signal-to-noise ratio and spatial resolution. Deep learning approaches, particularly convolutional neural networks (CNNs), have demonstrated remarkable capabilities for learning complex mappings between undersampled k-space data and fully sampled images, enabling significant reductions in scan time while maintaining, or even improving, image quality (Hammernik et al., 2018).

The fundamental principle underlying deep learning reconstruction is to train neural networks on large datasets of paired undersampled and fully sampled MRI data. These networks learn to predict high-quality images directly from accelerated acquisitions by identifying patterns and relationships that traditional reconstruction algorithms cannot capture. U-Net architectures, initially developed for biomedical image segmentation, have been successfully adapted for MRI reconstruction tasks due to their ability to capture both local and global image features through encoder-decoder structures with skip connections (Ronneberger et al., 2015). These skip connections preserve spatial information across different resolution scales, which is crucial for maintaining fine anatomical details in reconstructed images.

One of the most significant applications of deep learning reconstruction is in compressed sensing MRI, where data is acquired using variable-density sampling patterns that violate the Nyquist sampling theorem. Traditional compressed sensing reconstruction requires solving complex optimisation problems with sparsity constraints, which can be computationally intensive. Deep learning networks can perform similar or superior reconstruction in a fraction of the time by learning the underlying manifold of MRI images during training. Studies have shown that deep learning methods can achieve acceleration factors of four to ten times while maintaining diagnostic image quality comparable to fully sampled acquisitions (Hammernik et al., 2018).

Generative adversarial networks (GANs) represent another promising approach to MRI reconstruction, utilising a competitive framework between a generator network that produces reconstructed images and a discriminator network that evaluates their authenticity. This adversarial training process encourages the generator to create images that are perceptually indistinguishable from fully sampled references, potentially capturing texture and fine details that may be lost with other reconstruction methods. However, GAN-based reconstruction also raises concerns about introducing artificial features or hallucinations that could mislead diagnostic interpretation, necessitating careful validation before clinical deployment (Dar et al., 2020).

The integration of physics-based models with deep learning, known as model-based deep learning or unrolled optimisation networks, represents a hybrid approach that combines the interpretability of traditional methods with the learning capacity of neural networks. These architectures incorporate known physical constraints of MRI signal formation, such as coil sensitivity profiles and k-space sampling patterns, directly into the network structure. By embedding domain knowledge into the learning process, model-based networks often require less training data and generalise better across different imaging protocols and anatomies than purely data-driven approaches. Variational networks and recurrent inference machines exemplify this paradigm, showing robust performance across various acceleration factors and anatomical regions (Hammernik et al., 2018). Table 15.1 compares deep learning reconstruction methods for MRI.

Table 15.1. Comparison of deep learning reconstruction methods for MRI

Method	Architecture	Acceleration Factor	Advantages	Limitations	Clinical Status
CNN-based	U-Net, ResNet	2-6x	Fast inference, well-established	May over-smooth details	FDA-approved systems available
GAN-based	DCGAN, StyleGAN	4-10x	Preserves texture, perceptually sharp	Risk of hallucinations, training instability	Research stage
Model-based	Variational Networks, Unrolled	3-8x	Physics-informed, interpretable	Complex implementation	Early clinical adoption
Recurrent	ConvLSTM, GRU	4-8x	Temporal consistency for dynamic imaging	Higher computational cost	Research stage
Hybrid	Combined approaches	5-12x	Leverages multiple strengths	Increased model complexity	Emerging technology

Real-time MRI applications, such as cardiac imaging and MRI-guided interventions, particularly benefit from deep learning reconstruction techniques. These applications require high temporal resolution to capture rapidly changing anatomical structures and physiological processes, which traditionally necessitates significant trade-offs among spatial, temporal, and image quality. Deep learning networks trained on temporal sequences can exploit spatiotemporal correlations to reconstruct dynamic images from highly undersampled data, enabling frame rates that were previously unattainable. This capability is especially valuable in cardiac MRI, where capturing rapid cardiac motion with adequate spatial detail is essential for assessing myocardial function and detecting subtle abnormalities (Bai et al., 2018).

The clinical translation of deep learning reconstruction presents several significant challenges that must be addressed for its widespread adoption. Generalisation across different scanner manufacturers, field strengths, and imaging protocols remains a considerable concern, as networks trained on data from specific acquisition parameters may not perform optimally when applied to different settings. Transfer learning and domain adaptation techniques are being explored to enhance model robustness and minimise the need for extensive retraining when deploying models across diverse clinical environments. Additionally, regulatory approval processes require comprehensive validation demonstrating that AI-reconstructed images maintain diagnostic equivalence to traditional methods across various pathologies and patient populations (Finlayson et al., 2021).

15.2. Automated Segmentation and Analysis

Automated segmentation of anatomical structures and pathological tissues in MRI represents a critical application of machine learning that addresses one of the most time-consuming and subjective aspects of medical image analysis. Manual segmentation by radiologists or trained technicians can require hours of painstaking labour for complex three-dimensional anatomies, introducing inter-observer variability that can affect diagnostic consistency and treatment planning accuracy. Deep learning algorithms, particularly fully convolutional networks and their variants, have achieved near-human or superhuman performance in segmenting various anatomical structures, dramatically reducing analysis time while improving reproducibility (Ronneberger et al., 2015).

The U-Net architecture and its numerous derivatives have become the de facto standard for medical image segmentation tasks, including MRI analysis. The symmetric encoder-decoder architecture of the U-Net, combined with skip connections that preserve spatial information across different resolution levels, enables precise boundary delineation even for structures with complex geometries and variable appearances. The encoder pathway captures contextual information through progressive downsampling, while the decoder pathway recovers spatial resolution for pixel-wise classification. This architecture has been successfully applied to segment brain structures, cardiac chambers, abdominal organs, tumours, and many other anatomical and pathological features across diverse MRI sequences and protocols (Ronneberger et al., 2015).

Brain MRI segmentation represents one of the most mature applications of automated analysis, with algorithms capable of accurately delineating Grey matter, white matter, cerebrospinal fluid, and numerous subcortical structures. These segmentations enable quantitative assessment of brain volumes, which is crucial for monitoring neurodegenerative diseases such as Alzheimer's disease and multiple sclerosis. Longitudinal studies tracking disease progression rely heavily on accurate, reproducible measurements of structural changes over time, making automated segmentation an essential tool for both clinical practice and research studies. Modern deep learning approaches can segment dozens of brain structures in minutes, compared to hours required for manual annotation, while achieving superior consistency across repeated scans and different operators (Akkus et al., 2017).

Cardiac MRI segmentation presents unique challenges due to the heart's complex anatomy and the continuous motion it undergoes throughout the cardiac cycle. Automated segmentation of the left and right ventricles, myocardium, and atria from cine MRI sequences enables calculation of clinically significant functional parameters such as ejection fraction, cardiac output, and myocardial mass. These quantitative biomarkers are essential for diagnosing and monitoring cardiovascular diseases, which remain the leading cause of mortality worldwide. Deep learning networks trained on large annotated cardiac MRI datasets can segment cardiac chambers across all phases of the cardiac cycle with high accuracy, facilitating comprehensive functional assessment that would be impractical with manual methods. The temporal consistency of automated segmentation across the cardiac cycle also improves the reliability of derived functional measurements (Bernard et al., 2018).

Tumour segmentation in MRI poses particular challenges due to the heterogeneous appearance of neoplastic tissues, infiltrative growth patterns, and variable contrast enhancement. Glioblastoma segmentation from multi-parametric brain MRI, for instance, requires delineating multiple tumour components, including the enhancing tumour, the non-enhancing tumour core, and the surrounding oedema, each with distinct therapeutic and prognostic implications. The annual Brain Tumour Segmentation (BraTS) challenge has driven significant advances in this domain, with top-performing methods now achieving Dice coefficients exceeding 0.90 for enhancing tumour segmentation. These automated segmentation tools are being integrated into radiation therapy planning systems, where accurate tumour delineation is crucial for targeting treatment while minimising damage to healthy tissue (Bakas et al., 2018).

Multi-organ segmentation in abdominal MRI exemplifies the complexity of anatomical variability and the challenge of segmenting structures with similar signal intensities. The liver, spleen, kidneys, pancreas, and gastrointestinal organs are all visible on abdominal scans, often with overlapping intensity profiles that make differentiation difficult. Advanced network architectures incorporating attention mechanisms and multi-scale feature fusion have improved performance on these challenging tasks by enabling the model to focus on relevant features while suppressing background information. Automated abdominal organ segmentation supports various clinical applications, including surgical planning, disease staging, and assessment of organ volumes and fat distribution patterns associated with metabolic diseases (Akkus et al., 2017).

The integration of uncertainty estimation into segmentation algorithms represents an essential advancement for clinical translation, as it provides confidence measures for each prediction that can alert clinicians to potentially problematic results. Bayesian deep learning approaches and ensemble methods can quantify prediction uncertainty, highlighting regions where the model is less confident and may require human review for further refinement. This capability is particularly valuable in challenging cases with unusual anatomy, artefacts, or pathology that deviates from the training distribution. Uncertainty-aware segmentation systems can improve clinical trust and safety by explicitly acknowledging the limitations of automated analysis rather than presenting potentially erroneous results with unwarranted confidence (Bernard et al., 2018).

15.3. AI-Based Diagnosis and Classification

The application of artificial intelligence to MRI diagnostic classification has demonstrated impressive capabilities for detecting and characterising diseases across multiple organ systems and pathological conditions. Deep learning models trained on large, annotated datasets can learn complex patterns associated with specific diseases, often identifying subtle features that may be overlooked by human observers or that reflect relationships too intricate for explicit rule-based algorithms. These diagnostic support systems have the potential to improve detection rates, reduce interpretation errors, and provide consistent second opinions that enhance diagnostic confidence, particularly in settings with limited access to subspecialty expertise (Lundervold & Lundervold, 2019).

Neurological disease classification is among the most extensively studied applications of AI in MRI diagnostics. Convolutional neural networks have been trained to differentiate between various types of dementia, classify brain tumours by histological grade and molecular subtype, detect multiple sclerosis lesions, and identify acute ischemic stroke. In Alzheimer's disease detection, deep learning models analysing structural MRI can predict conversion from mild cognitive impairment to

Alzheimer's dementia with accuracy exceeding traditional biomarker-based approaches, potentially enabling earlier intervention when disease-modifying treatments may be most effective. The ability to extract prognostic information from routine imaging studies adds significant clinical value beyond traditional diagnostic classification (Akkus et al., 2017).

Oncological applications of AI-based classification encompass tumour detection, characterisation, and assessment of treatment response across diverse anatomical sites. In prostate MRI, deep learning algorithms have demonstrated performance comparable to that of expert radiologists in detecting clinically significant prostate cancer, using multi-parametric imaging protocols that combine T2-weighted, diffusion-weighted, and dynamic contrast-enhanced sequences. These systems can help standardise interpretation using structured reporting frameworks such as PI-RADS, thereby reducing inter-observer variability, a persistent challenge in prostate cancer diagnosis. Similarly, in breast MRI, AI algorithms can distinguish between benign and malignant lesions, prioritise suspicious findings for review, and potentially reduce false-positive rates that lead to unnecessary biopsies (Litjens et al., 2014). Table 15.2 shows performance metrics of AI diagnostic systems in MRI applications.

Table 15.2. Performance metrics of AI diagnostic systems in MRI applications

Application	Disease/ Condition	Dataset Size	Sensitivity (%)	Specificity (%)	AUC	Reference Standard	Clinical Impact
Brain	Alzheimer's Disease	1,200 patients	92.5	89.7	0.96	Clinical diagnosis + CSF biomarkers	Early detection support
Brain	Glioblastoma vs. Metastases	850 cases	88.3	91.2	0.94	Histopathology	Treatment planning guidance
Prostate	Clinically Significant Cancer	1,500 patients	91.8	87.4	0.93	Biopsy/ Pathology	Biopsy decision support
Cardiac	Myocardial Infarction	980 patients	94.2	88.9	0.95	Clinical outcomes	Risk stratification
Musculoskeletal	ACL Tear Detection	1,750 cases	93.7	89.5	0.94	Arthroscopy/ Surgery	Pre-surgical assessment
Liver	Cirrhosis Stageing	680 patients	86.5	84.3	0.91	Biopsy/Clinical staging	Non-invasive monitoring

The classification of musculoskeletal pathology on MRI has benefited substantially from deep learning, with applications ranging from detecting meniscal and ligament tears in knee MRIs to assessing rotator cuff injuries in shoulder imaging. These algorithms can analyse multiple MRI sequences simultaneously, integrating information from different imaging contrasts to improve diagnostic accuracy. In a landmark study, a deep learning model trained on knee MRI scans achieved diagnostic performance statistically equivalent to that of board-certified musculoskeletal radiologists in detecting anterior cruciate ligament tears, meniscal tears, and cartilage abnormalities. Such systems could serve as decision-support tools in emergency departments or primary care settings where immediate access to subspecialty radiology expertise may be limited (Bien et al., 2018).

Cardiac MRI classification applications address various aspects of cardiovascular disease, including the detection of myocardial infarction, characterisation of cardiomyopathy, and assessment of congenital heart disease. Deep learning models can analyse both structural images and functional parameters derived from cine sequences to classify cardiac pathology and predict clinical outcomes. For instance, algorithms trained to identify patterns of delayed gadolinium enhancement in cardiac MRI can detect myocardial scar tissue indicative of previous infarction and predict risk of future adverse cardiac events. The integration of multiple imaging biomarkers through deep learning may provide more comprehensive risk assessment than traditional clinical scoring systems (Bai et al., 2018).

The challenge of algorithmic interpretability is a significant consideration in diagnostic AI, as clinicians need to understand the basis for AI-generated predictions to integrate them into clinical decision-making appropriately. Black-box neural networks, although highly accurate, do not inherently provide explanations for their classifications, which can potentially limit clinical acceptance and trust. Explainable AI techniques, such as gradient-weighted class activation mapping (Grad-CAM) and attention mechanisms, can visualise which image regions most significantly influence the network's decision, providing valuable insights into the model's reasoning process. These visualisation tools help validate that the network is focusing on clinically relevant features rather than spurious correlations or artefacts, and they can serve as educational tools by highlighting subtle findings that may warrant closer human review (Selvaraju et al., 2017).

The performance of AI diagnostic systems in controlled research settings often exceeds their effectiveness in real-world clinical deployment, a phenomenon known as the AI chasm. Factors contributing to this gap include differences between carefully curated research datasets and heterogeneous clinical data, variations in imaging protocols across institutions, the evolution of disease definitions and diagnostic criteria, and the challenge of integrating AI outputs into existing clinical workflows. Prospective clinical trials evaluating AI diagnostic tools in actual practice settings, rather than retrospective analyses of historical data, are essential for demonstrating real-world utility and identifying implementation barriers that must be addressed for successful clinical translation (Finlayson et al., 2021).

15.4. Predictive Modelling and Prognosis

Predictive modelling using machine learning extends beyond diagnostic classification to estimate future clinical outcomes, disease progression trajectories, and treatment responses based on MRI features. These prognostic models integrate quantitative imaging biomarkers with clinical variables to generate personalised risk assessments that can inform treatment selection and intensity. Radiomics approaches, which extract large numbers of quantitative features describing image texture, shape, and intensity distributions, combined with machine learning classifiers, have shown promise in predicting outcomes across various diseases. The ability to extract prognostic information from routine clinical imaging could transform MRI from a purely diagnostic modality to a tool for precision medicine and individualised patient management (Gillies et al., 2016).

In oncology, predictive models trained on MRI data can estimate tumour aggressiveness, the likelihood of metastatic spread, and the probability of treatment response, all of which influence therapeutic decisions. For glioblastoma, the most aggressive primary brain tumour, machine learning models analysing pre-treatment MRI features have predicted overall survival with modest but clinically useful accuracy, potentially identifying patients who may benefit from more intensive treatment regimens. Similarly, in rectal cancer, MRI-based predictive models can estimate the likelihood of complete response to neoadjuvant chemoradiotherapy, information that may support consideration of organ-preserving approaches in selected patients rather than mandatory surgery. These applications exemplify how predictive modelling can facilitate more nuanced, patient-specific treatment planning rather than one-size-fits-all protocols (Kickingereder et al., 2016).

Cardiovascular prognostic models leverage cardiac MRI to predict adverse events such as heart failure hospitalisation, arrhythmias, and mortality. Beyond traditional functional parameters, such as ejection fraction, machine learning algorithms can incorporate tissue characterisation data, including patterns of myocardial fibrosis detected on late gadolinium enhancement imaging and quantitative T1- and T2-mapping parameters. These comprehensive assessments of cardiac structure and tissue composition provide a more complete picture of cardiovascular health than conventional measures alone. Studies have demonstrated that AI models integrating multiple cardiac MRI biomarkers can outperform established clinical risk scores in predicting outcomes, potentially enabling more accurate risk stratification for preventive interventions such as implantable cardioverter-defibrillator placement (Bai et al., 2018).

Neurodegenerative disease progression modelling is another critical application, in which longitudinal MRI studies tracking structural brain changes over time can be analysed using machine learning to predict cognitive decline trajectories. In Alzheimer's disease research, models incorporating patterns of brain atrophy, white matter lesion burden, and connectivity changes from diffusion MRI can estimate the rate of future cognitive deterioration and time to conversion from mild cognitive impairment to dementia. These predictive capabilities are particularly valuable in clinical trial design, enabling enrichment strategies that identify participants most likely to show measurable progression during the trial, thereby improving statistical power and potentially accelerating drug development timelines (Akkus et al., 2017).

The integration of radiomics with genomics and other omics data creates opportunities for truly multimodal predictive models that capture disease characteristics across different biological scales. In cancer research, radiogenomics studies have identified correlations between MRI features and molecular characteristics, including gene expression patterns and mutational profiles. Machine learning models that integrate imaging and molecular data can predict which tumours harbour specific genetic alterations associated with treatment response or prognosis, potentially enabling non-invasive molecular profiling that guides targeted therapy selection. This convergence of imaging and molecular biomarkers exemplifies the potential for AI to advance precision medicine by synthesising diverse data sources into actionable clinical predictions (Kickingereder et al., 2016).

Treatment response assessment during therapy represents an actionable application of predictive modelling, in which early MRI changes can be analysed to predict ultimate treatment outcomes before they become clinically apparent. In cancer immunotherapy, for example, conventional response assessment criteria may not capture the complex patterns of tumour response and pseudoprogression that can occur with immune checkpoint inhibitors. Machine learning models that analyse longitudinal MRI studies during treatment can potentially distinguish actual progression from inflammatory pseudoprogression earlier than traditional methods, enabling more timely decisions about treatment continuation or modification. Similar approaches in stroke rehabilitation can predict functional recovery based on early post-stroke MRI findings, informing rehabilitation intensity and discharge planning (Gillies et al., 2016).

The clinical utility of prognostic models depends not only on predictive accuracy but also on how the predictions change clinical management and ultimately patient outcomes. Decision curve analysis and other methods that quantify the net benefit of using predictive models compared to default strategies provide essential insights into clinical value beyond statistical performance metrics, such as the area under the receiver operating characteristic curve. A highly accurate model that does not lead to different treatment decisions or improved outcomes may have limited practical utility despite impressive performance statistics. Prospective studies demonstrating that AI-based prognostic models improve patient outcomes by enabling better treatment selection or risk stratification are essential for establishing their clinical value and justifying their integration into routine practice (Finlayson et al., 2021).

15.5. Quality Control and Artefact Detection

Quality control represents a critical but often overlooked application of artificial intelligence in MRI, addressing the challenge of ensuring consistent image quality across diverse scanning protocols, equipment, and patient populations. Poor image quality due to motion artefacts, an insufficient signal-to-noise ratio, improper patient positioning, or technical malfunctions can compromise diagnostic accuracy and necessitate repeat scans, which waste resources and inconvenience patients. AI-based quality control systems can automatically assess image quality in real-time or immediately post-acquisition, flagging problematic scans for technologist review or automated correction. These systems have the potential to reduce repeat scan rates, improve workflow efficiency, and ensure that referring physicians receive diagnostic images that are adequate for their purposes (Reuter et al., 2015).

Motion artefacts are among the most common causes of degraded MRI quality, arising from patient movement during the relatively long acquisition times required for most MRI sequences. Deep learning networks can be trained to detect various types of motion artefacts, including ghosting from periodic motion, blurring from continuous motion, and ringing from abrupt movement. Beyond detection, some AI systems can actually correct motion artefacts through image post-processing, effectively recovering diagnostic image quality without requiring repeat scans. Motion-corrected reconstruction networks, which estimate and compensate for motion during reconstruction, integrate quality control and image reconstruction, demonstrating how AI can address multiple challenges simultaneously (Duffy et al., 2021).

Automated protocol compliance checking is another valuable quality control application that verifies that acquired images meet the specifications required for specific diagnostic tasks or multicenter research studies. In clinical trials, protocol deviations represent a significant source of unusable data and can compromise study validity. AI systems can automatically review imaging parameters, coverage, and quality metrics to ensure compliance with study protocols, providing immediate feedback to technologists so that any deficiencies can be corrected during the same scanning session. This real-time quality assurance capability is particularly valuable in multicenter studies, where maintaining standardisation across sites with different equipment and practices is challenging (Reuter et al., 2015). Table 15.3 shows AI applications in MRI quality control and artefact detection.

Table 15.3. AI applications in MRI quality control and artefact detection

Quality Issue	Detection Method	Correction Capability	Implementation Stage	Clinical Impact	Reduction in Repeat Scans
Patient Motion	CNN-based classifiers	Retrospective motion correction	Clinical deployment	High - common artefact	15-25% reduction
Insufficient SNR	Image quality metrics + ML	Limited - may suggest protocol adjustment	Clinical trials	Moderate	5-10% reduction
Aliasing/Wrap-around	Feature detection algorithms	Automated unwrapping	Mature technology	Moderate	3-5% reduction
Susceptibility artifacts	Spatial distortion analysis	Field map correction	Clinical deployment	Variable by anatomy	N/A - correction primary
Incomplete coverage	3D volume analysis	None - requires re-scan	Early clinical adoption	Moderate	8-12% reduction
Contrast timing errors	Dynamic series analysis	Limited - may estimate optimal phase	Research stage	Low - protocol-dependent	2-4% reduction

Artefact detection systems can identify a wide range of image quality problems beyond motion, including aliasing artefacts resulting from an inadequate field of view, susceptibility artefacts near air-tissue interfaces, radiofrequency inhomogeneity causing uneven signal across the image, and various technical artefacts related to gradient performance or radiofrequency coil malfunction. Training neural networks to recognise these diverse artefact types requires large datasets annotated by expert reviewers, as artefact appearance can be subtle and varied. Transfer learning approaches, where networks pre-trained on general image classification tasks are fine-tuned for artefact detection, can help address the challenge of limited training data by leveraging features learned from other domains (Duffy et al., 2021).

The integration of quality control AI into MRI scanner consoles or picture archiving and communication systems (PACS) enables automated quality assessment as part of the routine clinical workflow. Real-time quality metrics can be displayed during scanning, allowing technologists to identify problems immediately rather than discovering them only after the patient has left. For outpatients, this capability avoids the need to recall patients for repeat scans, improving patient satisfaction and reducing costs. For inpatients or patients under sedation, preventing the need for repeat scanning is even more valuable given the complexity of patient transport and sedation administration. The seamless integration of quality control AI into existing infrastructure represents a vital usability consideration for successful clinical adoption (Reuter et al., 2015).

Quality control AI also has essential applications in ensuring consistent image quality in longitudinal studies, such as monitoring disease progression or treatment response. Automated co-registration and comparison of serial scans can detect subtle changes in image quality, patient positioning, or acquisition parameters that might affect the accuracy of longitudinal measurements. This capability is critical in clinical trials where quantitative imaging biomarkers serve as endpoints, as changes in image quality over time could be misinterpreted as disease progression or treatment effects. AI-based quality control provides an objective, reproducible assessment, thereby enhancing the reliability of longitudinal imaging studies (Reuter et al., 2015).

The economic value of AI quality control extends beyond the direct costs of repeat scans to include factors such as scanner utilisation efficiency, patient satisfaction, and radiologist productivity. Reducing the proportion of non-diagnostic scans that reach radiologists for interpretation saves reading time that can be redirected to other cases. Moreover, by catching quality problems at the point of acquisition rather than after the fact, AI quality control prevents delays in diagnosis that can occur when poor-quality images necessitate repeat studies. These indirect benefits, while more challenging to quantify than direct cost savings, contribute substantially to the overall value proposition of AI quality control systems (Finlayson et al., 2021).

15.6. Ethical Considerations and Clinical Implementation

The integration of artificial intelligence into clinical MRI practice raises profound ethical considerations that must be carefully addressed to ensure that these powerful technologies benefit patients and society while minimising potential harms. Issues of algorithmic bias, data privacy, informed consent, clinical validation, liability, and equitable access all require thoughtful consideration and the development of appropriate governance frameworks. The development and deployment of AI systems in healthcare carry unique responsibilities given the high stakes of medical decision-making and the vulnerability of patient populations. Ensuring that AI technologies align with core medical ethics principles, including beneficence, non-maleficence, autonomy, and justice, is essential for maintaining public trust and realising the potential benefits of these innovations (Char et al., 2020).

Algorithmic bias is one of the most significant ethical concerns in medical AI. When training datasets fail to adequately reflect the diversity of the patient populations these systems will ultimately serve, these systems will ultimately serve. If AI models are trained predominantly on data from certain demographic groups, they may perform poorly on underrepresented populations, potentially exacerbating existing healthcare disparities. Studies have documented performance differences in AI diagnostic systems across racial and ethnic groups, age ranges, and between male and female patients, often reflecting imbalances in the training data composition. Ensuring diverse and representative training datasets and rigorously testing AI systems across different patient subgroups are crucial steps toward the fair and equitable deployment of AI. Ongoing monitoring of AI performance across demographic categories in clinical use is also necessary to detect and address bias that may emerge over time (Obermeyer et al., 2019).

Data privacy and security considerations are particularly acute in medical AI, given the sensitivity of health information and the large datasets required for training robust models. The aggregation of imaging data from multiple institutions for AI development creates risks of data breaches, unauthorised access, and potential re-identification of supposedly de-identified images. Federated learning approaches, where models are trained on distributed datasets without centralising the data itself, offer a possible solution to privacy concerns by allowing institutions to contribute to model development while retaining their data locally. Differential privacy techniques, which add controlled noise to prevent the identification of individual data points, represent another approach to protecting patient privacy in AI training datasets. Clear policies regarding data ownership, use restrictions, and patient consent for AI development are necessary to maintain ethical standards (Char et al., 2020).

Informed consent for AI-assisted diagnosis and treatment planning poses complex challenges, as patients may not fully understand how AI algorithms arrive at their predictions or the level of evidence supporting their use in specific clinical contexts. Should patients be explicitly informed when AI systems contribute to their diagnosis or treatment decisions, and if so, what level of detail is appropriate and meaningful? The concept of algorithmic transparency conflicts with the inherent complexity of many deep learning models, where even developers cannot fully explain individual predictions. Developing appropriate consent frameworks that respect patient autonomy while acknowledging the technical complexity of AI systems requires ongoing dialogue among clinicians, ethicists, patients, and AI developers (Char et al., 2020).

Clinical validation of AI systems presents unique challenges compared to traditional medical devices, as AI algorithms can continue learning and evolving after initial deployment, potentially changing their behaviour over time. The distinction between locked algorithms that remain fixed after regulatory approval and adaptive algorithms that continuously update raises questions about appropriate validation standards and regulatory oversight. Prospective clinical trials demonstrating that AI systems improve patient outcomes, not just diagnostic accuracy metrics, represent the gold standard for validation; however, they are resource-intensive and may slow innovation. Balancing the need for rigorous evidence with the pace of AI advancement requires thoughtful regulatory frameworks that ensure safety and efficacy without stifling innovation (Finlayson et al., 2021).

Liability and accountability questions arise when AI systems contribute to diagnostic errors or adverse patient outcomes. If an AI algorithm fails to detect a significant finding that a human radiologist also misses, should liability be shared between the human and algorithmic components of the diagnostic process? If an AI system produces a false positive that leads to unnecessary invasive procedures, who bears responsibility? Legal frameworks have not yet fully addressed these questions, leaving healthcare providers and AI developers in uncertainty. Clear documentation of AI's involvement in clinical decision-making, along with well-defined roles for AI as a decision-support system rather than an autonomous decision-maker, can help clarify accountability and responsibility. However, more comprehensive legal and regulatory guidance is needed (Char et al., 2020).

The impact of AI on the radiologist workforce and professional practice represents another critical consideration. While some have feared that AI will replace radiologists, the more likely scenario is that AI will augment radiologists' capabilities and transform their role. Radiologists may shift their focus from routine image interpretation tasks, which are increasingly handled by AI, toward complex cases that require expert judgment, effective communication with referring physicians and patients, image-guided procedures, and oversight of AI systems. Medical education will need to evolve to prepare future radiologists for this AI-augmented practice environment, incorporating training in AI principles, validation methods, and appropriate integration of AI tools into clinical workflows. Professional societies and training programs are beginning to address these educational needs, but significant work remains (Lundervold & Lundervold, 2019).

Equitable access to AI technologies represents a justice consideration, as advanced AI capabilities may initially be available only at well-resourced academic medical centres, potentially widening disparities between these institutions and community hospitals or practices in underserved areas. The cost of developing, validating, and implementing AI systems creates barriers to widespread adoption that could disadvantage patients without access to advanced care centres. Conversely, AI could potentially reduce disparities by bringing expert-level diagnostic capabilities to settings that lack subspecialty expertise, if implemented thoughtfully with attention to accessibility and affordability. Ensuring that the benefits of AI in MRI are broadly distributed rather than concentrated among privileged populations should be an explicit goal of health policy and AI development efforts (Obermeyer et al., 2019).

Conclusion

Artificial intelligence and machine learning have already demonstrated transformative potential across the entire spectrum of MRI applications, from image acquisition and reconstruction through diagnosis, prognosis, and quality assurance. Deep learning techniques have achieved remarkable performance in tasks ranging from accelerating imaging to detecting subtle pathology, often matching or exceeding human expert capabilities in controlled research settings. The continued rapid advancement of AI methods, combined with the growing availability of large annotated imaging datasets and increasing computational resources, suggests that AI's impact on MRI will continue to expand and deepen in the years to come.

The successful translation of AI innovations from research prototypes to routine clinical tools requires addressing multiple technical, clinical, ethical, and regulatory challenges. Ensuring that AI systems generalise robustly across diverse patient populations, imaging equipment, and clinical settings remains a significant technical challenge. Establishing appropriate validation frameworks that demonstrate not just accuracy but actual improvement in patient outcomes will be essential for widespread clinical adoption. Addressing ethical concerns related to bias, privacy, consent, and accountability through thoughtful governance and ongoing vigilance is crucial to maintaining public trust and ensuring equitable access to AI benefits (Char et al., 2020).

The evolution of MRI practice in an AI-augmented future will likely involve a collaborative partnership between human expertise and machine intelligence, leveraging the complementary strengths of each. AI systems excel at consistently processing large volumes of data, detecting subtle patterns, and performing repetitive tasks with precision and accuracy. In contrast, human clinicians bring contextual understanding, clinical judgment, communication skills, and ethical reasoning that current AI cannot replicate. The optimal integration of AI into the MRI workflow should enhance, rather than replace, human capabilities, enabling radiologists and other clinicians to focus their expertise where it provides the most value (Lundervold & Lundervold, 2019).

The alignment of AI applications in MRI with broader global health goals, particularly Sustainable Development Goal 3, which focuses on health and well-being, highlights the potential for these technologies to address pressing healthcare challenges. By improving diagnostic accuracy, reducing costs, accelerating image interpretation, and potentially democratizing access to expert-level analysis, AI could contribute to more effective and equitable healthcare delivery globally. Realising this potential will require intentional efforts to ensure that AI development and deployment prioritise patient benefit, address healthcare disparities, and align with the fundamental ethical principles that guide medical practice. As the field continues to mature, ongoing collaboration among AI researchers, clinicians, ethicists, regulators, and patient advocates will be essential to navigate the complex landscape of AI in medical imaging and ensure that these powerful technologies serve humanity's best interests (Finlayson et al., 2021).

Acknowledgments

The authors would like to extend our appreciation to those who offered helpful commentary during the drafting process of this manuscript. We also acknowledge the role the Nova Publishing department played in enabling the work described herein.

References

Akkus, Z., Galimzianova, A., Hoogi, A., Rubin, D. L., & Erickson, B. J. (2017). Deep learning for brain MRI segmentation: State of the art and future directions. *Journal of Digital Imaging*, 30(4), 449-459. https://doi.org/10.1007/s10278-017-9983-4.

Bai, W., Sinclair, M., Tarroni, G., Oktay, O., Rajchl, M., Vaillant, G., Lee, A. M., Aung, N., Lukaschuk, E., Sanghvi, M. M., Zemrak, F., Fung, K., Paiva, J. M., Carapella, V., Kim, Y. J., Suzuki, H., Kainz, B., Matthews, P. M., Petersen, S. E., Rueckert, D. (2018). Automated cardiovascular magnetic resonance image analysis with fully convolutional networks. *Journal of Cardiovascular Magnetic Resonance*, 20(1), 65. https://doi.org/10.1186/s12968-018-0471-x.

Bakas, S., Reyes, M., Jakab, A., Bauer, S., Rondina, M., Crimi, A., Shinohara, R. T., Berger, C., Ha, S. M., Rozycki, M., Prastawa, M., Alberts, E., Lipkova, J., Freymann, J., Kirby, J., Bilello, M., Fathallah-Shaykh, H., Wiest, R., Kirschke, J., Menze, B. (2018). *Identifying the best machine learning algorithms for brain tumor segmentation, progression assessment, and overall survival prediction in the BRATS challenge.* arXiv preprint. https://arxiv.org/abs/1811.02629.

Bernard, O., Lalande, A., Zotti, C., Cervenansky, F., Yang, X., Heng, P. A., Cetin, I., Lekadir, K., Camara, O., Gonzalez Ballester, M. A., Sanroma, G., Napel, S., Petersen, S., Tziritas, G., Grinias, E., Khened, M., Kollerathu, V. A., Krishnamurthi, G., Rohe, M. M., Jodoin, P. M. (2018). Deep learning techniques for automatic MRI cardiac multi-structures segmentation and diagnosis: Is the problem solved? *IEEE Transactions on Medical Imaging*, 37(11), 2514-2525. https://doi.org/10.1109/TMI.
2018.2837502.

Bien, N., Rajpurkar, P., Ball, R. L., Irvin, J., Park, A., Jones, E., Bereket, M., Patel, B. N., Yeom, K. W., Shpanskaya, K., Halabi, S., Zucker, E., Fanton, G., Amanatullah, D. F., Beaulieu, C. F., Riley, G. M., Stewart, R. J., Blankenberg, F. G., Larson, D. B., Lungren, M. P. (2018). Deep-learning-assisted diagnosis for knee magnetic resonance imaging: Development and retrospective validation of MRNet. *PLOS Medicine,* 15(11), e1002699. https://doi.org/10.1371/journal.pmed.1002699.

Char, D. S., Shah, N. H., & Magnus, D. (2020). Implementing machine learning in health care—Addressing ethical challenges. *New England Journal of Medicine*, 378(11), 981-983. https://doi.org/10.1056/NEJMp1714229.

Dar, S. U., Yurt, M., Karacan, L., Erdem, A., Erdem, E., & Çukur, T. (2020). Image synthesis in multi-contrast MRI with conditional generative adversarial networks. *IEEE Transactions on Medical Imaging*, 38(10), 2375-2388. https://doi.org/10.1109/TMI.2019.2901750.

Duffy, B. A., Zhang, L., Dahan, H., & Daftary, A. (2021). Retrospective motion artifact correction of structural MRI images using deep learning improves the quality of cortical surface reconstructions. *NeuroImage*, 230, 117756. https://doi.org/10.1016/j.neuroimage.2021.117756.

Finlayson, S. G., Subbaswamy, A., Singh, K., Bowers, J., Kupke, A., Zittrain, J., Kohane, I. S., & Saria, S. (2021). The clinician and dataset shift in artificial intelligence. New *England Journal of Medicine*, 385(3), 283-286. https://doi.org/10.1056/NEJMc2104626.

Gillies, R. J., Kinahan, P. E., & Hricak, H. (2016). Radiomics: Images are more than pictures, they are data. *Radiology*, 278(2), 563-577. https://doi.org/10.1148/radiol.2015151169.

Hammernik, K., Klatzer, T., Kobler, E., Recht, M. P., Sodickson, D. K., Pock, T., & Knoll, F. (2018). Learning a variational network for reconstruction of accelerated MRI data. *Magnetic Resonance in Medicine*, 79(6), 3055-3071. https://doi.org/10.1002/mrm.26977.

Kickingereder, P., Bonekamp, D., Nowosielski, M., Kratz, A., Sill, M., Burth, S., Wick, A., Eidel, O., Schlemmer, H. P., Radbruch, A., Debus, J., Herold-Mende, C., Unterberg, A., Platten, M., Winkler, F., Wick, W., Bendszus, M., & Radbruch, A. (2016). Radiogenomics of glioblastoma: Machine learning-based classification of molecular characteristics by using multiparametric and multiregional MR imaging features. *Radiology*, 281(3), 907-918. https://doi.org/10.1148/radiol.2016161382.

Litjens, G., Debats, O., Barentsz, J., Karssemeijer, N., & Huisman, H. (2014). Computer-aided detection of prostate cancer in MRI. *IEEE Transactions on Medical Imaging,* 33(5), 1083-1092. https://doi.org/10.1109/TMI.2014.2303821.

Lundervold, A. S., & Lundervold, A. (2019). An overview of deep learning in medical imaging focusing on MRI. *Zeitschrift für Medizinische Physik*, 29(2), 102-127. https://doi.org/10.1016/j.zemedi.2018.11.002.

Obermeyer, Z., Powers, B., Vogeli, C., & Mullainathan, S. (2019). Dissecting racial bias in an algorithm used to manage the health of populations. *Science*, 366(6464), 447-453. https://doi.org/10.1126/science.aax2342.

Reuter, M., Tisdall, M. D., Qureshi, A., Buckner, R. L., van der Kouwe, A. J., & Fischl, B. (2015). Head motion during MRI acquisition reduces Grey matter volume and thickness estimates. *NeuroImage*, 107, 107-115. https://doi.org/10.1016/j.neuroimage.2014.12.006.

Ronneberger, O., Fischer, P., & Brox, T. (2015). U-Net: Convolutional networks for biomedical image segmentation. In *Medical Image Computing and Computer-Assisted Intervention* (pp. 234-241). Springer. https://doi.org/10.1007/978-3-319-24574-4_28.

Selvaraju, R. R., Cogswell, M., Das, A., Vedantam, R., Parikh, D., & Batra, D. (2017). Grad-CAM: Visual explanations from deep networks via gradient-based localisation. In *Proceedings of the IEEE International Conference on Computer Vision* (pp. 618-626). https://doi.org/10.1109/ICCV.2017.74.

Chapter 16

Compressed Sensing and Accelerated Imaging

Maajid Mohi Ud Din Malik*
Radiology and Imaging Technology, Dr. D. Y. Patil School of Allied Health Sciences,
Dr. D. Y. Patil Vidyapeeth (Deemed to be University), Sant Tukaram Nagar, Pimpri, Pune, India

Abstract

Compressed sensing and accelerated imaging techniques have revolutionised magnetic resonance imaging by dramatically reducing scan times while maintaining diagnostic image quality. This chapter explores the mathematical foundations of compressed sensing theory, including sparsity, incoherent sampling, and nonlinear reconstruction algorithms. We examine parallel imaging techniques such as SENSE and GRAPPA, which exploit spatial encoding from multiple receiver coils to accelerate data acquisition. Advanced methods, including simultaneous multi-slice imaging, Wave-CAIPI, and synthetic MRI, are discussed in detail, highlighting their clinical applications and current limitations. The integration of compressed sensing with parallel imaging and deep learning reconstruction represents the cutting edge of acceleration technology, enabling routine clinical protocols that were previously impractical. This chapter provides a comprehensive overview of acceleration principles, implementation strategies, and clinical validation studies across diverse anatomical applications. These innovations align with Sustainable Development Goal 3 (Good Health and Well-being) by improving patient comfort, increasing scanner throughput, and enabling wider access to advanced MRI diagnostics.

Keywords: compressed sensing, parallel imaging, SENSE, GRAPPA, simultaneous multi-slice, wave-CAIPI, image acceleration, k-space sampling, SDG 3 - good health and well-being

* Corresponding Author's Email: maajid.malik@dpu.edu.in

In: Recent Advances in Magnetic Resonance Imaging in Neuroimaging
Editors: Maajid Mohi Ud Din Malik, Purnachandra Kawdu Lamghare and R. S. Kuber
ISBN: 979-8-90134-244-2

Introduction

The fundamental challenge in magnetic resonance imaging has always been the inherent trade-off between acquisition speed, spatial resolution, signal-to-noise ratio, and anatomical coverage. Traditional MRI sequences require complete k-space sampling, as per the Nyquist-Shannon sampling theorem, resulting in scan times ranging from several minutes to over an hour for high-resolution three-dimensional acquisitions. These lengthy scan times increase patient discomfort, limit throughput, exacerbate motion artefacts, and restrict the clinical utility of MRI, particularly in pediatric, claustrophobic, or critically ill patients who cannot tolerate prolonged imaging sessions. The development of compressed sensing and other acceleration techniques over the past two decades has fundamentally transformed this landscape, enabling dramatic reductions in scan time while maintaining or even improving diagnostic image quality (Lustig et al., 2007).

Compressed sensing emerged from mathematical signal processing theory, demonstrating that signals with sparse representations can be accurately recovered from far fewer measurements than the Nyquist criterion requires. When applied to MRI, compressed sensing exploits the inherent compressibility of medical images in appropriate transform domains, such as wavelets or total variation, combined with incoherent undersampling patterns and iterative reconstruction algorithms. Parallel imaging techniques, which preceded compressed sensing by several years, take a complementary approach by utilising the spatial encoding inherent in arrays of multiple receiver coils to reduce the number of required phase-encoding steps. The combination of compressed sensing and parallel imaging, along with recent advances in simultaneous multi-slice acquisition and deep learning reconstruction, has enabled acceleration factors of 5 to 10 times or more for many clinical applications (Sodickson & Manning, 1997).

These acceleration technologies have moved beyond research laboratories to become integral components of routine clinical imaging protocols worldwide. Modern MRI systems from all major manufacturers incorporate various forms of parallel imaging as standard features, while compressed sensing implementations are increasingly available for clinical use. The practical impact extends across all anatomical regions and clinical indications, from pediatric neuroimaging, where reduced scan times minimise sedation requirements, to cardiac MRI, where real-time imaging enables the assessment of dynamic cardiac function, to musculoskeletal imaging, where increased throughput improves access to care. This chapter provides a comprehensive examination of the principles underlying these acceleration techniques, their clinical implementation and validation, current limitations, and emerging developments that promise even greater acceleration in the future (Jaspan et al., 2015).

16.1. Principles of Compressed Sensing

Compressed sensing theory, introduced by Candès, Romberg, Tao, and Donoho in the mid-2000s, revolutionised signal processing by demonstrating that specific signals can be perfectly reconstructed from significantly fewer samples than required by traditional Nyquist-Shannon sampling theory. The application of this mathematical framework to MRI, pioneered by Lustig and colleagues in 2007, opened the door to significantly reducing scan time. The fundamental premise of compressed sensing rests on three key requirements: sparsity, incoherent sampling, and nonlinear reconstruction. Understanding these principles is essential for appreciating both the power and limitations of compressed sensing in clinical MRI applications (Lustig et al., 2007).

Sparsity represents the first pillar of compressed sensing theory, asserting that the signal of interest must have a sparse representation in some transform domain. In the context of MRI, while images themselves are not sparse in the pixel domain, they often exhibit sparsity when transformed to appropriate domains such as wavelets, finite differences, or other mathematical representations. Medical images typically contain large regions of relatively uniform intensity with sharp boundaries between different tissue types, making them amenable to sparse representation through total variation or wavelet transforms. The degree of sparsity directly influences the achievable acceleration factor, as sparser signals allow for greater undersampling. This sparsity requirement explains why compressed sensing works particularly well for angiography, where vessels appear bright against a dark background. Still, it may be less effective for images with more complex texture patterns (Lustig et al., 2008).

Incoherent sampling constitutes the second essential requirement, which demands that the undersampling pattern be designed so that artefacts appear noise-like rather than coherent. In traditional Cartesian MRI with regular undersampling, aliasing artefacts appear as structured, coherent replications of the anatomy that cannot be distinguished from the actual signal. Compressed sensing employs variable-density random or pseudo-random sampling patterns that violate the regular sampling condition, spreading aliasing energy incoherently throughout the image. This incoherence transforms aliasing from structured artefacts into noise-like interference that can be separated from the actual signal during reconstruction. Variable-density sampling typically maintains denser sampling near the centre of k-space, where most image energy is concentrated, while undersampling more aggressively in the periphery. Poisson disk sampling and other sophisticated patterns have been developed to optimise this incoherence while maintaining practical implementation on clinical scanners (Vasanawala et al., 2011).

Nonlinear reconstruction algorithms form the third pillar of compressed sensing, replacing simple inverse Fourier transforms with iterative optimisation procedures that simultaneously enforce data consistency and promote sparsity. These algorithms typically minimise a cost function that combines a data fidelity term, which ensures consistency between reconstructed images and acquired k-space data, with regularisation terms that promote sparsity in the appropriate transform domains. The optimisation problem is formulated as finding the image that best matches the acquired data while minimising the total variation or wavelet coefficients. Solving this optimisation requires iterative algorithms, such as the conjugate gradient method, the alternating direction method of multipliers, or the fast iterative shrinkage-thresholding algorithm, which can be computationally intensive but have become increasingly practical with modern computing hardware (Feng et al., 2014).

The mathematical formulation of compressed sensing reconstruction can be expressed as the minimisation of an objective function that combines data consistency and sparsity constraints. The data consistency term ensures that the Fourier transform of the reconstructed image matches the acquired k-space samples. In contrast, the sparsity term, typically implemented as L1 norm minimisation in the transform domain, encourages a compact representation. The relative weighting between these terms, controlled by regularisation parameters, must be carefully adjusted to balance artefact suppression against image quality. Too much regularisation produces over-smoothed images that lack fine detail, while insufficient regularisation fails to adequately suppress undersampling artefacts. This optimisation represents a fundamentally different paradigm from traditional MRI reconstruction, where the inverse Fourier transform provides a closed-form analytical solution.

The clinical implementation of compressed sensing necessitates careful consideration of multiple practical factors beyond theoretical requirements. The choice of transform domain significantly impacts reconstruction quality, with wavelets commonly used for structural imaging and temporal Fourier transforms or principal component analysis for dynamic imaging. Sampling pattern design must balance theoretical incoherence requirements with practical hardware constraints, as some theoretically optimal sampling patterns may be challenging to implement on clinical scanners with finite gradient performance. Reconstruction time represents another critical consideration, as iterative algorithms can require minutes or hours of computation for three-dimensional datasets. Recent advances in GPU-accelerated reconstruction and online reconstruction integrated into scanner hardware have reduced this bottleneck, making compressed sensing increasingly practical for routine clinical use (Jaspan et al., 2015).

16.2. Parallel Imaging Techniques

Parallel imaging exploits the spatially varying sensitivity profiles of multiple receiver coils to reduce the number of phase-encoding steps required for image formation, providing an alternative acceleration mechanism that predates compressed sensing. The fundamental insight underlying parallel imaging is that each coil in a phased array sees the imaging object from a different spatial perspective, with sensitivity that varies smoothly across the field of view. This spatial information can substitute for some phase-encoding steps that would traditionally be acquired through gradient encoding, enabling acceleration by skipping lines in k-space. The two dominant parallel imaging methods, SENSE (Sensitivity Encoding) and GRAPPA (Generalised Autocalibrating Partially Parallel Acquisitions), differ in whether reconstruction occurs in image space or k-space but achieve similar acceleration performance (Pruessmann et al., 1999; Griswold et al., 2002).

SENSE reconstruction operates in image space, utilising coil sensitivity maps to unfold aliased images acquired with reduced phase encoding. When a factor of R undersamples k-space, the resulting image from each coil contains R overlapped copies of the anatomy, spatially shifted according to the undersampling pattern. If coil sensitivities are known, this represents a system of linear equations with R unknowns (the actual pixel values at R aliased locations) and as many equations as available coils. With sufficient coils and appropriate geometry, this system can be inverted to recover unaliased images. The quality of SENSE reconstruction depends critically on the accuracy of sensitivity maps and the conditioning of the unfolding matrix, which is determined by the spatial arrangement of receiver coils relative to the imaging volume. Regions with similar coil sensitivities exhibit poor conditioning, leading to noise amplification, which is quantified by the geometry factor, also known as the g-factor (Pruessmann et al., 1999).

GRAPPA reconstruction operates in k-space, synthesising missing k-space lines from acquired data through linear combinations determined by coil sensitivities. Rather than requiring explicit sensitivity maps, GRAPPA learns interpolation weights from a small number of fully sampled autocalibration signal (ACS) lines acquired near the centre of k-space. These weights characterise how k-space data from different coils relate to each other, enabling the prediction of missing lines from neighbouring acquired lines. The reconstructed k-space for each coil is then Fourier transformed and combined to produce the final image. GRAPPA's self-calibrating nature eliminates errors caused by imperfect sensitivity estimation, but it requires the acquisition of additional ACS lines, which slightly reduces the achievable acceleration. Various GRAPPA variants have been developed for specific applications, including GRAPPA-2 for improved artefact suppression and slice-GRAPPA for simultaneous multi-slice imaging (Griswold et al., 2002).

The geometry factor quantifies noise amplification inherent in parallel imaging reconstruction, providing a spatially varying measure of reconstruction conditioning. In ideal conditions where coil sensitivities are perfectly orthogonal, the g-factor equals 1, and noise is not amplified. In practice, g-factors increase with the acceleration factor and are similar across regions with identical sensitivity patterns. Peripheral areas of the field of view typically exhibit better conditioning than central regions due to greater spatial variation in coil sensitivities. The g-factor imposes practical limits on achievable acceleration, as areas with g-factors exceeding two to three suffer significant noise amplification that may degrade diagnostic quality. Modern coil designs, featuring larger numbers of elements and sophisticated coil geometries, aim to minimise g-factors across the imaging volume, enabling higher acceleration factors while maintaining an adequate signal-to-noise ratio (Robson et al., 2008).

Calibration strategies critically impact parallel imaging performance and workflow. SENSE requires separate acquisition of coil sensitivity maps, which are typically obtained from low-resolution reference scans or body coil images. These sensitivity maps must match the geometry and position of the diagnostic scan, requiring careful quality control and potentially limiting the technique's robustness to patient motion between reference and diagnostic acquisitions. Self-calibrating methods, such as GRAPPA, eliminate the need for separate reference scans by incorporating autocalibration data directly into the diagnostic acquisition, thereby enhancing workflow and robustness. However, the need for fully sampled ACS lines reduces the achievable acceleration slightly from the theoretical maximum. Hybrid approaches combining SENSE and GRAPPA-type reconstructions aim to leverage the advantages of both methods while minimising their respective limitations (Blaimer et al., 2004).

Clinical applications of parallel imaging span virtually all anatomical regions and contrast mechanisms, with acceleration factors of two to four routinely employed in clinical practice. The choice of parallel imaging method often depends on the specific application, available hardware, and institutional preferences. Cardiac imaging, particularly when using parallel imaging acceleration, benefits from improved temporal resolution, enabling breath-hold cine sequences and real-time imaging for stress studies. Neuroimaging applications utilise parallel imaging to reduce geometric distortion in echo-planar imaging for functional MRI and diffusion imaging. Abdominal and pelvic imaging employ parallel imaging to shorten breath holds, thereby reducing motion artefacts. The widespread availability and robust performance of parallel imaging have made it a foundational technology in modern MRI, often combined synergistically with other acceleration techniques to achieve even greater speed-ups (Deshmane et al., 2012).

16.3. Simultaneous Multi-Slice (SMS) Imaging

Simultaneous multi-slice imaging represents a revolutionary acceleration technique that excites and acquires multiple slices simultaneously rather than sequentially, multiplying scan speed by the number of simultaneously excited slices. Initially developed for functional MRI to enhance temporal resolution in brain mapping studies, SMS imaging has been expanded to include anatomical, diffusion, and perfusion imaging across multiple anatomical regions. The technique exploits the fact that slices separated along the slice-select direction can be distinguished by their different spatial locations using parallel imaging principles, even when excited simultaneously. By acquiring multiple slices in the time traditionally required for one, SMS imaging achieves dramatic acceleration without the noise amplification penalties typically associated with in-plane parallel imaging (Barth et al., 2016).

The implementation of SMS imaging requires specialised radiofrequency pulses that simultaneously excite multiple slices with controlled phase relationships. Multiband radiofrequency pulses are constructed by summing individual slice-selective pulses with appropriate frequency offsets corresponding to the desired slice separations. The resulting composite pulse excites all target slices essentially simultaneously; however, the increased bandwidth and peak power of multiband pulses impose practical limits on the number of slices that can be excited simultaneously. Phase cycling strategies, such as CAIPIRINHA (Controlled Aliasing in Parallel Imaging Results in Higher Acceleration), introduce additional phase modulation across simultaneously

excited slices to improve separability during reconstruction. These phase offsets effectively shift the aliasing pattern of overlapped slices, thereby optimising the conditioning for parallel imaging unfolding (Setsompop et al., 2012).
Slice-GRAPPA and split-slice-GRAPPA represent the predominant reconstruction approaches for SMS imaging, extending conventional GRAPPA principles to separate simultaneously acquired slices. Slice-GRAPPA learns reconstruction kernels from single-band reference data or embedded autocalibration, allowing for the synthesis of individual slice data from the superimposed multi-slice acquisition. Split-slice-GRAPPA extends basic slice-GRAPPA by dividing k-space into sub-blocks, reconstructing them separately before combination, thereby reducing computational complexity and improving artefact suppression. Alternative reconstruction methods, including SENSE-based approaches and regularised reconstructions incorporating sparsity constraints, have been developed, each offering different trade-offs between reconstruction quality, computation time, and calibration requirements (Cauley et al., 2014).

The application of SMS imaging to diffusion-weighted imaging has been particularly transformative, enabling clinically practical acquisition of high-resolution diffusion tensor imaging and advanced diffusion models that would be prohibitively time-consuming with conventional methods. Diffusion imaging benefits especially from SMS acceleration because each diffusion direction and b-value must be acquired separately, multiplying the scan time. SMS acceleration by factors of 3 to 8 enables the acquisition of tens of diffusion directions at multiple b-values within reasonable scan times, allowing advanced techniques such as diffusion kurtosis imaging, neurite orientation dispersion and density imaging, and high-angular-resolution diffusion imaging. Whole-brain high-resolution diffusion imaging, which once required 30 to 60 minutes, can now be completed in 5 to 10 minutes, dramatically improving clinical feasibility (Setsompop et al., 2012).

Functional MRI represents the original application domain for SMS imaging, where improved temporal resolution enables better characterisation of brain hemodynamics and greater statistical power to detect activation. Conventional fMRI typically acquires whole-brain coverage in 2 to 3 seconds, which is adequate for many studies but suboptimal for capturing rapid hemodynamic responses or studying brain networks with high temporal precision. SMS acceleration reduces repetition times to 500 milliseconds or less, capturing four to six times as many time points in the same scan duration. This improved temporal resolution benefits resting-state connectivity studies, event-related designs, and the modelling of physiological noise. The combination of high spatial and temporal resolution enabled by SMS has yielded new insights into brain network dynamics that were previously inaccessible (Feinberg & Setsompop, 2013).

The clinical implementation of SMS imaging requires careful optimisation of multiple interrelated parameters, including the multiband factor, in-plane acceleration, and slice separation. Higher multiband factors provide greater acceleration but increase radiofrequency power deposition, potentially approaching specific absorption rate limits, particularly at higher field strengths. Combined SMS and in-plane parallel imaging can achieve very high net acceleration factors, but must be carefully managed to minimise cumulative noise amplification and artefact propagation. Slice separation influences reconstruction conditioning, with larger separations generally improving separability but potentially reducing anatomical coverage or increasing minimum repetition time. Modern SMS implementations incorporate adaptive parameter selection and online reconstruction, making the technique increasingly accessible for routine clinical use across diverse applications (Barth et al., 2016). Table 16.1 compares primary acceleration techniques in MRI.

Table 16.1. Comparison of major acceleration techniques in MRI

Technique	Acceleration Mechanism	Typical Acceleration Factor	Primary Advantages	Main Limitations	Clinical Maturity
Parallel Imaging (SENSE/GRAPPA)	Multi-coil spatial encoding	2-4x	Well-established, robust, vendor-neutral	g-factor noise amplification requires multiple coils	Mature - routine clinical use
Compressed Sensing	Sparse representation + incoherent sampling	2-8x	High acceleration, flexible sampling	Iterative reconstruction time, image-dependent performance	Emerging - increasing clinical adoption
Simultaneous Multi-Slice	Multi-band RF excitation	3-8x (slice direction)	Minimal noise penalty, high acceleration	SAR constraints require specialised RF pulses	Established for neuro, expanding
Wave-CAIPI	Sinusoidal gradient waveforms	9-12x (combined)	Very high acceleration, good SNR efficiency	Complex reconstruction, hardware requirements	Research/early clinical
Combined CS + PI	Synergistic multi-technique	6-12x	Highest acceleration, leverages multiple mechanisms	Computational complexity, parameter optimisation	Rapidly evolving

16.4. Wave-CAIPI and Other Advanced Methods

Wave-CAIPI (Wave-Controlled Aliasing in Parallel Imaging) represents the cutting edge of MRI acceleration technology, combining parallel imaging, controlled aliasing, and sinusoidal gradient waveforms during readout to achieve unprecedented acceleration factors with excellent image quality. Introduced by Bilgic and colleagues in 2015, Wave-CAIPI extends the CAIPIRINHA concept by using oscillatory readout gradients to generate corkscrew k-space trajectories that spread aliasing across three dimensions. This three-dimensional point spread function provides superior coil separability compared to conventional parallel imaging, enabling routine acceleration factors of 9-12 for three-dimensional acquisitions with acceptable g-factors. The technique has been successfully applied to neuroimaging, including structural imaging, magnetic resonance angiography, and susceptibility-weighted imaging (Bilgic et al., 2015).

The implementation of Wave-CAIPI requires sinusoidal gradient waveforms applied during readout in the phase-encoding and slice-encoding directions, creating a corkscrew trajectory through k-space. These sinusoidal gradients cause position-dependent phase accumulation that varies smoothly across the three-dimensional field of view, effectively spreading each point in the object to multiple locations in the aliased image according to a three-dimensional point spread function. This spreading dramatically improves the conditioning of parallel imaging reconstruction by ensuring that aliased points originate from spatial locations with maximally different coil sensitivities. The amplitude and frequency of the sinusoidal gradients must be carefully optimised to maximise conditioning while remaining within the hardware gradient performance specifications (Polak et al., 2018).

Reconstruction of Wave-CAIPI data requires accounting for the additional phase introduced by sinusoidal gradient waveforms, typically implemented via a wave-encoding operator in the forward model. The reconstruction problem is formulated similarly to standard parallel imaging, but it includes an additional encoding term that maps between image space and the acquired data. Iterative algorithms solve this inverse problem, which may also incorporate additional regularisation terms to further improve image quality. The computational demands of Wave-CAIPI reconstruction exceed those of standard parallel imaging due to the more complex forward model. However, GPU-accelerated implementations have reduced reconstruction times to clinically acceptable levels. Some implementations integrate wave encoding with compressed sensing to achieve even higher acceleration (Cauley et al., 2015).

Synthetic MRI represents a fundamentally different acceleration paradigm that acquires quantitative tissue parameters rather than conventional contrast-weighted images, then synthesises arbitrary contrast weightings retrospectively without additional scanning. A single multi-echo, multi-saturation-delay acquisition quantifies T1, T2, and proton density for each voxel within a clinically acceptable scan time of 5 to 6 minutes. These quantitative maps can then generate an unlimited number of synthetic images with any desired T1-, T2-, or inversion-recovery contrast, including contrasts that would be impractical to acquire separately. This approach significantly enhances workflow efficiency by eliminating the need for multiple separate acquisitions, while also providing quantitative information valuable for longitudinal monitoring and texture analysis (Warntjes et al., 2007).

Magnetic resonance fingerprinting (MRF) extends the concept of quantitative multiparametric imaging even further, utilising pseudorandom acquisition patterns and template matching to simultaneously quantify multiple tissue properties from highly undersampled data. MRF sequences employ varying flip angles, repetition times, and other parameters in a seemingly random manner, generating unique signal-evolution fingerprints for different tissue types. Pattern recognition algorithms match measured signals to a pre-computed dictionary of possible signals corresponding to varying combinations of T1, T2, proton density, and other parameters. MRF can quantify multiple parameters in acquisition times comparable to or shorter than those of single conventional scans. However, the technique remains primarily in the research domain, with ongoing efforts to optimise sequences, accelerate reconstruction, and validate clinical utility (Ma et al., 2013).

Zero echo time (ZTE) and ultrashort echo time (UTE) imaging employ alternative encoding strategies that enable imaging of tissues with extremely short T2 relaxation times, such as cortical bone, ligaments, and lung parenchyma, which produce negligible signal in conventional sequences. These techniques utilise non-Cartesian k-space trajectories that initiate data acquisition immediately after radiofrequency excitation, before appreciable T2 decay has occurred. Radial or spiral trajectories sample k-space from the centre to the periphery, with encoding achieved through rotating or varying readout gradients rather than phase-encoding gradients. The radial acquisition pattern provides inherent motion robustness and enables highly undersampled acquisition with compressed sensing reconstruction. ZTE imaging has found applications in neuroimaging and musculoskeletal imaging, and, more recently, in generating pseudo-CT images for radiation therapy planning (Weiger & Pruessmann, 2012).

16.5. Clinical Applications and Limitations

The clinical implementation of acceleration techniques has transformed MRI workflow across virtually all anatomical regions and clinical indications. However, successful deployment requires careful consideration of application-specific factors and potential limitations (Table 16.2). Neuroimaging represents the most mature application domain, with parallel imaging routinely used in clinical brain and spine protocols and SMS imaging increasingly adopted for diffusion and functional imaging. Acceleration has enabled previously impractical protocols such as whole-brain three-dimensional T2-FLAIR with isotropic submillimeter resolution, high-b-value diffusion imaging with multiple b-values and directions, and high-temporal-resolution dynamic contrast-enhanced perfusion imaging. However, the benefits must be weighed against potential image quality trade-offs, including altered noise characteristics, subtle artefact patterns, and modified tissue contrast, which may affect diagnostic confidence (Deshmane et al., 2012).

Cardiac MRI has particularly benefited from acceleration technologies, addressing the fundamental challenge of imaging a constantly moving organ within breath-hold constraints. Parallel imaging with acceleration factors of two to three has become standard for cine imaging, enabling improved temporal resolution and reduced breath-hold duration. Real-time imaging for stress testing and free-breathing acquisitions for patients unable to hold their breath relies heavily on parallel imaging acceleration. Compressed sensing combined with parallel imaging enables single-breath-hold whole-heart coronary MRI angiography and advanced perfusion sequences with improved spatial and temporal resolution. The integration of SMS imaging for multi-slice first-pass perfusion offers excellent coverage without the time delays inherent in sequential slice acquisition. Despite these advances, cardiac acceleration faces unique challenges, including sensitivity to cardiac and respiratory motion, blood flow artefacts, and the need to maintain an adequate signal-to-noise ratio in inherently low-SNR sequences (Vincenti et al., 2014).

Musculoskeletal imaging applications prioritise high spatial resolution for visualising fine anatomical details, such as cartilage, ligaments, and small bone structures. This makes acceleration particularly valuable for reducing the lengthy scan times traditionally required for high-resolution sequences. Parallel imaging acceleration of two to four times has become routine in knee, shoulder, and spine imaging protocols, enabling submillimeter isotropic three-dimensional sequences that allow reformatting in arbitrary planes. Compressed sensing has shown promise for further accelerating isotropic sequences, although careful validation of subtle pathology visibility is essential. The combination of multiple acceleration techniques enables comprehensive joint protocols to be completed in 15 to 20 minutes, rather than the 45 to 60 minutes typically required, thereby improving patient comfort and scanner efficiency. However, the impact of acceleration on the detection of subtle cartilage defects, meniscal tears, and ligament injuries requires ongoing validation to ensure that speed gains do not compromise diagnostic accuracy (Fritz et al., 2012).

Body imaging applications face additional challenges from respiratory and bowel motion, heterogeneous tissues with varying T1 and T2 values, and the need for ample anatomical coverage. Parallel imaging has become integral to abdominal and pelvic imaging protocols, shortening breath-holds to 15 to 20 seconds and enabling breath-hold three-dimensional sequences that were previously acquired during free breathing with respiratory gating. Compressed sensing shows particular promise for free-breathing abdominal imaging, where the temporal sparsity of respiratory motion can be leveraged to achieve high acceleration factors. Dynamic contrast-enhanced imaging of the liver and kidneys benefits from the combination of parallel imaging and compressed sensing, achieving improved temporal and spatial resolution for assessing enhancement patterns. Diffusion-weighted imaging of the abdomen and pelvis utilises parallel imaging to reduce echo train length and geometric distortion, although maintaining an adequate signal-to-noise ratio remains challenging (Chandarana et al., 2013).

Pediatric imaging represents an application area where acceleration techniques offer particularly high clinical value by reducing or eliminating the need for sedation. Young children often cannot remain still for the 30 to 60 minutes required for comprehensive MRI examinations, necessitating general anaesthesia with associated risks and costs. Accelerated protocols can reduce total examination time to 15-20 minutes, making imaging feasible in many children without sedation. Fast sequences utilising combined acceleration techniques enable motion-robust imaging, even in uncooperative patients, thereby improving diagnostic yield. However, the developing brain, smaller anatomical structures, and differences in tissue relaxation properties in children require careful adaptation of acceleration parameters optimised for adults. The potential for differential effects of acceleration on pediatric tissue contrast, as well as the need for age-specific reference standards, must be considered when implementing accelerated protocols in pediatric populations (Jaimes et al., 2016).

Artefact patterns associated with acceleration techniques differ from those of conventional imaging artefacts and require radiologists' familiarity for appropriate interpretation. Parallel imaging can produce spatially varying noise amplification with regional hotspots corresponding to poor coil conditioning, residual aliasing if reconstruction fails, and altered noise texture that may affect the conspicuity of subtle lesions. Compressed sensing may introduce blurring or patchy signal variations, particularly in regions of low sparsity, and can create subtle edge artefacts at tissue boundaries. SMS imaging can produce slice-to-slice intensity variations if reconstruction is imperfect and may show increased artefact sensitivity to head motion in neuroimaging. These artefact patterns generally differ from pathology and decrease with increasing radiologist experience; however, rigorous validation and quality control protocols are essential when implementing new acceleration techniques in clinical practice (Jaspan et al., 2015). Table 16.2 shows clinical applications and recommendations for acceleration factors by anatomical region.

Table 16.2. Clinical applications and recommended acceleration factors by anatomical region

Anatomical Region	Primary Applications	Recommended Techniques	Typical Acceleration	Key Clinical Benefits
Brain	Structural, fMRI, DTI, perfusion	PI (2-3x) + SMS (3-8x) + CS (2-4x)	4-10x combined	Reduced motion artefacts, higher resolution DTI, and improved fMRI temporal resolution.
Spine	Morphological, myelography	PI (2-4x) + CS (2-3x)	3-6x combined	Shorter scan times, reduced motion, isotropic 3D imaging
Cardiac	Cine, perfusion, LGE, flow	PI (2-3x) + CS (3-6x)	4-8x combined	Shorter breath-holds, real-time imaging, improved temporal resolution
Abdomen/Pelvis	Morphological, DWI, DCE	PI (2-3x) + CS (2-4x)	3-6x combined	Breath-hold reduction, motion robustness, and improved DCE temporal resolution
Musculoskeletal	Morphological, cartilage mapping	PI (2-4x) + CS (2-3x)	3-6x combined	High-resolution 3D imaging, reduced scan time, improved patient comfort
Angiography	CE-MRA, time-of-flight	PI (2-3x) + CS (4-8x)	6-12x combined	Reduced contrast dose, improved temporal resolution, faster coverage

16.6. Future Acceleration Techniques

The future of MRI acceleration lies in integrating multiple complementary approaches, particularly the combination of advanced sampling strategies with artificial intelligence-powered reconstruction. Deep learning reconstruction methods, which learn optimal reconstruction mappings from large training datasets rather than relying on hand-crafted priors, are enabling acceleration factors that exceed what is achievable with traditional compressed sensing while maintaining superior image quality. These AI-based approaches can leverage both k-space and image-space information, learning complex regularisations that capture anatomical structure more effectively than wavelets or total variation methods. The combination of physics-based models with data-driven learning, often referred to as hybrid or model-based deep learning, promises to achieve the best of both worlds: the generalizability and interpretability of physics-based methods, along with the performance of deep learning (Hammernik et al., 2018).

Low-field MRI systems operating at 0.5 Tesla or below represent an emerging area where advanced acceleration techniques may have a particularly significant impact. These systems offer reduced cost, improved portability, and enhanced safety profiles compared to high-field systems, potentially democratizing MRI access in resource-limited settings and enabling point-of-care imaging. However, the inherently lower signal-to-noise ratio at low field necessitates aggressive acceleration strategies to maintain clinically acceptable image quality within reasonable scan times. Deep learning reconstruction, explicitly trained for low-field data, shows promise in compensating for SNR deficits, while optimised pulse sequences and receive array designs maximise the available signal. The combination of these technologies could enable low-field systems to approach the image quality of high-field systems for many clinical applications (Sarracanie & Salameh, 2020).

Scan-time adaptive and intelligent MRI represents a paradigm shift from predetermined acquisition protocols to systems that optimise acquisition parameters in real-time based on preliminary image data. Machine learning algorithms can predict optimal acceleration factors, sampling patterns, and reconstruction parameters for individual patients based on initial scout images or early-acquired data. Adaptive protocols could automatically adjust spatial resolution, field of view, and contrast weighting based on detected anatomy or pathology, ensuring optimal allocation of scan time. Reinforcement learning agents could learn optimal acquisition strategies through interaction with the MRI system, potentially discovering novel acceleration approaches that human designers might not conceive. These intelligent systems promise to maximise diagnostic yield per unit scan time while maintaining robust image quality across diverse patient populations and clinical scenarios (Loktyushin et al., 2019).

Quantum computing and neuromorphic computing represent speculative but potentially transformative technologies for MRI reconstruction. The massive parallelism of quantum algorithms could dramatically accelerate the solution of large-scale optimisation problems inherent in compressed sensing reconstruction, potentially enabling real-time reconstruction of highly accelerated three-dimensional datasets. Neuromorphic processors that mimic brain architecture might allow more efficient deep learning reconstruction with reduced power consumption and latency. While these technologies remain in early research stages with uncertain timelines for practical implementation, they illustrate the potential for fundamental computational advances to remove remaining barriers to real-time, ultra-high-acceleration imaging (Schuld & Petruccione, 2018).

Integrated diagnostics, combining MRI with other modalities in hybrid systems such as PET-MRI or MRI-guided radiotherapy, particularly benefit from acceleration techniques that enable high-quality image acquisition within the workflow constraints of multimodal procedures. Simultaneous PET-MRI faces the challenge of acquiring diagnostic-quality MRI. At the same time, PET data are being collected, necessitating the use of silent or quiet MRI sequences with aggressive acceleration to minimise acoustic noise and maintain a reasonable total examination time. MRI-guided radiation therapy requires rapid imaging for target localisation and motion monitoring, with image quality sufficient for treatment planning but updated frequently enough to track anatomical changes accurately. These applications are driving the development of specialised acceleration techniques optimised for hybrid imaging constraints (Gatidis et al., 2016).

Standardisation and validation of acceleration techniques across vendors and institutions are critical for the widespread clinical adoption and meaningful comparison of research results. Currently, different implementations of nominally similar techniques, such as compressed sensing or SMS imaging, may produce subtly different image characteristics across vendors. The development of standardised phantoms, quantitative image quality metrics, and validation protocols would facilitate objective comparison of techniques and inform optimal parameter selection. Collaborative efforts among vendors, regulatory agencies, and clinical researchers are necessary to establish evidence-based guidelines for acceleration techniques across various clinical applications. Machine learning approaches for harmonising multi-vendor data show promise for improving reproducibility and enabling large-scale multi-institutional studies using accelerated protocols (Deshmane et al., 2012). Table 16.3 shows performance metrics and trade-offs of acceleration techniques.

Table 16.3. Performance metrics and Trade-offs of acceleration techniques

Metric	Parallel Imaging	Compressed Sensing	SMS Imaging	Wave-CAIPI	Deep Learning
SNR Efficiency	Decreased (g-factor)	Maintained (sparsity-dependent)	Maintained (slice direction)	Good (3D spreading)	Variable (training-dependent)
Reconstruction Time	Fast (<1 sec)	Slow (minutes)	Fast (<5 sec)	Moderate (10-30 sec)	Fast after training (<5 sec)
Robustness to Motion	Good	Moderate	Good	Moderate	Good (if trained)
Vendor Availability	Universal	Expanding	Major vendors	Limited	Emerging
Training/ Calibration	Coil sensitivity maps	None (self-calibrating)	Single-band reference	Coil calibration	Large training datasets
Regulatory Status	FDA approved	FDA approved (limited)	FDA approved (neuro)	Research	Investigational

Conclusion

Compressed sensing and accelerated imaging techniques have fundamentally transformed magnetic resonance imaging from a slow modality to an increasingly rapid diagnostic tool. The combination of parallel imaging, compressed sensing, simultaneous multi-slice acquisition, and emerging deep learning reconstruction methods enables acceleration factors of 5-12 times across diverse clinical applications, dramatically reducing scan times while maintaining diagnostic image quality. These technologies have expanded clinical utility for populations previously limited by time constraints, including pediatric and cardiac imaging and comprehensive whole-body examinations. Successful implementation requires an understanding of the underlying physics and mathematics, as well as practical considerations for clinical deployment, parameter optimisation, artefact recognition, and quality control protocols. Future developments will be driven by artificial intelligence and machine learning for optimised reconstruction and acquisition planning, hardware innovations including high-channel-count receiver arrays and advanced gradient systems, novel encoding strategies exploiting inherent MRI data redundancy, and standardisation efforts enabling reproducible multi-institutional research and clinical protocols, ultimately improving patient access, experience, and healthcare outcomes.

Acknowledgments

The authors would like to extend our appreciation to those who offered helpful commentary during the drafting process of this manuscript. We also acknowledge the role the Nova Publishing department played in enabling the work described herein.

References

Barth, M., Breuer, F., Koopmans, P. J., Norris, D. G., & Poser, B. A. (2016). Simultaneous multislice (SMS) imaging techniques. *Magnetic Resonance in Medicine*, 75(1), 63-81. https://doi.org/10.1002/mrm.25897.

Bilgic, B., Gagoski, B. A., Cauley, S. F., Fan, A. P., Polimeni, J. R., Grant, P. E., Wald, L. L., & Setsompop, K. (2015). Wave-CAIPI for highly accelerated 3D imaging. *Magnetic Resonance in Medicine*, 73(6), 2152-2162. https://doi.org/10.1002/mrm.25347.

Blaimer, M., Breuer, F., Mueller, M., Heidemann, R. M., Griswold, M. A., & Jakob, P. M. (2004). SMASH, SENSE, PILS, GRAPPA: How to choose the optimal method. *Topics in Magnetic Resonance Imaging*, 15(4), 223-236. https://doi.org/10.1097/01.rmr.0000136558.09801.dd.

Cauley, S. F., Polimeni, J. R., Bhat, H., Wald, L. L., & Setsompop, K. (2014). Interslice leakage artifact reduction technique for simultaneous multislice acquisitions. *Magnetic Resonance in Medicine*, 72(1), 93-102. https://doi.org/10.1002/mrm.24898.

Cauley, S. F., Setsompop, K., Bilgic, B., Bhat, H., Gagoski, B., & Wald, L. L. (2015). Autocalibrated wave-CAIPI reconstruction: Joint optimization of k-space trajectory and parallel imaging reconstruction. *Magnetic Resonance in Medicine*, 78(4), 1093-1099. https://doi.org/10.1002/mrm.26499.

Chandarana, H., Block, T. K., Rosenkrantz, A. B., Lim, R. P., Kim, D., Mossa, D. J., Babb, J. S., Kiefer, B., & Sodickson, D. K. (2013). Free-breathing radial 3D fat-suppressed T1-weighted gradient echo sequence: A viable alternative for contrast-enhanced liver imaging in patients unable to suspend respiration. *Investigative Radiology*, 46(10), 648-653. https://doi.org/10.1097/RLI.0b013e31821eea45.

Deshmane, A., Gulani, V., Griswold, M. A., & Seiberlich, N. (2012). Parallel MR imaging. *Journal of Magnetic Resonance Imaging*, 36(1), 55-72. https://doi.org/10.1002/jmri.23639.

Feinberg, D. A., & Setsompop, K. (2013). Ultra-fast MRI of the human brain with simultaneous multi-slice imaging. *Journal of Magnetic Resonance*, 229, 90-100. https://doi.org/10.1016/j.jmr.2013.02.002.

Feng, L., Grimm, R., Block, K. T., Chandarana, H., Kim, S., Xu, J., Axel, L., Sodickson, D. K., & Otazo, R. (2014). Golden-angle radial sparse parallel MRI: Combination of compressed sensing, parallel imaging, and golden-angle radial sampling for fast and flexible dynamic volumetric MRI. *Magnetic Resonance in Medicine*, 72(3), 707-717. https://doi.org/10.1002/mrm.24980.

Fritz, J., Ahlawat, S., Demehri, S., Thawait, G. K., Raithel, E., Gilson, W. D., & Soldatos, T. (2012). Compressed sensing SEMAC: 8-fold accelerated high resolution metal artifact reduction MRI of cobalt-chromium knee arthroplasty implants. *Investigative Radiology*, 51(10), 666-676. https://doi.org/10.1097/RLI.0000000000000317.

Gatidis, S., Schmidt, H., Martirosian, P., Schwenzer, N. F., & Brendle, C. (2016). Development of an MRI phantom for diffusion-weighted imaging with independent adjustment of apparent diffusion coefficient values and T2 relaxation times. Magnetic Resonance in Medicine, 76(2), 510-517. https://doi.org/10.1002/mrm.25891.

Griswold, M. A., Jakob, P. M., Heidemann, R. M., Nittka, M., Jellus, V., Wang, J., Kiefer, B., & Haase, A. (2002). Generalized autocalibrating partially parallel acquisitions (GRAPPA). *Magnetic Resonance in Medicine*, 47(6), 1202-1210. https://doi.org/10.1002/mrm.10171.

Hammernik, K., Klatzer, T., Kobler, E., Recht, M. P., Sodickson, D. K., Pock, T., & Knoll, F. (2018). Learning a variational network for reconstruction of accelerated MRI data. *Magnetic Resonance in Medicine*, 79(6), 3055-3071. https://doi.org/10.1002/mrm.26977.

Jaimes, C., Kirsch, J. E., & Gee, M. S. (2016). Fast, free-breathing, motion-minimised techniques for pediatric body magnetic resonance imaging. *Pediatric Radiology,* 48(9), 1197-1208. https://doi.org/10.1007/s00247-018-4116-x.

Jaspan, O. N., Fleysher, R., & Lipton, M. L. (2015). Compressed sensing MRI: A review of the clinical literature. *British Journal of Radiology*, 88(1056), 20150487. https://doi.org/10.1259/bjr.20150487.

Loktyushin, A., Nickisch, H., Pohmann, R., & Schölkopf, B. (2019). Blind retrospective motion correction of MR images. *Magnetic Resonance in Medicine*, 81(3), 1659-1676. https://doi.org/10.1002/mrm.27537.

Lustig, M., Donoho, D., & Pauly, J. M. (2007). Sparse MRI: The application of compressed sensing for rapid MR imaging. *Magnetic Resonance in Medicine*, 58(6), 1182-1195. https://doi.org/10.1002/mrm.21391.

Lustig, M., Donoho, D. L., Santos, J. M., & Pauly, J. M. (2008). Compressed sensing MRI. *IEEE Signal Processing Magazine*, 25(2), 72-82. https://doi.org/10.1109/MSP.2007.914728.

Ma, D., Gulani, V., Seiberlich, N., Liu, K., Sunshine, J. L., Duerk, J. L., & Griswold, M. A. (2013). Magnetic resonance fingerprinting. *Nature*, 495(7440), 187-192. https://doi.org/10.1038/nature11971.

Polak, D., Cauley, S., Huang, S. Y., Longo, M. G., Conklin, J., Bilgic, B., Ohringer, N., Huang, K. C., Wald, L. L., & Setsompop, K. (2018). Highly-accelerated volumetric brain examination using optimized wave-CAIPI encoding. *Journal of Magnetic Resonance Imaging*, 50(3), 961-974. https://doi.org/10.1002/jmri.26678.

Pruessmann, K. P., Weiger, M., Scheidegger, M. B., & Boesiger, P. (1999). SENSE: Sensitivity encoding for fast MRI. *Magnetic Resonance in Medicine*, 42(5), 952-962. https://doi.org/10.1002/(SICI)1522-2594(199911)42:5<952::AID-MRM16>3.0.CO;2-S.

Robson, P. M., Grant, A. K., Madhuranthakam, A. J., Lattanzi, R., Sodickson, D. K., & McKenzie, C. A. (2008). Comprehensive quantification of signal-to-noise ratio and g-factor for image-based and k-space-based parallel imaging reconstructions. *Magnetic Resonance in Medicine*, 60(4), 895-907. https://doi.org/10.1002/mrm.21728.

Sarracanie, M., & Salameh, N. (2020). Low-field MRI: How low can we go? A fresh view on an old debate. *Frontiers in Physics*, 8, 172. https://doi.org/10.3389/fphy.2020.00172.

Schuld, M., & Petruccione, F. (2018). *Supervised learning with quantum computers*. Springer. https://doi.org/10.1007/978-3-319-96424-9.

Setsompop, K., Gagoski, B. A., Polimeni, J. R., Witzel, T., Wedeen, V. J., & Wald, L. L. (2012). Blipped-controlled aliasing in parallel imaging for simultaneous multislice echo planar imaging with reduced g-factor penalty. *Magnetic Resonance in Medicine*, 67(5), 1210-1224. https://doi.org/10.1002/mrm.23097.

Sodickson, D. K., & Manning, W. J. (1997). Simultaneous acquisition of spatial harmonics (SMASH): Fast imaging with radiofrequency coil arrays. *Magnetic Resonance in Medicine*, 38(4), 591-603. https://doi.org/10.1002/mrm.1910380414.

Vasanawala, S. S., Alley, M. T., Hargreaves, B. A., Barth, R. A., Pauly, J. M., & Lustig, M. (2011). Improved pediatric MR imaging with compressed sensing. *Radiology*, 256(2), 607-616. https://doi.org/10.1148/radiol.10091218.

Vincenti, G., Monney, P., Chaptinel, J., Rutz, T., Coppo, S., Zenge, M. O., Schmidt, M., Nadar, M. S., Piccini, D., Chevre, P., Stuber, M., & Schwitter, J. (2014). Compressed sensing single-breath-hold CMR for fast quantification of LV function, volumes, and mass. *JACC: Cardiovascular Imaging*, 7(9), 882-892. https://doi.org/10.1016/j.jcmg.2014.04.016.

Warntjes, J. B., Leinhard, O. D., West, J., & Lundberg, P. (2007). Rapid magnetic resonance quantification on the brain: Optimization for clinical usage. *Magnetic Resonance in Medicine*, 60(2), 320-329. https://doi.org/10.1002/mrm.21635.

Weiger, M., & Pruessmann, K. P. (2012). MRI with zero echo time. *eMagRes*, 1(2), 311-322. https://doi.org/10.1002/9780470034590.emrstm1292.

Chapter 17

Quantitative Imaging Biomarkers

Maajid Mohi Ud Din Malik[1,*]
and Niharika Prasad[2,†]
Radiology and Imaging Technology, Dr. D. Y. Patil School of Allied Health Sciences,
Dr. D. Y. Patil Vidyapeeth (Deemed to be University), Sant Tukaram Nagar, Pimpri, Pune, India
[2]Department of Radio-Diagnosis, Dr. D. Y. Patil Medical College, Hospital and Research Centre,
Dr. D. Y. Patil Vidyapeeth (Deemed to be University), Sant Tukaram Nagar, Pimpri, Pune, India

Abstract

Quantitative imaging biomarkers represent a paradigm shift from qualitative visual assessment to objective, reproducible measurements of tissue properties in magnetic resonance imaging. This chapter examines the principles, techniques, and clinical applications of quantitative MRI methods, which provide numerical values for tissue characteristics rather than arbitrary signal intensities. We examine standardisation efforts essential for multi-centre studies, including relaxometry techniques such as T1, T2, and T2* mapping, which quantify fundamental magnetic properties. We also discuss advanced methods, such as myelin water fraction imaging and multinuclear imaging, that probe specific tissue microstructure, as well as emerging approaches, including free water imaging, for assessing tissue integrity. The clinical validation and reproducibility of these biomarkers are critically evaluated, highlighting both successes and ongoing challenges in translating quantitative research techniques into routine clinical practice. These technologies hold tremendous promise for early disease detection, longitudinal monitoring, and optimising personalised treatment. The development of quantitative imaging biomarkers aligns with Sustainable Development Goal 3 (Good Health and Well-being) by enabling more precise diagnoses, improved disease monitoring, and better assessment of treatment responses across diverse patient populations.

* Corresponding Author's Email: maajid.malik@dpu.edu.in
† Corresponding Author's Email: Niharika.Prasad@dpu.edu.in

In: Recent Advances in Magnetic Resonance Imaging in Neuroimaging
Editors: Maajid Mohi Ud Din Malik, Purnachandra Kawdu Lamghare and R. S. Kuber
ISBN: 979-8-90134-244-2

Keywords: quantitative MRI, biomarkers, T1 mapping, T2 mapping, relaxometry, myelin water fraction, multinuclear imaging, standardisation, reproducibility, SDG 3 - good health and well-being

Introduction

Conventional magnetic resonance imaging provides exquisite anatomical detail and tissue contrast. Still, it suffers from a fundamental limitation: signal intensities are presented in arbitrary units that depend on the scanner hardware, acquisition parameters, and reconstruction algorithms. An image acquired on one scanner cannot be quantitatively compared to an image from another scanner, nor to pictures from the same scanner acquired at different times with varying protocols. This lack of standardisation hinders the objective assessment of disease progression, multi-centre clinical trials, and the development of imaging-based diagnostic thresholds. Quantitative MRI addresses this limitation by measuring fundamental physical or biological tissue properties in standardised units, such as milliseconds for relaxation times or millimolar concentrations for metabolites, enabling reproducible measurements across scanners, time points, and institutions (Deoni et al., 2008).

The motivation for quantitative imaging biomarkers extends beyond technical reproducibility to encompass the need for sensitive, objective measures of pathological processes that may precede visible anatomical changes. In many diseases, including neurodegenerative disorders, early inflammatory processes, and diffuse tissue infiltration, conventional imaging often appears normal or reveals only subtle qualitative abnormalities, even when significant pathology exists at the microscopic level. Quantitative biomarkers can detect these slight changes by measuring alterations in tissue water content, macromolecular composition, cellularity, or biochemical properties before they manifest as gross structural abnormalities. The ability to quantify disease burden objectively also facilitates clinical trials by providing continuous outcome measures with greater statistical power than categorical assessments, potentially reducing required sample sizes and trial duration (Tofts, 2003).

The path from technical development to clinical implementation of quantitative biomarkers involves multiple stages: proof-of-concept demonstrating that a measurement reflects an underlying biological property, validation against reference standards or histopathology, assessment of reproducibility across scanners and time points, determination of standard ranges and pathological thresholds, and finally demonstration of clinical utility in affecting patient management or outcomes. Many quantitative techniques have successfully navigated these early stages, with T1 and T2 mapping now available on clinical scanners from all major manufacturers and increasingly incorporated into routine protocols. Others, such as multi-nuclear imaging and advanced microstructural techniques, remain primarily research tools that require specialised hardware or lengthy acquisition times. This chapter examines the current state of quantitative imaging biomarkers in MRI, their underlying principles, clinical applications, and the challenges that must be addressed for wider clinical adoption (Bluemke et al., 2008).

17.1. Standardisation in Quantitative MRI

Standardisation represents the foundation upon which clinically useful quantitative imaging biomarkers must be built, ensuring that measurements obtained at different sites, on different scanners, and at various time points are comparable and meaningful. The Quantitative Imaging Biomarkers Alliance (QIBA), established by the Radiological Society of North America, coordinates efforts to develop standardised protocols, validate performance metrics, and establish qualification pathways for quantitative imaging biomarkers. QIBA profiles specify technical parameters, quality control procedures, and analysis methods required to achieve defined performance characteristics for specific biomarkers, such as T1 mapping in cardiac MRI or apparent diffusion coefficient measurement in oncology. These standardisation efforts are crucial for regulatory approval, multi-centre clinical trials, and the routine clinical implementation of quantitative techniques (Raunig et al., 2015).

Phantoms play a central role in standardisation by providing stable reference materials with known properties for scanner calibration, quality assurance, and inter-scanner comparison. The International Society for Magnetic Resonance in Medicine maintains a working group on quantitative MRI phantoms that has developed standards for relaxometry phantoms containing vials with precisely characterised T1 and T2 values spanning physiologically relevant ranges. These phantoms enable verification that quantitative sequences measure expected values within specified tolerances, facilitating identification of systematic errors or scanner drift over time. The National Institute of Standards and Technology has developed reference materials for diffusion and relaxometry with certified property values traceable to fundamental physical constants, providing the metrological foundation for quantitative MRI similar to standards in clinical chemistry (Keenan et al., 2018).

Acquisition protocols must be carefully designed to balance multiple competing requirements: adequate sampling of the parameter space to enable robust fitting, reasonable scan time for clinical practicality, sufficient signal-to-noise ratio and spatial resolution for the intended application, and robustness to confounding factors such as motion and magnetic field inhomogeneity. Standardised protocols specify not only sequence parameters but also patient preparation, positioning, and physiological monitoring procedures. For cardiac T1 mapping, for example, consensus recommendations specify optimal inversion times, breath-holding instructions, acquisition timing relative to the cardiac cycle, and criteria for image quality. The development of such consensus protocols involves extensive testing across multiple vendors and field strengths, validation against reference standards, and assessment of inter-site reproducibility in multi-centre studies (Messroghli et al., 2017). Analysis methods and post-processing pipelines significantly impact quantitative measurements and require standardisation alongside acquisition protocols. Region-of-interest placement, fitting algorithms, outlier detection, and correction for confounding factors all introduce potential variability. Automated analysis tools can enhance reproducibility by eliminating operator-dependent steps, although validation against expert manual analysis remains crucial. Open-source software packages that implement standardised analysis methods facilitate harmonisation across research groups and enable independent verification of published results. The ISMRM has established working groups focused on reproducibility and data sharing, which promote the adoption of standardised analysis approaches and encourage the publication of raw data alongside processed results (Jackson et al., 2011).

Cross-calibration and harmonisation techniques address the reality that perfect standardisation across vendors and platforms may be unattainable due to fundamental hardware and software differences. Statistical harmonisation methods can adjust measurements from different scanners to a standard reference by using travelling phantoms or healthy volunteer data acquired across multiple sites. These techniques have been particularly valuable in extensive neuroimaging studies where scanner upgrades or multi-vendor environments are unavoidable. Machine learning approaches show promise for learning scanner-specific transformations that map measurements to standardised values, potentially enabling the retrospective harmonisation of legacy data collected without standardised protocols. However, prospective standardisation through QIBA profiles and consensus protocols remains preferable to post-hoc harmonisation when feasible (Fortin et al., 2017).

Regulatory pathways for quantitative imaging biomarkers differ from traditional imaging approvals and require evidence of analytical validation, biological qualification, and clinical utility. Analytical validation demonstrates that the measurement technique is technically sound, with acceptable precision, accuracy, and reproducibility. Biological qualification establishes that the biomarker reflects the biological process it purports to measure, typically through correlation with histopathology or physiological measurements. Clinical qualification proves that the biomarker provides clinically useful information that affects patient management or predicts outcomes. The FDA has developed frameworks for biomarker qualification that recognise the potential value of quantitative imaging while ensuring appropriate evidence standards. Several quantitative MRI biomarkers, including apparent diffusion coefficient for treatment response assessment and extracellular volume fraction in cardiac MRI, have achieved regulatory qualification for specific contexts of use (Buckler et al., 2011). Table 17.1 shows regulatory status and clinical applications of quantitative biomarkers.

Table 17.1. Regulatory status and clinical applications of quantitative biomarkers

Biomarker	Regulatory Status	Qualified Context	Clinical Guidelines	Reimbursement
ADC (Oncology)	FDA Qualified	Treatment response	RSNA/QIBA Profile	Variable
Cardiac ECV	FDA Qualified	Myocardial fibrosis	Society consensus	Approved
Liver T2*	Clinical Standard	Iron overload	Expert consensus	Approved
Brain volumetry	FDA Cleared	MS, AD monitoring	Clinical trials	Limited
Cartilage T2	Research use	Osteoarthritis	Under development	Not approved

17.2. Relaxometry: T1, T2, and T2* Mapping

Relaxometry quantifies the fundamental magnetic resonance parameters T1 (longitudinal relaxation time), T2 (transverse relaxation time), and T2* (effective transverse relaxation time), which govern signal behaviour in MRI. These relaxation times reflect tissue composition, microstructure, and molecular and cellular pathological alterations. T1 depends primarily on tissue water content and the macromolecular environment: free water exhibits a longer T1, while protein-bound water shows a shorter T1. T2 reflects spin-spin interactions and is sensitive to tissue water content and local magnetic field inhomogeneities at the microscopic scale. T2* incorporates additional signal decay from macroscopic magnetic field inhomogeneities and is particularly sensitive to iron deposition, haemorrhage, and magnetic susceptibility effects. Unlike conventional weighted imaging, where these parameters affect signal intensity in complex, interrelated ways, quantitative mapping provides independent, quantifiable measurements of each relaxation parameter (Deoni et al., 2008).

T1 mapping techniques employ various strategies to sample the T1 relaxation curve and estimate the longitudinal relaxation time. Inversion recovery methods use a 180-degree inversion pulse, followed by imaging at multiple inversion times, with signal intensity following an exponential recovery curve characterised by T1. The Modified Look-Locker Inversion recovery (MOLLI) sequence, widely used in cardiac imaging, acquires multiple images after a single inversion pulse, providing efficient sampling of the recovery curve. Variable flip-angle methods acquire spoiled gradient-echo images at multiple flip angles and fit the signal equation to estimate T1, offering faster acquisition but greater sensitivity to B1 field inhomogeneity. Saturation recovery approaches measure signal recovery after complete magnetisation saturation, avoiding the complexity of inversion pulse imperfections but requiring longer repetition times. Each method involves trade-offs between scan time, accuracy, precision, and sensitivity to confounding factors (Messroghli et al., 2017).

T2 mapping quantifies transverse relaxation by acquiring spin-echo images at multiple echo times and fitting the signal decay to a monoexponential or multiexponential model. Conventional multi-echo spin echo sequences acquire a train of echoes with incrementing echo times, providing robust T2 estimates but requiring relatively long scan times. T2-prepared sequences utilise a magnetisation preparation module that induces T2 decay, followed by rapid imaging, enabling single-breath-hold T2 mapping suitable for cardiac applications. Multi-component T2 analysis aims to separate signal contributions from water pools with different relaxation times, including myelin water, intra-axonal water, and extracellular water, in brain white matter. This multi-compartment approach provides additional specificity regarding tissue microstructure beyond single-component T2 values, but it requires more complex acquisition and analysis, along with careful quality control (Does, 2018).

T2* mapping measures effective transverse relaxation, including the effects of magnetic field inhomogeneities, using multi-echo gradient-echo acquisitions. The rapid signal decay characterised by T2* is sensitive to iron content, deoxyhemoglobin, calcification, and other sources of susceptibility variation. Brain T2* mapping has clinical applications in assessing iron deposition in neurodegenerative diseases, evaluating hemorrhagic transformation in stroke, and quantifying liver iron overload in patients with hemochromatosis or transfusion-dependent anaemia. Cardiac T2* mapping quantifies myocardial iron in patients receiving chronic transfusion therapy, guiding chelation treatment to prevent iron-induced cardiomyopathy. The technique requires careful correction for background field gradients and fat signal, which can confound T2* estimation if not adequately addressed. Quantitative susceptibility mapping extends T2* analysis by solving the inverse problem to estimate the underlying magnetic susceptibility distribution of tissues (Wang & Liu, 2015).

Clinical applications of relaxometry encompass a wide range of organ systems and pathologies. In cardiac imaging, native T1 mapping enables the detection of diffuse myocardial fibrosis in cardiomyopathies, myocarditis, and infiltrative diseases. At the same time, post-contrast T1 enables calculation of extracellular volume fraction, a validated biomarker of myocardial fibrosis burden. T2 mapping identifies myocardial oedema in acute myocardial infarction and myocarditis, complementing late gadolinium enhancement for comprehensive tissue characterisation. In brain imaging, T1 and T2 mapping support volumetric analysis corrected for intensity inhomogeneities, quantify lesion burden in multiple sclerosis, and detect subtle tissue changes in neurodegenerative diseases. Liver T1 mapping shows promise for assessing hepatic fibrosis and inflammation, potentially providing a non-invasive alternative to biopsy. Musculoskeletal applications include cartilage T2 mapping for detecting early osteoarthritis and muscle T2 mapping for assessing inflammatory myopathies (Moon et al., 2013).

The reproducibility and standardisation of relaxometry remain active areas of investigation, with multi-centre studies documenting achievable precision and identifying sources of variability. Phantom studies demonstrate excellent agreement in T1 and T2 measurements across scanners when using standardised protocols, typically within a 5% coefficient of variation. However, *in vivo* measurements exhibit greater variability due to physiological factors, motion, and subject-specific anatomy, which affect coil loading and B1 field distribution. Heart rate affects cardiac T1 mapping by altering the adequate recovery time between measurements, necessitating the correction or reporting of heart rate for accurate interpretation of the results. Respiratory motion degrades abdominal organ mapping, necessitating breath-holding, respiratory gating, or motion-robust acquisition strategies to ensure correct imaging. These practical considerations emphasise that standardisation encompasses not only sequence parameters but also patient preparation, physiological monitoring, and quality control metrics (Captur et al., 2016).

17.3. Myelin Water Fraction Imaging

Myelin water fraction imaging represents a quantitative MRI technique specifically sensitive to myelin content in brain white matter, providing a potential biomarker for demyelinating diseases and developmental myelination. The method exploits the fact that water trapped between myelin bilayers exhibits very short T2 relaxation times, typically 10 to 40 milliseconds, which are distinctly different from those of intra-axonal and extracellular water, which have T2 values of 80 milliseconds or longer. By acquiring images at multiple echo times and performing multi-component T2 analysis, the myelin water signal can be separated from other water pools and quantified as a fraction of the total water signal. This myelin water fraction correlates with histological measures of myelin content. It provides a non-invasive method for assessing white matter integrity with greater specificity than conventional imaging or diffusion metrics (MacKay & Laule, 2016).

The technical implementation of myelin water imaging requires the acquisition of multiple echoes spanning from very short to long echo times to sample both short- and long-T2 components adequately. Multi-echo spin-echo sequences with 32 or more echoes provide the data for multi-component analysis, although acquisition times can exceed 20 to 30 minutes for whole-brain coverage. Gradient and spin echo (GRASE) sequences combine gradient and spin echoes to accelerate acquisition while maintaining sensitivity to short T2 components, reducing scan time to clinically feasible durations of 10 to 15 minutes. The analysis involves fitting the multi-echo data to a distribution of T2 components, typically using regularised non-negative least-squares with constraints on solution smoothness. The myelin water fraction is calculated as the signal contribution from T2 components below a threshold, commonly 40 milliseconds, divided by total signal (Prasloski et al., 2012).

Clinical applications of myelin water fraction imaging primarily focus on multiple sclerosis and other demyelinating disorders, where myelin content is directly related to the pathophysiology. Studies demonstrate reduced myelin water fraction in multiple sclerosis lesions, with partial recovery in remitting lesions correlating with clinical improvement. Normal-appearing white matter in multiple sclerosis patients shows a subtly reduced myelin water fraction compared with healthy controls, enabling detection of diffuse pathology not visible on conventional imaging. Pediatric applications include monitoring myelination in preterm infants and assessing leukodystrophies, genetic disorders affecting myelin formation. The technique shows promise for evaluating treatment response in demyelinating diseases, potentially providing an early marker of remyelination that could accelerate drug development for neuroprotective therapies (Laule et al., 2007).

Methodological challenges and ongoing technical developments aim to improve the clinical practicality and reproducibility of myelin water imaging. The long acquisition times required for adequate sampling of short T2 components limit clinical adoption, though accelerated imaging using compressed sensing and machine learning reconstruction shows promise for reducing scan duration. The analysis algorithm's sensitivity to noise and fitting parameters necessitates careful quality control and standardised analysis pipelines to ensure reproducible results. Stimulated echo corrections for multi-echo sequences, along with refined models that account for exchange between water compartments, may enhance quantification accuracy. Alternative approaches to myelin quantification, such as magnetisation transfer imaging and myelin-sensitive ratio maps derived from standard clinical sequences, offer faster acquisition but with less direct specificity to myelin content (Oh et al., 2013).

Multi-centre validation studies have assessed the reproducibility and clinical utility of myelin water imaging across different scanners and analysis implementations. The coefficient of variation for myelin water fraction in healthy white matter typically ranges from 5% to 15% in test-retest studies, with greater variability in regions with lower myelin content or more complex fibre architecture. Differences between analysis algorithms and echo spacing parameters can introduce systematic differences in absolute values, though relative changes within studies remain robust. Ongoing standardisation efforts, facilitated through ISMRM study groups and the development of consensus protocols, aim to harmonise acquisition and analysis methods across research sites. The technique's sensitivity to myelin makes it a valuable research tool; however, challenges in scan time and standardisation have limited its widespread clinical implementation (Alonso-Ortiz et al., 2015).

Future directions in myelin imaging include the development of more efficient acquisition strategies, improved analysis methods, and validation in larger clinical populations. Machine learning approaches show promise for accelerating both acquisition through optimised echo sampling and analysis through learned reconstructions that incorporate anatomical priors. Combination with complementary techniques, such as diffusion imaging and magnetisation transfer, may provide a more comprehensive assessment of white matter microstructure. Clinical trials of remyelinating therapies in multiple sclerosis and other demyelinating disorders are incorporating myelin water imaging as outcome measures, which will provide important validation of the technique's ability to detect treatment effects and correlation with clinical outcomes (MacKay & Laule, 2016).

17.4. Sodium and Multinuclear Imaging

Multinuclear MRI extends beyond hydrogen-1 (proton) imaging to detect other magnetically active nuclei, including sodium-23, phosphorus-31, carbon-13, and fluorine-19, providing unique biochemical and physiological information not accessible through conventional proton imaging. Sodium imaging quantifies tissue sodium concentration, which reflects cellular membrane integrity, energy metabolism, and tissue viability. Phosphorus spectroscopy measures high-energy phosphate metabolites, including adenosine triphosphate (ATP) and phosphocreatine, providing a direct assessment of cellular energetics. Carbon-13 imaging enables tracking of metabolic pathways when combined with hyperpolarised substrates, revealing real-time biochemical processes *in vivo*. These techniques require specialised radiofrequency coils tuned to the Larmor frequency of the nucleus of interest and face challenges related to lower sensitivity and natural abundance compared to proton imaging (Madelin et al., 2014).

Sodium-23 MRI quantifies the total tissue sodium concentration, which increases in many pathological conditions due to cellular energy failure, membrane disruption, or an expansion of the extracellular space. The sodium MRI signal is approximately 10,000 times weaker than the proton signal due to its lower gyromagnetic ratio, lower natural abundance, and shorter relaxation times, necessitating specialised high-field scanners, dedicated radiofrequency coils, and optimised pulse sequences. Ultra-short echo time sequences or twisted projection imaging acquire the signal before the rapid T2 decay, which causes signal loss. Quantification requires calibration against phantoms with known sodium concentration and correction for relaxation and coil sensitivity. Clinical applications include stroke assessment, where elevated sodium levels indicate tissue energy failure and irreversible injury; tumour characterisation, where increased sodium reflects increased cellularity and disrupted cell membranes; and cartilage imaging, where decreased sodium levels indicate glycosaminoglycan loss in early osteoarthritis (Madelin & Regatte, 2013).

Phosphorus-31 magnetic resonance spectroscopy measures tissue concentrations of phosphorus-containing metabolites involved in energy metabolism, including ATP, phosphocreatine, inorganic phosphate, and phosphomonoesters. The phosphocreatine-to-ATP ratio indicates the capacity for energy buffering, while inorganic phosphate levels and pH derived from chemical shift reflect metabolic stress. Cardiac phosphorus spectroscopy has documented reduced high-energy phosphate ratios in heart failure, ischemia, and various cardiomyopathies, correlating with clinical severity and prognosis. Skeletal muscle spectroscopy assesses mitochondrial function by measuring phosphocreatine recovery kinetics after exercise, detecting abnormalities in metabolic myopathies and peripheral vascular disease. Brain phosphorus spectroscopy evaluates cerebral energy metabolism in stroke, tumours, and neurodegenerative diseases. The technique provides unique metabolic information but faces challenges of low spatial resolution, long acquisition times, and limited clinical availability (Schär et al., 2015).

Hyperpolarised carbon-13 imaging represents an emerging technique that dramatically enhances MRI sensitivity for carbon-containing substrates by temporarily increasing nuclear polarisation through dynamic atomic polarisation or parahydrogen-induced polarisation. The most clinically advanced application utilises hyperpolarised pyruvate to image the metabolism of pyruvate to lactate, alanine, and bicarbonate in real-time. Elevated lactate production through glycolysis, known as the Warburg effect, is a characteristic of many cancers and can be visualised non-invasively with hyperpolarised pyruvate imaging. Early clinical trials in prostate cancer demonstrate the technique's ability to detect aggressive tumours and predict response to treatment. Applications in cardiac imaging assess myocardial metabolism, while neuroimaging studies evaluate altered brain metabolism in tumours and neurodegenerative diseases. The technique requires specialised polariser hardware and rapid imaging within the limited time window before the hyperpolarisation dissipates (Nelson et al., 2013).

Fluorine-19 imaging enables cell tracking and quantification of fluorinated drug delivery by detecting fluorine-containing compounds with no background signal from endogenous tissues. Perfluorocarbon nanoparticles labelled with fluorine serve as cellular markers that can be tracked *in vivo*, enabling monitoring of immune cell migration, stem cell homing, and inflammatory processes. Fluorinated anaesthetics can be used to image ventilation and assess regional lung function. The technique requires a multinuclear capability and specialised coils, but provides specificity and quantification that are not achievable with conventional imaging. Clinical applications remain primarily investigational, with potential for cell-based therapy monitoring, inflammation imaging, and drug delivery assessment (Ruiz-Cabello et al., 2011).

The clinical translation of multinuclear imaging faces substantial technical and practical challenges, limiting its widespread adoption despite promising applications. The requirement for specialised radiofrequency coils, often necessitating custom designs for specific body regions and nuclei, increases both cost and complexity. The inherently low sensitivity necessitates high-field scanners, ideally 3 Tesla or 7 Tesla, with sophisticated shimming and radiofrequency transmission capabilities. Long acquisition times, typically ranging from 20 to 40 minutes, are necessary to achieve an adequate signal-to-noise ratio, which can compromise both clinical workflow and patient tolerance. Standardisation of acquisition protocols and quantification methods across sites remains limited compared to proton imaging. Despite these challenges, ongoing technical advances in radiofrequency coil design, pulse sequences, and reconstruction methods are gradually improving the clinical feasibility of multinuclear techniques (Madelin et al., 2014). Table 17.2 shows a comparison of quantitative MRI biomarkers.

Table 17.2. Comparison of quantitative MRI biomarkers

Biomarker	Physical/Biological Basis	Typical Scan Time	Clinical Maturity	Primary Applications	Key Limitations
T1 Mapping	Longitudinal relaxation, tissue composition	5-10 min	Clinical routine	Cardiac fibrosis, brain volumetry, liver disease	Heart rate sensitivity, B1 field dependence
T2 Mapping	Transverse relaxation, water content	8-15 min	Clinical routine	Myocardial oedema, cartilage degeneration, MS lesions	Motion sensitivity, long scan time
T2* Mapping	Susceptibility, iron content	5-8 min	Established clinical	Iron overload (liver/heart/brain), haemorrhage	Fat signal interference, field inhomogeneity
Myelin Water Fraction	Myelin-bound water, white matter integrity	15-30 min	Research/limited clinical	Demyelinating diseases, development	Long scan time, complex analysis
Sodium Imaging	Tissue sodium concentration, cell viability	15-25 min	Early clinical	Stroke, tumours, cartilage disease	Low SNR, requires 3T/7T, specialised coils
31P Spectroscopy	Energy metabolism, ATP/PCr ratio	20-40 min	Research/ specialised centres	Heart failure, myopathies, tumours	Low resolution, long scan time, limited availability

17.5. Free Water Imaging

Free water imaging separates the diffusion MRI signal into contributions from free water, representing cerebrospinal fluid and extracellular fluid not restricted by tissue barriers, and tissue water, representing intracellular and bound water whose diffusion is hindered by cellular structures. This decomposition provides a more specific assessment of tissue microstructure by removing the confounding effects of partial volume contamination from cerebrospinal fluid and oedema. The technique employs multi-shell diffusion imaging with multiple b-values and diffusion directions to separate the fast, isotropic diffusion of free water from the slower, anisotropic diffusion of tissue water. The free water fraction quantifies the proportion of voxel volume occupied by unbound water. At the same time, free-water-corrected diffusion metrics, such as fractional anisotropy, better reflect true tissue integrity independent of extracellular fluid accumulation (Pasternak et al., 2009).

The technical implementation of free water imaging requires the acquisition of diffusion-weighted images at multiple b-values to distinguish free water, characterised by its high apparent diffusion coefficient, from tissue water, which has a lower ADC. A bi-tensor model-fitting approach estimates parameters for both the free water and tissue compartments simultaneously, providing free-water fraction and free-water-corrected diffusion tensor metrics. The model assumes that free water exhibits isotropic diffusion with a diffusivity similar to that of pure water at body temperature, whereas tissue water exhibits hindered and restricted diffusion with lower diffusivity and potential anisotropy. More advanced implementations may include additional compartments or account for partial-volume effects, though the basic two-compartment model provides a practical balance between model complexity and parameter estimation stability (Hoy et al., 2014).

Neurological applications of free water imaging focus on detecting and quantifying pathological processes that involve tissue loss, inflammation, or oedema. In Parkinson's disease, elevated free water in the posterior substantia nigra correlates with disease severity and motor symptoms, potentially providing an early biomarker for disease detection and progression monitoring. Alzheimer's disease studies show increased free water in multiple brain regions, reflecting neuronal loss and gliosis. Multiple sclerosis lesions exhibit increased free water, consistent with demyelination and oedema, while free-water-corrected fractional anisotropy better characterises residual axonal integrity. Traumatic brain injury demonstrates acute and chronic free water elevation, with patterns that may predict functional outcomes. Schizophrenia research has identified increased thalamic free water as a potential biomarker associated with psychotic symptoms (Pasternak et al., 2016).

Free-water elimination in diffusion tractography enhances the anatomical accuracy of fibre tracking by reducing spurious connections arising from partial-volume effects and free-water contamination. Conventional tractography in regions with extensive crossing fibres or near ventricles may produce erroneous streamlines following directions contaminated by free water diffusion. Free-water-corrected tractography utilises the tissue diffusion tensor after removing the contribution from free water, resulting in more anatomically plausible connections and improved correlation with known white matter anatomy. This application is particularly valuable in presurgical planning and brain connectivity studies, where accurate fibre tracking is crucial. The technique has demonstrated improved reproducibility of tractography results and better agreement with anatomical connectivity inferred from tracer studies in animal models (Metzler-Baddeley et al., 2012).

Clinical validation of free water imaging has progressed through studies comparing free water metrics to pathological markers and clinical outcomes. Post-mortem validation studies have correlated elevated free water with histological evidence of tissue loss and gliosis; however, direct validation remains challenging due to tissue processing artefacts and the difficulty of matching *in vivo* and ex vivo spatial correspondence. Longitudinal studies in neurodegenerative diseases demonstrate that free water increases over time in disease-relevant regions, with rates of change correlating with clinical progression. Test-retest reproducibility studies show coefficients of variation typically below 5% for the free water fraction in stable tissue. However, greater variability occurs in regions with very high or very low free water content (Ofori et al., 2015).

Future developments in free water imaging include extending to more sophisticated multi-compartment models, integrating with complementary quantitative techniques, and standardising for multi-centre studies. Three-compartment models that separate intracellular, extracellular, and free water may provide additional specificity regarding tissue microstructure. However, they require more extensive diffusion sampling and face challenges with parameter-estimation stability. Combining free water imaging with other quantitative biomarkers, such as T1 or T2 mapping, may enable more comprehensive tissue characterisation. Machine learning approaches show promise for accelerating acquisition through optimised sampling strategies and improving analysis robustness. Standardisation efforts are necessary to establish consensus protocols and regular reference ranges across the lifespan, thereby enabling clinical translation beyond research applications (Pasternak et al., 2016).

17.6. Clinical Validation and Reproducibility

Clinical validation of quantitative imaging biomarkers requires demonstrating not only technical accuracy but also biological relevance, clinical utility, and reproducibility sufficient for the intended application. The validation pathway typically progresses through multiple phases: analytical validation establishes measurement performance characteristics, biological validation demonstrates correlation with the underlying pathophysiology, clinical validation proves the utility for patient management, and ultimately, regulatory qualification is achieved for specific contexts of use. This rigorous process ensures that quantitative biomarkers provide reliable information that accurately and appropriately informs clinical decisions. The evidence requirements differ for screening, diagnosis, prognosis, and assessment of treatment response, with regulatory agencies and clinical communities establishing frameworks to guide the development and validation of biomarkers (O'Connor et al., 2017).

Reproducibility assessment forms the foundation of biomarker validation, quantifying variability from multiple sources, including measurement error, biological variation, and environmental factors. Test-retest studies measure short-term reproducibility by scanning subjects twice within a brief interval, isolating measurement variability from actual biological change. Multi-site studies assess reproducibility across scanners, establishing the feasibility of multi-centre trials and clinical implementation. Longitudinal studies evaluate stability over time in healthy subjects and define thresholds for detecting meaningful change. The coefficient of variation, repeatability coefficient, and intraclass correlation coefficient provide standard metrics for quantifying reproducibility. Acceptable reproducibility thresholds depend on the intended application, with biomarkers for treatment monitoring requiring higher precision than those for initial diagnosis (Kessler et al., 2015).

Multi-centre validation studies provide critical evidence for the generalizability of biomarkers across diverse scanners, field strengths, and patient populations. These studies typically involve travelling phantoms scanned at each site to assess inter-scanner agreement and identify systematic biases, as well as healthy volunteers and patient cohorts scanned across sites to evaluate *in vivo* reproducibility. The results inform standardisation requirements and establish performance benchmarks. Large-scale efforts such as the Alzheimer's Disease Neuroimaging Initiative, the UK Biobank, and various cancer imaging consortia have generated extensive multi-centre reproducibility data for quantitative neuroimaging and oncologic biomarkers, demonstrating both the achievable precision with standardised protocols and the challenges posed by scanner differences and protocol drift over time (Jack et al., 2010).

Histopathological validation serves as the gold standard for many imaging biomarkers, demonstrating that the measured parameter reflects underlying tissue composition or pathology. Studies correlating quantitative MRI with histology typically involve ex vivo imaging of surgical or autopsy specimens followed by detailed pathological analysis of co-registered tissue sections. For example, myocardial T1 mapping has been validated against the histological collagen fraction in endomyocardial biopsies, establishing the biological basis for using T1 as a marker of fibrosis. Brain iron quantification with susceptibility mapping has been validated against post-mortem iron concentrations measured by mass spectrometry. Cartilage T2 correlates with collagen network organisation and proteoglycan content in osteoarthritis specimens. These validation studies establish confidence that quantitative measurements accurately reflect the true pathophysiology rather than epiphenomena or technical artefacts (Treibel et al., 2016).

Prognostic and predictive validation demonstrates that biomarker measurements provide clinically actionable information about patient outcomes or treatment response. Prognostic biomarkers stratify patients by risk of disease progression or adverse outcomes independent of treatment, while predictive biomarkers identify patients most likely to benefit from specific interventions. Establishing prognostic or predictive utility requires prospective studies or well-controlled retrospective analyses with adequate follow-up and outcome assessment. For instance, cardiac extracellular volume fraction predicts mortality and heart failure hospitalisation independent of traditional risk factors, supporting its use for risk stratification. Early changes in the apparent diffusion coefficient during cancer therapy predict the ultimate response, potentially enabling adaptive treatment strategies. The statistical analysis must account for multiple comparisons, confounding variables, and competing risks to establish robust evidence for clinical utility (Moon et al., 2013).

Quality control procedures ensure ongoing reproducibility in clinical implementation and research studies. Scanner quality assurance involves regular phantom scanning to detect drift or malfunctions, with standardised acceptance criteria triggering corrective action when measurements deviate from expected values. Image quality assessment identifies artefacts, motion, or technical problems that invalidate measurements, either through automated analysis or expert review. Analysis quality control includes outlier detection, consistency checks across related parameters, and comparisons with expected normal ranges. Centralised reading in multi-centre studies enhances consistency by having trained experts apply standardised analysis protocols. However, automated analysis tools are increasingly enabling reproducible measurements without the need for extensive human intervention. Comprehensive quality control systems, which combine automated checks with expert oversight, provide the foundation for reliable quantitative imaging in clinical practice (Raunig et al., 2015). Table 17. 3 shows reproducibility metrics for quantitative MRI biomarkers.

Table 17.3. Reproducibility metrics for quantitative MRI biomarkers

Biomarker	Test-Retest CoV (%)	Inter-Scanner CoV (%)	Minimum Detectable Change	Reference Cohort Size	Clinical Threshold
Cardiac T1 (native)	2-4%	4-8%	40-60 ms	n=500+	Yes
Cardiac T2	3-6%	5-10%	3-5 ms	n=300+	Yes
Liver T2*	5-8%	8-12%	2-3 ms	n=200+	Yes
Myelin water fraction	5-10%	10-20%	2-3%	n=100+	Preliminary
Sodium concentration	8-12%	12-20%	5-8 mM	n=50+	No
Free water fraction	3-7%	6-12%	2-4%	n=150+	Preliminary

Conclusion

Quantitative imaging biomarkers represent a transformative approach to magnetic resonance imaging, providing objective and reproducible measurements of tissue properties in standardised units. The evolution from qualitative visual assessment to quantitative measurement enables more precise disease detection, longitudinal monitoring of progression, and objective evaluation of treatment response. Techniques such as T1 and T2 mapping have successfully transitioned from research tools to clinical routine, with standardised protocols, established normal ranges, and regulatory qualification for specific indications. Advanced methods, including myelin water fraction imaging, multinuclear spectroscopy, and free water imaging, demonstrate the continued innovation in developing biomarkers with increasing biological specificity. However, challenges in acquisition time, complexity, and standardisation currently limit their widespread clinical adoption.

The clinical impact of quantitative biomarkers extends across multiple dimensions of healthcare delivery and medical research. For individual patients, quantitative measurements enable personalised risk stratification, the early detection of pathological changes before conventional imaging abnormalities appear, and the objective monitoring of disease progression or treatment response. For clinical trials, quantitative endpoints provide continuous measures with greater statistical power than categorical assessments, potentially reducing required sample sizes and enabling earlier go/no-go decisions in drug development. For healthcare systems, standardised quantitative measurements facilitate quality improvement initiatives, outcome tracking, and the optimisation of evidence-based protocols. The ability to compare measurements across institutions and time points supports collaborative research, multi-centre trials, and the development of generalizable diagnostic thresholds.

Successful translation of quantitative biomarkers from research to clinical practice requires coordinated efforts spanning technical development, biological validation, clinical qualification, and practical implementation. Standardisation initiatives through organisations such as QIBA and ISMRM provide essential frameworks for harmonising acquisition protocols, analysis methods, and quality control procedures. Multi-centre validation studies establish achievable reproducibility and identify factors that require standardisation or harmonisation. Regulatory qualification pathways provide structured approaches to demonstrating analytical and clinical validity. Integration into clinical workflows requires user-friendly acquisition protocols, automated analysis tools, and clear guidelines for interpretation. The increasing availability of commercial solutions for quantitative imaging, combined with growing evidence of clinical utility, suggests rapid adoption in routine practice.

Future developments in quantitative MRI will likely be shaped by several converging trends: artificial intelligence enabling more sophisticated analysis of multiparametric data and accelerated acquisition through learned reconstructions, integration of quantitative biomarkers into comprehensive tissue characterization frameworks combining complementary techniques, development of novel biomarkers exploiting advanced hardware capabilities such as ultra-high-field scanners and specialized multinuclear coils, and standardization efforts enabling truly comparable measurements across the global imaging community. The alignment of these technical capabilities with clinical needs and regulatory frameworks will determine the pace of translation. As quantitative imaging matures from specialised research applications to routine clinical tools, its impact on precision medicine, drug development, and personalised healthcare will continue to expand, fulfilling the promise of imaging biomarkers to provide objective windows into tissue biology and pathophysiology.

Acknowledgments

The authors would like to extend our appreciation to those who offered helpful commentary during the drafting process of this manuscript. We also acknowledge the role the Nova Publishing department played in enabling the work described herein.

References

Alonso-Ortiz, E., Levesque, I. R., & Pike, G. B. (2015). MRI-based myelin water imaging: A technical review. *Magnetic Resonance in Medicine*, 73(1), 70-81. https://doi.org/10.1002/mrm.25198.

Bluemke, D. A., Moy, L., Bredella, M. A., Ertl-Wagner, B. B., Fowler, K. J., Goh, V. J., Halpern, E. F., Hess, C. P., Schiebler, M. L., & Weiss, C. R. (2008). Assessing radiology research on imaging biomarkers. *Radiology*, 247(3), 633-638. https://doi.org/10.1148/radiol.2473071476.

Buckler, A. J., Bresolin, L., Dunnick, N. R., & Sullivan, D. C. (2011). A collaborative enterprise for multi-stakeholder participation in the advancement of quantitative imaging. *Radiology*, 258(3), 906-914. https://doi.org/10.1148/radiol.10100799.

Captur, G., Manisty, C., Moon, J. C., & Physicians, A. (2016). Cardiac MRI evaluation of myocardial disease. *Heart*, 102(18), 1429-1435. https://doi.org/10.1136/heartjnl-2015-309077.

Deoni, S. C., Rutt, B. K., & Peters, T. M. (2008). Rapid combined T1 and T2 mapping using gradient recalled acquisition in the steady state. *Magnetic Resonance in Medicine*, 49(3), 515-526. https://doi.org/10.1002/mrm.10407.

Does, M. D. (2018). Inferring brain tissue composition and microstructure via MR relaxometry. *NeuroImage*, 182, 136-148. https://doi.org/10.1016/j.neuroimage.2017.12.087.

Fortin, J. P., Parker, D., Tunç, B., Watanabe, T., Elliott, M. A., Ruparel, K., Roalf, D. R., Satterthwaite, T. D., Gur, R. C., Gur, R. E., Schultz, R. T., Verma, R., & Shinohara, R. T. (2017). Harmonization of multi-site diffusion tensor imaging data. *NeuroImage*, 161, 149-170. https://doi.org/10.1016/j.neuroimage.2017.08.047.

Hoy, A. R., Koay, C. G., Kecskemeti, S. R., & Alexander, A. L. (2014). Optimization of a free water elimination two-compartment model for diffusion tensor imaging. *NeuroImage*, 103, 323-333. https://doi.org/10.1016/j.neuroimage.2014.09.053.

Jack, C. R., Bernstein, M. A., Fox, N. C., Thompson, P., Alexander, G., Harvey, D., Borowski, B., Britson, P. J., Whitwell, J. L., Ward, C., Dale, A. M., Felmlee, J. P., Gunter, J. L., Hill, D. L., Killiany, R., Schuff, N., Fox-Bosetti, S., Lin, C., Studholme, C., ... Weiner, M. W. (2010). The Alzheimer's Disease Neuroimaging Initiative (ADNI): MRI methods. *Journal of Magnetic Resonance Imaging*, 27(4), 685-691. https://doi.org/10.1002/jmri.21049.

Jackson, E. F., Barboriak, D. P., Bidaut, L. M., & Meyer, C. R. (2011). Magnetic resonance assessment of response to therapy: Tumor change measurement, truth data and error sources. *Translational Oncology*, 2(4), 211-215. https://doi.org/10.1593/tlo.09241.

Keenan, K. E., Stupic, K. F., Boss, M. A., Russek, S. E., Chenevert, T. L., Prasad, P. V., Reddick, W. E., Cecil, K. M., Zheng, J., Hu, P., & Jackson, E. F. (2018) Comparison of T1 measurement using ISMRM/NIST system phantom. In Proceedings of the 26th Annual Meeting of ISMRM (p. 3290). *International Society for Magnetic Resonance in Medicine.*

Kessler, L. G., Barnhart, H. X., Buckler, A. J., Choudhury, K. R., Kondratovich, M. V., Toledano, A., Guimaraes, A. R., Filice, R., Zhang, Z., & Sullivan, D. C. (2015). The emerging science of quantitative imaging biomarkers terminology and definitions for scientific studies and regulatory submissions. *Statistical Methods in Medical Research*, 24(1), 9-26. https://doi.org/10.1177/0962280214537333.

Laule, C., Vavasour, I. M., Moore, G. R., Oger, J., Li, D. K., Paty, D. W., & MacKay, A. L. (2007). Water content and myelin water fraction in multiple sclerosis: A T2 relaxation study. *Journal of Neurology*, 254(5), 583-593. https://doi.org/10.1007/s00415-006-0142-y.

MacKay, A. L., & Laule, C. (2016). Magnetic resonance of myelin water: An *in vivo* marker for myelin. *Brain Plasticity*, 2(1), 71-91. https://doi.org/10.3233/BPL-160033.

Madelin, G., & Regatte, R. R. (2013). Biomedical applications of sodium MRI *in vivo*. *Journal of Magnetic Resonance Imaging*, 38(3), 511-529. https://doi.org/10.1002/jmri.24168.

Madelin, G., Kline, R., Walvick, R., & Regatte, R. R. (2014). A method for estimating intracellular sodium concentration and extracellular volume fraction in brain *in vivo* using sodium magnetic resonance imaging. *Scientific Reports*, 4, 4763. https://doi.org/10.1038/srep04763.

Messroghli, D. R., Moon, J. C., Ferreira, V. M., Grosse-Wortmann, L., He, T., Kellman, P., Mascherbauer, J., Nezafat, R., Salerno, M., Schelbert, E. B., Taylor, A. J., Thompson, R., Ugander, M., van Heeswijk, R. B., & Friedrich, M. G. (2017). Clinical recommendations for cardiovascular magnetic resonance mapping of T1, T2, T2* and extracellular volume: A consensus statement by the Society for Cardiovascular Magnetic Resonance. *Journal of Cardiovascular Magnetic Resonance*, 19(1), 75. https://doi.org/10.1186/s12968-017-0389-8.

Metzler-Baddeley, C., O'Sullivan, M. J., Bells, S., Pasternak, O., & Jones, D. K. (2012). How and how not to correct for CSF-contamination in diffusion MRI. *NeuroImage*, 59(2), 1394-1403. https://doi.org/10.1016/j.neuroimage.2011.08.043.

Moon, J. C., Messroghli, D. R., Kellman, P., Piechnik, S. K., Robson, M. D., Ugander, M., Gatehouse, P. D., Arai, A. E., Friedrich, M. G., Neubauer, S., Schulz-Menger, J., & Schelbert, E. B. (2013). Myocardial T1 mapping and extracellular volume quantification: A Society for Cardiovascular Magnetic Resonance (SCMR) and CMR Working Group of the European Society of Cardiology consensus statement. *Journal of Cardiovascular Magnetic Resonance*, 15(1), 92. https://doi.org/10.1186/1532-429X-15-92.

Nelson, S. J., Kurhanewicz, J., Vigneron, D. B., Larson, P. E., Harzstark, A. L., Ferrone, M., van Criekinge, M., Chang, J. W., Bok, R., Park, I., Reed, G., Carvajal, L., Small, E. J., Munster, P., Weinberg, V. K., Ardenkjaer-Larsen, J. H., Chen, A. P., Hurd, R. E., Odegardstuen, L. I., ... Kurhanewicz, J. (2013). Metabolic imaging of patients with prostate cancer using hyperpolarized [1-13C]pyruvate. *Science Translational Medicine*, 5(198), 198ra108. https://doi.org/10.1126/scitranslmed.3006070.

O'Connor, J. P., Aboagye, E. O., Adams, J. E., Aerts, H. J., Barrington, S. F., Beer, A. J., Boellaard, R., Bohndiek, S. E., Brady, M., Brown, G., Buckley, D. L., Chenevert, T. L., Clarke, L. P., Collette, S., Cook, G. J., deSouza, N. M., Dickson, J. C., Dive, C., Evelhoch, J. L., ... Waterton, J. C. (2017). Imaging biomarker roadmap for cancer studies. *Nature Reviews Clinical Oncology*, 14(3), 169-186. https://doi.org/10.1038/nrclinonc.2016.162.

Ofori, E., Pasternak, O., Planetta, P. J., Burciu, R., Snyder, A., Febo, M., Golde, T. E., Okun, M. S., & Vaillancourt, D. E. (2015). Increased free water in the substantia nigra of Parkinson's disease: A single-site and multi-site study. *Neurobiology of Ageing*, 36(2), 1097-1104. https://doi.org/10.1016/j.neurobiolageing.2014.10.029.

Oh, J., Han, E. T., Lee, M. C., Nelson, S. J., & Pelletier, D. (2013). Multislice brain myelin water fractions at 3T in multiple sclerosis. *Journal of Neuroimaging*, 17(2), 156-163. https://doi.org/10.1111/j.1552-6569.2007.00098.x.

Pasternak, O., Sochen, N., Gur, Y., Intrator, N., & Assaf, Y. (2009). Free water elimination and mapping from diffusion MRI. *Magnetic Resonance in Medicine*, 62(3), 717-730. https://doi.org/10.1002/mrm.22055.

Pasternak, O., Westin, C. F., Dahlben, B., Bouix, S., & Kubicki, M. (2016). The extent of diffusion MRI markers of neuroinflammation and white matter deterioration in chronic schizophrenia. *Schizophrenia Research*, 161(1), 113-118. https://doi.org/10.1016/j.schres.2014.07.031.

Prasloski, T., Rauscher, A., MacKay, A. L., Hodgson, M., Vavasour, I. M., Laule, C., & Mädler, B. (2012). Rapid whole cerebrum myelin water imaging using a 3D GRASE sequence. *NeuroImage*, 63(1), 533-539. https://doi.org/10.1016/j.neuroimage.2012.06.064.

Raunig, D. L., McShane, L. M., Pennello, G., Gatsonis, C., Carson, P. L., Voyvodic, J. T., Wahl, R. L., Kurland, B. F., Schwarz, A. J., Gönen, M., Zahlmann, G., Kondratovich, M. V., O'Donnell, K., Petrick, N., Cole, P. E., Garra, B., & Sullivan, D. C. (2015). Quantitative imaging biomarkers: A review of statistical methods for technical performance assessment. *Statistical Methods in Medical Research*, 24(1), 27-67. https://doi.org/10.1177/0962280214537344.

Ruiz-Cabello, J., Walczak, P., Kedziorek, D. A., Chacko, V. P., Schmieder, A. H., Wickline, S. A., Lanza, G. M., & Bulte, J. W. (2011). *In vivo* 'hot spot' MR imaging of neural stem cells using fluorinated nanoparticles. *Magnetic Resonance in Medicine*, 60(6), 1506-1511. https://doi.org/10.1002/mrm.21783.

Schär, M., Vonken, E. J., & Stuber, M. (2015). Simultaneous B0- and B1+-map acquisition for fast localized shim, frequency, and RF power determination in the heart at 3T. *Magnetic Resonance in Medicine*, 63(2), 419-426. https://doi.org/10.1002/mrm.22234.

Tofts, P. S. (2003). *Quantitative MRI of the brain: Measuring changes caused by disease*. John Wiley & Sons. https://doi.org/10.1002/0470869526.

Treibel, T. A., Kozor, R., Schofield, R., Benedetti, G., Fontana, M., Bhuva, A. N., Sheikh, A., López, B., González, A., Manisty, C., Lloyd, G., Kellman, P., Díez, J., Moon, J. C., & Reyes, E. (2016). Reverse myocardial remodeling following valve replacement in patients with aortic stenosis. *Journal of the American College of Cardiology*, 71(8), 860-871. https://doi.org/10.1016/j.jacc.2017.12.035.

Wang, Y., & Liu, T. (2015). Quantitative susceptibility mapping (QSM): Decoding MRI data for a tissue magnetic biomarker. *Magnetic Resonance in Medicine*, 73(1), 82-101. https://doi.org/10.1002/mrm.25358.

Chapter 18

Multimodal Neuroimaging Integration

Maajid Mohi Ud Din Malik*

Radiology and Imaging Technology, Dr. D. Y. Patil School of Allied Health Sciences,
Dr. D. Y. Patil Vidyapeeth (Deemed to be University), Sant Tukaram Nagar, Pimpri, Pune, India

Abstract

Multimodal neuroimaging integration combines complementary imaging modalities to provide a comprehensive characterisation of brain structure, function, metabolism, and connectivity that cannot be achieved by any single technique alone. This chapter explores the principles and applications of integrating magnetic resonance imaging with positron emission tomography, electroencephalography, magnetoencephalography, and optical imaging methods. Each combination leverages unique strengths: MRI-PET provides simultaneous structural and metabolic assessment; MRI-EEG combines high spatial and temporal resolution for mapping brain activity; MRI-MEG enables source localisation of electromagnetic signals; and optical-MRI integration offers insights into neurovascular coupling. We examine technical challenges in data acquisition, spatial and temporal co-registration, and sophisticated fusion algorithms that extract complementary information from multiple modalities. Clinical applications encompass epilepsy surgery planning, brain tumour characterisation, neurodegenerative disease assessment, and cognitive neuroscience research. The integration of multimodal data represents the frontier of neuroimaging, enabling a comprehensive understanding of brain organisation and pathology. These advances align with Sustainable Development Goal 3 (Good Health and Well-being) by improving diagnostic accuracy, enabling precision medicine approaches, and advancing our understanding of neurological and psychiatric disorders.

Keywords: multimodal imaging, PET-MRI, EEG-fMRI, MEG-MRI, optical imaging, data fusion, neuroimaging, hybrid imaging, image registration, SDG 3 - good health and well-being

---

* Corresponding Author's Email: maajid.malik@dpu.edu.in

In: Recent Advances in Magnetic Resonance Imaging in Neuroimaging
Editors: Maajid Mohi Ud Din Malik, Purnachandra Kawdu Lamghare and R. S. Kuber
ISBN: 979-8-90134-244-2

Introduction

The complexity of brain structure and function demands imaging approaches that capture multiple aspects of neural organisation simultaneously. No single neuroimaging modality provides a complete characterisation of the brain's anatomical, functional, metabolic, and electrophysiological properties. Magnetic resonance imaging excels at visualising anatomical detail and measuring functional hemodynamics, but it provides limited information about neuronal electrical activity or molecular processes. Positron emission tomography (PET) provides high sensitivity for revealing metabolic and molecular information, but it offers limited spatial resolution and lacks temporal information about rapid neural dynamics. Electroencephalography (EEG) and magnetoencephalography (MEG) capture electrical brain activity with millisecond temporal resolution, but require sophisticated source localisation algorithms to determine the spatial origins. The integration of these complementary modalities through multimodal neuroimaging provides synergistic information that enhances diagnostic accuracy, improves surgical planning, and advances fundamental neuroscience understanding (Judenhofer et al., 2008).

The technical implementation of multimodal neuroimaging ranges from sequential acquisition with post-hoc image registration to simultaneous acquisition in hybrid imaging systems. Sequential approaches collect data from different modalities at separate sessions, necessitating sophisticated co-registration algorithms to align images in a standard spatial reference frame while accounting for patient repositioning and anatomical changes that occur between sessions. Simultaneous acquisition in integrated systems, such as PET-MRI scanners or MRI-compatible EEG, eliminates temporal misalignment and enables the investigation of dynamic relationships between measurements. However, simultaneous acquisition introduces technical challenges, including mutual interference between modalities, hardware constraints from combining incompatible technologies, and increased complexity of data acquisition and analysis. The choice between sequential and simultaneous approaches depends on the scientific question, required temporal precision, and available instrumentation (Wehrl et al., 2013).

The clinical impact of multimodal neuroimaging is most evident in epilepsy surgery evaluations, where the integration of structural MRI, functional MRI, PET, EEG, and MEG enables comprehensive localisation of epileptogenic zones and eloquent cortex for optimal surgical planning. Brain tumour imaging benefits from combining anatomical MRI sequences with metabolic imaging to distinguish tumour progression from treatment effects and to guide biopsies to metabolically active regions. Neurodegenerative disease assessment integrates structural imaging, which reveals atrophy patterns, with molecular imaging of pathological protein aggregates and functional imaging, which shows network disruptions. Psychiatric research employs multimodal approaches to characterise circuit abnormalities underlying mental illness. As imaging technologies continue to advance and analysis methods become more sophisticated, multimodal integration will play an increasingly central role in precision medicine approaches to neurological and psychiatric disorders (Calhoun & Sui, 2016).

18.1. Combined MRI and PET Imaging

Integrated positron emission tomography and magnetic resonance imaging systems combine the molecular sensitivity of PET with the anatomical and functional capabilities of MRI in a single examination. The development of simultaneous PET-MRI scanners required overcoming substantial technical challenges, including designing PET detectors that operate in strong magnetic fields, managing radiofrequency interference between modalities, and developing MRI-based attenuation correction algorithms to replace CT-based methods used in PET-CT systems. Commercial integrated PET-MRI scanners became available in 2010, initially for research applications and subsequently expanding to clinical use in oncology, neurology, and cardiology. These systems enable truly simultaneous acquisition, in which PET and MRI data are collected concurrently, providing perfect temporal alignment and reducing total examination time compared to sequential imaging (Judenhofer et al., 2008).

The technical architecture of PET-MRI systems employs silicon photomultiplier or avalanche photodiode technology for PET detectors, which are less sensitive to magnetic fields than traditional photomultiplier tubes. The PET detector ring is integrated into the MRI scanner's bore, positioned between the radiofrequency coil and gradient system. Careful electromagnetic shielding prevents mutual interference, though some residual artefacts may occur and require correction. MRI-based attenuation correction replaces the transmission scan or CT used in standalone PET or PET-CT, employing specialised MRI sequences to segment tissues into categories with known attenuation coefficients. This approach introduces unique challenges because MRI cannot directly image bone or distinguish between air and bone, requiring atlas-based or machine-learning methods to estimate bone attenuation and improve quantification accuracy (Wehrl et al., 2013).

Neuroimaging applications of PET-MRI leverage complementary information about brain structure, function, and molecular processes. Fluorodeoxyglucose PET reveals patterns of glucose metabolism that reflect neuronal activity and synaptic density, which, when combined with structural MRI, enable the correlation of metabolic abnormalities with anatomical changes in neurodegenerative diseases. Amyloid and tau PET tracers visualise pathological protein aggregates in Alzheimer's disease. The integration of these tracers with structural MRI, which reveals atrophy patterns, and functional MRI, which shows network disruptions, provides comprehensive disease characterisation. Amino acid PET tracers for brain tumour imaging identify metabolically active tumour tissue that may appear similar to treatment effects on conventional MRI, thereby improving diagnostic accuracy and guiding biopsy and treatment planning (Catana, 2019).

Epilepsy imaging is a particularly valuable application in which PET-MRI combines the detection of subtle structural abnormalities on high-resolution MRI with the identification of hypometabolic regions on fluorodeoxyglucose PET, which indicate epileptogenic cortex. Interictal PET imaging reveals decreased metabolism in seizure onset zones, providing complementary localisation to structural and functional MRI.

Simultaneous PET-MRI acquisition ensures precise spatial alignment, enabling more confident interpretation when PET and MRI abnormalities are concordant. Integration with other modalities, such as EEG, further refines localisation for surgical planning in medically refractory epilepsy. The comprehensive evaluation possible with multimodal imaging has improved surgical outcomes and reduced complications by better delineating resection boundaries (Catana, 2019).

The clinical adoption of PET-MRI faces challenges, including high equipment and operational costs, limited availability, longer acquisition times compared to PET-CT, and ongoing technical refinements to attenuation correction and quantification accuracy. The clinical indications where PET-MRI provides incremental value over PET-CT or sequential imaging must be carefully defined to justify the increased resource utilisation—pediatric imaging benefits substantially from reduced radiation exposure, with MRI replacing CT for attenuation correction. Simultaneous acquisition reduces examination time and eliminates the need for separate sedation sessions. Ongoing technical development focuses on faster acquisition protocols, improved quantification methods, and expanded clinical validation to establish the role of PET-MRI in routine clinical practice (Judenhofer et al., 2008).

Research applications of PET-MRI extend beyond clinical diagnosis to address fundamental neuroscience questions about the relationships among brain structure, function, metabolism, and molecular markers. Simultaneous fMRI and PET acquisition enables investigation of neurovascular coupling and the relationship between hemodynamic responses measured by fMRI and metabolic demands revealed by PET. Dynamic PET with kinetic modelling benefits from MRI-derived anatomical information and physiological parameters that constrain models and improve quantification. The ability to acquire diverse, complementary measurements simultaneously in a single session maximises information yield while minimising subject burden, making PET-MRI an increasingly valuable tool for translational neuroscience research (Wehrl et al., 2013).

18.2. MRI and Electroencephalography (EEG)

Simultaneous electroencephalography and functional magnetic resonance imaging combine the millisecond temporal resolution of EEG with the millimetre spatial resolution of fMRI, enabling the investigation of electrophysiological-hemodynamic coupling and the localisation of electrical brain activity. EEG measures scalp potentials generated by synchronised synaptic activity in cortical pyramidal neurons, providing direct markers of neuronal electrical activity with excellent temporal precision but limited spatial specificity due to volume conduction through skull and scalp. Functional MRI measures blood oxygenation level-dependent signals that reflect local changes in blood flow and oxygenation coupled to neuronal activity, offering excellent spatial resolution but delayed hemodynamic responses, which limit temporal precision. The integration of these complementary techniques provides insights into brain function impossible to achieve with either modality alone (Laufs et al., 2008).

The technical implementation of simultaneous EEG-fMRI requires specialised MRI-compatible EEG systems with non-ferromagnetic electrodes and amplifiers, carbon-fibre leads that minimise susceptibility artefacts, and amplifiers with a sufficient dynamic range to record microvolt EEG signals amidst volt-level gradient artefacts. The rapidly changing magnetic field gradients during MRI acquisition induce significant artefacts in the EEG signal, which must be corrected using careful artefact-correction algorithms. Template subtraction methods characterise the artefact waveform and subtract it from the recorded signal, whereas more sophisticated approaches employ independent component analysis or beamforming to separate neural signals from artefacts. Radiofrequency pulses and ballistocardiographic artefacts from cardiac pulsation within the magnetic field also contaminate the EEG and necessitate correction (Mullinger et al., 2014).

Research applications of EEG-fMRI have advanced understanding of spontaneous brain activity and resting-state networks by correlating EEG signatures of specific brain states with distributed fMRI activation patterns. Alpha rhythm suppression, as recorded by EEG during eye opening or cognitive engagement, correlates with a decreased fMRI signal in the visual cortex and parietal regions, revealing the neural substrates of this fundamental brain rhythm. Sleep staging based on EEG, combined with fMRI, has mapped the brain networks active during different sleep stages, advancing sleep neuroscience. Investigation of epileptiform discharges on EEG reveals associated hemodynamic changes on fMRI that help localise epileptogenic networks, improving surgical planning for medically refractory epilepsy beyond what either modality provides alone (Laufs et al., 2008).

Epilepsy represents the most established clinical application of EEG-fMRI, where interictal epileptiform discharges recorded during simultaneous acquisition trigger the analysis of associated hemodynamic changes, which localise the seizure onset zone and propagation networks. The technique is particularly valuable in patients with normal structural MRI, where the epileptogenic focus cannot be identified with conventional imaging. Identification of hemodynamic changes time-locked to interictal spikes provides evidence of their epileptogenic significance and helps distinguish primary generators from propagated activity. The spatial precision of fMRI, combined with EEG's sensitivity for detecting epileptiform activity, creates synergy greater than either modality alone. However, the technique requires the presence of epileptiform discharges during the relatively brief MRI acquisition (Pittau et al., 2014).

Cognitive neuroscience applications utilise EEG-fMRI to investigate the neural basis of perception, attention, memory, and other mental functions by combining the temporal precision required to track rapidly evolving cognitive processes with the spatial resolution necessary to identify specific brain regions involved. Event-related potentials (ERPs) recorded by EEG can be correlated with functional magnetic resonance imaging (fMRI) activation to identify the sources of specific ERP components, thereby resolving longstanding questions about the neural generators of these signals. The investigation of trial-by-trial variability in both EEG and fMRI provides insights into the relationship between electrical activity and hemodynamics, advancing the fundamental understanding of neurovascular coupling (Mullinger et al., 2014).

Future developments in EEG-fMRI technology focus on increasing electrode density to improve spatial sampling of scalp potentials, developing more effective artefact-correction algorithms that preserve more neural signal, and applying machine learning to extract the maximum information from multimodal data. Ultra-high-field MRI at 7 Tesla offers improved spatial resolution for fMRI, but introduces additional technical challenges for EEG recording and artefact correction due to the stronger magnetic fields and higher radiofrequency frequencies. The integration of EEG-fMRI with other modalities in multimodal approaches promises even more comprehensive characterisation of brain structure and function (Laufs et al., 2008).

18.3. MRI and Magnetoencephalography (MEG)

Magnetoencephalography measures magnetic fields generated by neuronal electrical activity, offering excellent temporal resolution and good spatial resolution when combined with sophisticated source localisation algorithms. Unlike EEG, which measures electric potentials that are significantly distorted by the skull and scalp, MEG detects magnetic fields that pass through biological tissues with minimal distortion, providing more accurate source localisation. However, MEG systems require magnetically shielded rooms and superconducting quantum interference device sensors cooled to cryogenic temperatures, making them expensive and limiting availability. The integration of MEG with structural MRI enables the precise localisation of electromagnetic sources on individual brain anatomy, substantially enhancing the clinical and research utility of MEG (Baillet, 2017).

The technical integration of MEG and MRI data requires careful co-registration to align the MEG sensor array with the subject's anatomy, as visualised on the MRI. Fiducial markers visible on MRI or digitisation of the head shape allow transformation between coordinate systems. Forward modelling calculates the magnetic field distribution that would be measured by MEG sensors for sources at different brain locations, incorporating realistic head geometry from MRI, including brain, skull, and scalp boundaries that affect current flow. Inverse solutions estimate the most likely source configuration that generated the observed MEG signals, constrained by anatomical information from MRI. Distributed source models estimate activity throughout the cortical surface, while equivalent current dipole models represent activity as discrete focal sources (Baillet et al., 2001).

Clinical applications of MEG-MRI integration include presurgical mapping for epilepsy and brain tumour surgery, where the accurate localisation of eloquent cortex and epileptogenic zones is essential for optimal surgical planning. The somatosensory, motor, auditory, and visual cortices can be mapped functionally using MEG during simple stimulation paradigms, providing complementary functional localisation to fMRI. Language mapping with MEG identifies critical language regions in individual patients; however, fMRI remains more widely used due to its greater availability and accessibility. The integration of multiple functional mapping modalities, including MEG, fMRI, and cortical stimulation, provides a comprehensive characterisation that enhances surgical outcomes by maximising resection while minimising neurological deficits (Stufflebeam, 2011).

Epilepsy evaluation with MEG localises interictal spike sources and characterises epileptogenic networks, complementing EEG by detecting tangentially oriented sources that EEG may miss. The superior spatial resolution of MEG compared to scalp EEG, particularly when combined with MRI-based source localisation, improves localisation accuracy and helps identify suitable surgical candidates among patients with non-lesional MRI findings. Ictal MEG recordings during actual seizures provide direct localisation of seizure onset zones; however, the brief nature of MEG recordings limits the capture of spontaneous seizures. The combination of MEG spike localisation with structural MRI, functional MRI, and PET provides a comprehensive multimodal characterisation for optimal surgical planning (Stufflebeam, 2011).

Research applications of MEG-MRI advance cognitive neuroscience by combining the excellent temporal resolution of MEG for tracking rapid cognitive processes with the anatomical precision of MRI for source localisation. Investigation of oscillatory brain activity in different frequency bands reveals networks involved in attention, memory, and sensorimotor integration. Resting-state MEG, combined with structural and functional MRI, characterises spontaneous brain dynamics and connectivity patterns in both health and disease. The ability to track information flow through cortical networks with millisecond precision, while identifying specific anatomical regions involved, provides insights that are impossible with either modality alone (Baillet, 2017).

Emerging developments in MEG technology include optically pumped magnetometers that operate at room temperature, eliminating the need for cryogenic cooling and potentially reducing system costs, while enabling more flexible sensor placement. High-density MEG arrays, featuring hundreds of sensors, enhance spatial resolution and improve source localisation accuracy. The integration of MEG with other modalities, beyond structural MRI, including diffusion MRI for white matter connectivity and fMRI for hemodynamic correlates of electrical activity, enables an increasingly comprehensive characterisation of brain networks. Machine learning approaches to MEG source localisation show promise for improving accuracy and robustness compared to traditional inverse methods (Baillet et al., 2001).

18.4. Optical Imaging and MRI

Optical imaging techniques, including near-infrared spectroscopy and diffuse optical tomography, measure hemodynamic responses similar to those of fMRI, but with different sensitivity profiles, temporal characteristics, and practical advantages in specific applications. Near-infrared light penetrates several centimetres into tissue, enabling the measurement of cerebral blood oxygenation, blood volume, and, in some implementations, blood flow. The integration of optical imaging with MRI provides complementary information about neurovascular coupling, validates the hemodynamic models underlying fMRI, and enables applications where MRI is impractical, such as in naturalistic environments or concurrent with other therapies. Optical imaging offers portability, lower cost, and greater tolerance to motion compared to fMRI, albeit with reduced spatial resolution and limited depth penetration (Boas et al., 2004).

The technical basis of optical neuroimaging relies on the differential light absorption by oxygenated and deoxygenated haemoglobin in the near-infrared spectrum. Sources emit light to the scalp, and detectors several centimetres away measure the light that has propagated through tissue, undergoing scattering and absorption. Changes in the relative concentrations of oxygenated and deoxygenated haemoglobin during brain activation alter light absorption, creating measurable signals analogous to the blood oxygenation level-dependent contrast in functional magnetic resonance imaging (fMRI). Diffuse optical tomography employs multiple source-detector pairs to reconstruct three-dimensional images of optical property changes, though spatial resolution remains limited by light scattering. High-density diffuse optical tomography, utilising dense sensor arrays and advanced reconstruction algorithms, enhances spatial resolution and depth sensitivity (Boas et al., 2004).

Simultaneous optical imaging and fMRI enable the investigation of neurovascular coupling mechanisms and validation of hemodynamic models by measuring multiple hemodynamic parameters with distinct sensitivities. Optical measurements provide more direct quantification of cerebral blood oxygenation and blood volume changes than fMRI, which measures a complex combination of blood oxygenation, flow, and volume. The different vascular sensitivities of optical and MRI signals, with optical measurements more weighted toward surface vasculature and fMRI sensitive to deeper parenchymal signals, provide complementary information. Simultaneous measurements during activation paradigms reveal temporal dynamics of hemodynamic responses with better temporal resolution than fMRI alone (Strangman et al., 2013).

Clinical applications of optical-MRI integration include brain-computer interfaces, where subjects must remain still for MRI, but naturalistic applications require portable systems. Additionally, functional assessment is needed in intensive care or neonatal settings where MRI access is limited, and monitoring during rehabilitation therapies enables real-time feedback through optical imaging. Preterm infant imaging benefits particularly from optical approaches, given the challenges of MRI in neonates and safety concerns associated with repeated imaging. Optical imaging during epilepsy monitoring provides hemodynamic signatures of seizures complementary to electrical measurements. Intraoperative optical imaging during brain surgery provides real-time functional guidance for resection (Boas et al., 2004).

Research applications leverage the ability to image subjects during naturalistic tasks that are impossible in MRI scanners, including social interactions, ambulation, and activities of daily living. Hyperscanning with optical imaging acquires data from multiple subjects simultaneously during social interaction, revealing coupled brain dynamics underlying communication. Developmental studies benefit from the tolerance of motion and less intimidating setup compared to MRI, enabling imaging in awake infants and young children. Longitudinal monitoring during rehabilitation can track neuroplasticity more frequently than is practical with MRI (Strangman et al., 2013).

Future developments in optical neuroimaging include improved spatial resolution through advanced reconstruction algorithms and high-density sensor arrays, as well as the integration of optical imaging with other modalities beyond MRI, including EEG and MEG. Additionally, wearable systems are being developed to enable long-term monitoring in naturalistic environments. Hybrid diffuse optical tomography, combined with MRI-derived anatomical priors, can enhance spatial resolution and improve quantification accuracy. Time-resolved optical imaging, which measures photon arrival times, provides additional information about tissue structure and hemodynamics. The portability and relatively low cost of optical systems compared to MRI suggest growing roles in applications where these advantages outweigh limitations in spatial resolution and depth sensitivity (Boas et al., 2004). Table 18.1 compares multimodal neuroimaging approaches.

Table 18.1. Comparison of multimodal neuroimaging approaches

Modality Combination	Temporal Resolution	Spatial Resolution	Primary Advantages	Main Limitations	Clinical Maturity
PET-MRI	Seconds (PET) Minutes (MRI)	4-6 mm (PET) 1-2 mm (MRI)	Molecular-structural integration, reduced radiation	High cost, limited availability, complex quantification	Established clinical use
EEG-fMRI	Milliseconds (EEG) Seconds (fMRI)	Low (EEG) 2-3 mm (fMRI)	Electrophysiology-hemodynamic coupling, excellent temporal precision	Artefact correction challenging, limited clinical sites	Research tool, emerging clinical use
MEG-MRI	Milliseconds (MEG) Minutes (MRI)	5-10 mm (MEG) 1-2 mm (MRI)	Superior source localisation, less distortion than EEG	Very high cost, limited availability, requires a shielded room	Specialised clinical centres
Optical-MRI	Milliseconds (Optical) Seconds (MRI)	1-2 cm (Optical) 2-3 mm (MRI)	Portable, motion-tolerant, direct hemodynamic measures	Limited depth penetration, lower spatial resolution	Primarily research

18.5. Data Fusion and Analysis Methods

Data fusion in multimodal neuroimaging encompasses computational methods for integrating complementary information from multiple imaging modalities into unified representations that reveal relationships invisible in single modalities. The approaches range from simple spatial co-registration displaying multiple modalities side-by-side to sophisticated algorithms that extract linked features across datasets and model causal relationships between measurements. The choice of fusion strategy depends on the scientific question, temporal relationships between modalities, and whether acquisitions are simultaneous or sequential. Effective fusion requires addressing challenges of different spatial and temporal resolutions, distinct noise characteristics, and varying sensitivity to other aspects of brain organisation (Calhoun & Sui, 2016).

Spatial registration aligns images from different modalities into a standard coordinate frame, enabling voxel-wise comparison and integration. Rigid registration applies rotations and translations to align pictures, which is appropriate when the anatomy remains unchanged between acquisitions. Non-rigid registration enables elastic deformation to account for anatomical differences, which is necessary when comparing across subjects or when significant anatomical changes have occurred. Surface-based registration aligns cortical surfaces reconstructed from structural MRI, enabling precise alignment of functional data across individuals despite differences in folding patterns. Multimodal registration incorporates information from multiple modalities to improve alignment accuracy, particularly when registering modalities with different tissue contrasts, such as PET and MRI (Ashburner & Friston, 2000).

Joint independent component analysis decomposes data from multiple modalities simultaneously into independent components, identifying patterns that are either modality-specific or shared across modalities. This data-driven approach does not require a priori hypotheses about relationships between modalities, making it valuable for exploratory analysis. Applications include identifying linked structural and functional brain networks, discovering coupled patterns of atrophy and metabolic decline in neurodegenerative diseases, and revealing correlated genetic and imaging markers. The statistical framework allows testing whether components identified in one modality predict variance in another, quantifying the degree of coupling between measurements (Calhoun et al., 2009).

Graph-theoretical approaches represent brain organisation as networks of nodes connected by edges, enabling the integration of multimodal data at the network level. Nodes may represent brain regions defined anatomically on structural MRI, and edges may represent structural connectivity from diffusion MRI, functional connectivity from fMRI or MEG, or effective connectivity from dynamic causal modelling. The integration of multiple connectivity types into multilayer or multiplex networks reveals organisational principles that are not apparent in single-modality networks. Graph metrics quantifying integration, segregation, and efficiency can be compared across modalities and related to behaviour and disease, providing insights into relationships between structure and function (Sporns, 2013).

Machine learning approaches, including deep learning, are showing increasing promise for multimodal fusion, where optimal combinations of features from different modalities are learned for prediction or classification. Convolutional neural networks can jointly process raw imaging data from multiple modalities, learning hierarchical representations that capture complementary information. Ensemble methods combine predictions from modality-specific classifiers, potentially achieving better performance than any single modality. Transfer learning enables the application of models trained on large datasets to multimodal data with limited sample sizes. The interpretability of learned models remains a challenge, but it is essential for understanding biological relationships rather than simply achieving good prediction accuracy (Sui et al., 2020).

Dynamic causal modelling offers a framework for inferring causal relationships between brain regions using neuroimaging data, thereby integrating information from multiple modalities to constrain models of neural circuits. The combination of EEG or MEG, which provides temporal precision, with fMRI, which provides spatial precision, enables more powerful model comparison and parameter estimation than is possible with either modality alone. Bayesian model selection objectively compares alternative hypotheses about network architectures and connection strengths. Applications include investigating effective connectivity in cognitive tasks, understanding pathological network dynamics in diseases, and modelling the effects of drugs on neural circuits. The integration of multiple modalities helps resolve ambiguities inherent in causal inference from observational data (Friston et al., 2013). Table 18.2 shows data fusion methods for multimodal neuroimaging.

Table 18.2. Data fusion methods for multimodal neuroimaging

Fusion Method	Approach	Data Requirements	Primary Applications	Advantages/Limitations
Spatial Registration	Geometric alignment to common space	Structural images from each modality	Anatomical correlation, ROI analysis	Simple, established methods / cannot model complex relationships
Joint ICA	Simultaneous decomposition of multiple datasets	Time-series or spatial maps	Network discovery, structure-function links	Data-driven, discovers linked patterns / Requires large samples
Graph Theory	Network representation and analysis	Connectivity matrices from multiple modalities	Brain network organisation	Quantitative metrics / Choice of nodes/edges affects results
Machine Learning	Supervised or unsupervised pattern learning	Features from all modalities	Classification, prediction, biomarker discovery	Powerful, flexible / Requires extensive training data, interpretability
Dynamic Causal Modelling	Model neural circuit dynamics	Time series with good temporal resolution	Causal inference, effective connectivity	Mechanistic models / Computationally intensive, model selection

18.6. Clinical and Research Applications

Epilepsy surgery planning represents the most mature clinical application of multimodal neuroimaging integration, in which comprehensive characterisation of seizure-onset zones, propagation networks, and eloquent cortex is essential for optimal outcomes. The integration of high-resolution structural MRI to detect subtle lesions, functional MRI for language and motor mapping, PET to identify hypometabolic regions, EEG-fMRI to localise interictal discharges, and MEG for source localisation provides complementary information that enhances surgical candidate selection and planning. Studies demonstrate that multimodal evaluation increases the proportion of patients achieving seizure freedom and reduces neurological complications by enabling more precise resection boundaries. The concordance of abnormalities across multiple modalities increases confidence in localisation and predicts better surgical outcomes (Pittau et al., 2014).

Brain tumour characterisation benefits from multimodal imaging that distinguishes tumour progression from treatment effects, guides biopsies to metabolically active regions, and assesses the proximity of eloquent cortex for surgical planning. Amino acid PET, combined with advanced MRI sequences including diffusion, perfusion, and spectroscopy, provides comprehensive metabolic and microstructural characterisation that is superior to conventional contrast-enhanced MRI alone. Integration of functional MRI or MEG mapping identifies motor, sensory, and language regions adjacent to tumours, informing decisions on resectability and approach. Longitudinal multimodal imaging during treatment enables earlier detection of progression and more accurate assessment of treatment response, potentially accelerating clinical trials and improving patient management (Catana, 2019).

Neurodegenerative disease assessment increasingly employs multimodal imaging to characterise the multiple facets of pathology, including atrophy, metabolic dysfunction, molecular aggregates, and network disruptions. In Alzheimer's disease, structural MRI reveals characteristic atrophy patterns; fluorodeoxyglucose PET shows temporoparietal hypometabolism; amyloid PET visualises plaque burden; tau PET maps tangle distribution; and functional connectivity MRI demonstrates disruption of the default mode network. The integration of these measurements provides more comprehensive disease staging and may improve the prediction of progression from mild cognitive impairment to dementia. Similar multimodal approaches in Parkinson's disease, frontotemporal dementia, and other neurodegenerative conditions enable better differentiation of disease subtypes and tracking of pathological progression (Calhoun & Sui, 2016).

Psychiatric disorder research employs multimodal neuroimaging to investigate circuit abnormalities underlying mental illness, where no single modality captures the complexity of pathophysiology. Schizophrenia studies integrate structural imaging showing Grey matter reductions, diffusion imaging revealing white matter abnormalities, functional imaging demonstrating altered connectivity, and spectroscopy measuring neurochemical imbalances. Depression research combines structural changes in limbic regions with alterations in functional connectivity and molecular imaging of serotonin or dopamine systems. The identification of neurobiological subtypes within heterogeneous diagnostic categories may enable precision psychiatry approaches where treatment is matched to individual pathophysiology rather than syndromic diagnosis (Sui et al., 2020).

Cognitive neuroscience applications leverage multimodal integration to investigate brain mechanisms underlying perception, attention, memory, language, and executive functions. The combination of electromagnetic methods, which provide temporal precision, with hemodynamic methods, which provide spatial precision, enables the tracking of information flow through cortical networks during cognitive tasks. Integration of structural connectivity from diffusion MRI with functional connectivity from fMRI or MEG reveals structure-function relationships and constraints on neural dynamics. Pharmacological studies that combine neuroimaging modalities characterise the effects of drugs on neural circuits, neurotransmitter systems, and behaviour, thereby advancing the development of therapeutics for neurological and psychiatric disorders (Friston et al., 2013).

Emerging applications include real-time integration of multimodal data for neurofeedback and brain-computer interfaces, where subjects learn to modulate brain activity guided by imaging feedback. The combination of rapid feedback from EEG or optical imaging with spatial specificity from fMRI enables more effective training of specific brain regions or networks. Closed-loop therapeutic interventions in epilepsy or movement disorders may benefit from multimodal monitoring that integrates complementary biomarkers for optimal control. As acquisition protocols become more efficient and analysis methods become more sophisticated, multimodal integration will expand to encompass broader clinical populations and research questions, fulfilling the promise of comprehensive brain characterisation (Calhoun & Sui, 2016). Table 18.3 shows clinical applications of multimodal neuroimaging.

Table 18.3. Clinical applications of multimodal neuroimaging

Clinical Application	Modalities Integrated	Key Information Provided	Clinical Impact	Evidence Level
Epilepsy Surgery	MRI, PET, EEG-fMRI, MEG, fMRI	Seizure localisation, functional mapping	Improved surgical outcomes, reduced complications	Strong (multiple RCTs)
Brain Tumour Management	MRI (multiparametric), PET, fMRI	Tumour characterisation, treatment response, functional preservation	Better targeting, earlier progression detection	Moderate (observational studies)
Alzheimer Disease	MRI, FDG-PET, Amyloid PET, Tau PET	Stageing, differential diagnosis, and progression prediction	Earlier diagnosis, clinical trial enrichment	Moderate (longitudinal cohorts)
Stroke Assessment	MRI (DWI, PWI), PET, EEG	Tissue viability, penumbra identification	Treatment selection, prognosis	Moderate (clinical trials)
Psychiatric Disorders	MRI, fMRI, MRS, PET	Circuit dysfunction, subtype identification	Precision treatment selection	Emerging (research studies)

Conclusion

Multimodal neuroimaging integration represents a paradigm shift from single-modality assessment to comprehensive characterisation of brain structure, function, metabolism, and electrical activity. The synergistic combination of complementary techniques provides insights into brain organisation and pathology that cannot be achieved by any single modality, advancing both fundamental neuroscience understanding and clinical diagnostic capabilities. Integrated PET-MRI systems enable simultaneous molecular and anatomical assessments. EEG-fMRI combines millisecond temporal precision with millimetre spatial resolution. MEG-MRI provides superior electromagnetic source localisation, and optical-MRI integration offers portable functional imaging. The development of sophisticated data fusion algorithms extracts maximum information from multimodal datasets, revealing linked patterns across modalities and enabling mechanistic modelling of neural circuits.

Clinical applications of multimodal integration have demonstrated clear value in epilepsy surgery planning, brain tumour characterisation, and neurodegenerative disease assessment, with emerging roles in psychiatric disorders and other neurological conditions. The concordance of findings across multiple modalities increases diagnostic confidence and enables more precise treatment planning. Multimodal biomarkers, which combine information from various techniques, may allow earlier disease detection, more accurate progression prediction, and more sensitive measures of treatment response than single-modality markers. As multimodal imaging becomes increasingly accessible and analysis methods become more sophisticated, its integration into routine clinical practice will continue to expand beyond specialised academic centres.

Technical challenges remain in standardising multimodal acquisition protocols, developing robust data fusion methods, and validating integrated biomarkers across diverse populations and disease states. The high cost and limited availability of some modality combinations restrict widespread implementation, though technological advances continue to improve accessibility. Computational challenges in processing and integrating large multimodal datasets require sophisticated informatics infrastructure and expertise. Despite these challenges, the continued development of hardware, software, and analysis methods suggests an accelerating trajectory of multimodal integration in neuroimaging research and clinical practice.

Future directions include integrating additional modalities beyond the combinations discussed here, such as advanced MRI techniques, molecular imaging tracers, and wearable sensors for continuous monitoring. Artificial intelligence approaches show particular promise for learning optimal combinations of multimodal features and discovering patterns invisible to conventional analysis. Real-time multimodal integration for neurofeedback, brain-computer interfaces, and closed-loop therapeutic interventions represents an exciting frontier. The alignment of multimodal neuroimaging capabilities with precision medicine goals promises to transform diagnosis, treatment selection, and monitoring of neurological and psychiatric disorders, ultimately improving patient outcomes worldwide and advancing the Sustainable Development Goal of achieving health and well-being for all.

Acknowledgments

The authors would like to extend our appreciation to those who offered helpful commentary during the drafting process of this manuscript. We also acknowledge the role the Nova Publishing department played in enabling the work described herein.

References

Ashburner, J., & Friston, K. J. (2000). Voxel-based morphometry—The methods. *NeuroImage*, 11(6), 805-821. https://doi.org/10.1006/nimg.2000.0582.

Baillet, S. (2017). Magnetoencephalography for brain electrophysiology and imaging. Nature Neuroscience, 20(3), 327-339. https://doi.org/10.1038/nn.4504.

Baillet, S., Mosher, J. C., & Leahy, R. M. (2001). Electromagnetic brain mapping. *IEEE Signal Processing Magazine*, 18(6), 14-30. https://doi.org/10.1109/79.962275.

Boas, D. A., Dale, A. M., & Franceschini, M. A. (2004). Diffuse Optical Imaging of Brain Activation: Approaches to Optimising Image *Sensitivity, Resolution, and Accuracy NeuroImage*, 23(Suppl 1), S275-S288. https://doi.org/10.1016/j.neuroimage.2004.07.011.

Calhoun, V. D., Liu, J., & Adalı, T. (2009). A review of group ICA for fMRI data and ICA for joint inference of imaging, genetic, and ERP data. *NeuroImage*, 45(1 Suppl), S163-S172. https://doi.org/10.1016/j.neuroimage.2008.10.057.

Calhoun, V. D., & Sui, J. (2016). Multimodal fusion of brain imaging data: A key to finding the missing link(s) in complex mental illness. *Biological Psychiatry: Cognitive Neuroscience and Neuroimaging*, 1(3), 230-244. https://doi.org/10.1016/j.bpsc.2015.12.005.

Catana, C. (2019). Development of dedicated brain PET imaging devices: Recent advances and future perspectives. *Journal of Nuclear Medicine*, 60(8), 1044-1052. https://doi.org/10.2967/jnumed.118.217901.

Friston, K. J., Kahan, J., Biswal, B., & Razi, A. (2013). A DCM for resting state fMRI. *NeuroImage*, 94, 396-407. https://doi.org/10.1016/j.neuroimage.2013.12.009.

Judenhofer, M. S., Wehrl, H. F., Newport, D. F., Catana, C., Siegel, S. B., Becker, M., Thielscher, A., Kneilling, M., Lichy, M. P., Eichner, M., Klingel, K., Reischl, G., Widmaier, S., Röcken, M., Nutt, R. E., Machulla, H. J., Uludag, K., Cherry, S. R., Claussen, C. D., & Pichler, B. J. (2008). Simultaneous PET-MRI: A new approach for functional and morphological imaging. *Nature Medicine*, 14(4), 459-465. https://doi.org/10.1038/nm1700.

Laufs, H., Holt, J. L., Elfont, R., Krams, M., Paul, J. S., Krakow, K., & Kleinschmidt, A. (2008). Where the BOLD signal goes when alpha EEG leaves. *NeuroImage*, 31(4), 1408-1418. https://doi.org/10.1016/j.neuroimage.2006.02.002.

Mullinger, K. J., Yan, W. X., & Bowtell, R. (2014). Reducing the gradient artefact in simultaneous EEG-fMRI by adjusting the subject's axial position. *NeuroImage*, 54(3), 1942-1950. https://doi.org/10.1016/j.neuroimage.2010.09.079.

Pittau, F., Grova, C., Moeller, F., Dubeau, F., & Gotman, J. (2014). Patterns of altered functional connectivity in mesial temporal lobe epilepsy. *Epilepsia*, 53(6), 1013-1023. https://doi.org/10.1111/j.1528-1167.2012.03464.x.

Sporns, O. (2013). Network attributes for segregation and integration in the human brain. *Current Opinion in Neurobiology*, 23(2), 162-171. https://doi.org/10.1016/j.conb.2012.11.015.

Strangman, G. E., Li, Z., & Zhang, Q. (2013). Depth sensitivity and source-detector separations for near infrared spectroscopy based on the Colin27 brain template. *PLoS ONE*, 8(8), e66319. https://doi.org/10.1371/journal.pone.0066319.

Stufflebeam, S. M. (2011). Clinical magnetoencephalography for neurosurgery. *Neurosurgery Clinics of North America*, 22(2), 153-167. https://doi.org/10.1016/j.nec.2010.11.006.

Chapter 19

Emerging Technologies and Novel Contrasts

Niharika Prasad[1,*]
and Maajid Mohi Ud Din Malik[2,†]

[1]Department of Radio-Diagnosis, Dr. D. Y. Patil Medical College, Hospital and Research Centre, Dr. D. Y. Patil Vidyapeeth (Deemed to be University), Sant Tukaram Nagar, Pimpri, Pune, India
[2]Radiology and Imaging Technology, Dr. D. Y. Patil School of Allied Health Sciences, Dr. D. Y. Patil Vidyapeeth (Deemed to be University), Sant Tukaram Nagar, Pimpri, Pune, India

Abstract

Emerging magnetic resonance imaging technologies and novel contrast mechanisms are expanding MRI's capabilities beyond conventional structural and functional imaging to probe molecular composition, metabolic processes, and biomechanical properties of tissues. This chapter explores cutting-edge developments, including chemical exchange saturation transfer imaging that detects low-concentration metabolites and pH changes, molecular MRI with targeted contrast agents that bind to specific biomarkers, deuterium metabolic imaging that tracks glucose metabolism *in vivo*, hyperpolarised MRI that enhances sensitivity for real-time metabolic imaging, and MR elastography that quantifies tissue mechanical properties. We also examine the development of portable, low-field MRI systems that promise to democratise access to neuroimaging in resource-limited settings and for point of-care applications. These innovations leverage advances in physics, chemistry, engineering, and computational methods to create entirely new classes of image contrast, enabling applications previously impossible with conventional MRI. The clinical translation of these technologies holds promise for earlier disease detection, enhanced characterisation of pathology, and personalised treatment monitoring. These advances align with Sustainable Development Goal 3 (Good Health and Well-being) by expanding diagnostic capabilities and improving accessibility to advanced neuroimaging worldwide.

---

* Corresponding Author's Email: Niharika.Prasad@dpu.edu.in
† Corresponding Author's Email: maajid.malik@dpu.edu.in

In: Recent Advances in Magnetic Resonance Imaging in Neuroimaging
Editors: Maajid Mohi Ud Din Malik, Purnachandra Kawdu Lamghare and R. S. Kuber
ISBN: 979-8-90134-244-2

Keywords: CEST imaging, molecular MRI, deuterium imaging, hyperpolarised MRI, MR elastography, low-field MRI, metabolic imaging, novel contrasts, SDG 3 - good health and well-being

Introduction

The evolution of magnetic resonance imaging continues to accelerate through the development of novel physical principles, chemical agents, and technical implementations that extend imaging capabilities far beyond the anatomical and basic functional information provided by conventional techniques. While standard MRI excels at visualising anatomy and measuring blood flow-related signals, many pathological processes initially manifest through molecular and metabolic changes that precede structural abnormalities. The emerging technologies and novel contrasts described in this chapter address this gap by enabling the direct visualisation of molecular composition, metabolic activity, pH changes, protein aggregation, biomechanical properties, and other tissue characteristics directly relevant to disease pathophysiology. These innovations represent the frontier of MRI physics and chemistry, translating fundamental scientific discoveries into clinically applicable imaging methods (van Zijl & Yadav, 2011).

Chemical exchange saturation transfer (CEST) imaging leverages the exchange of saturated protons between mobile macromolecules and bulk water to generate contrast from low-concentration metabolites, proteins, and pH levels that are invisible to conventional MRI. Molecular MRI utilises targeted contrast agents that bind to specific cellular receptors, enzyme activities, or pathological protein aggregates, thereby enabling the visualisation of molecular processes *in vivo*. Deuterium metabolic imaging tracks glucose metabolism by detecting deuterium-labelled substrates, providing metabolic information similar to that of positron emission tomography (PET) without ionising radiation. Hyperpolarised MRI temporarily increases nuclear polarisation by several orders of magnitude, enabling real-time imaging of metabolic conversions with unprecedented sensitivity. MR elastography quantifies tissue mechanical properties by measuring the propagation of induced mechanical waves, revealing pathological changes in tissue stiffness. Portable low-field MRI systems reimagine scanner design to enable point-of-care neuroimaging at a fraction of the cost of conventional systems (Nelson et al., 2013).

The clinical impact of these emerging technologies spans early disease detection, improved characterisation of known pathologies, assessment of treatment response, and entirely new applications that are not possible with conventional imaging. In oncology, metabolic imaging using hyperpolarised substrates or deuterium labelling can distinguish aggressive tumours from indolent lesions and detect treatment responses before anatomical changes occur. In stroke, CEST imaging detecting pH changes can identify tissue at risk of infarction and guide reperfusion therapy. In neurodegenerative diseases, molecular imaging of protein aggregates provides specific biomarkers of Alzheimer's disease, Parkinson's disease, and related disorders. MR elastography identifies subtle mechanical property changes in brain tissue associated with ageing and disease. Low-field MRI could transform access to neuroimaging in emergency departments, intensive care units, and resource-limited regions where conventional scanners are unavailable. As these technologies mature and transition from research tools to clinical applications, they promise to fundamentally transform diagnostic imaging capabilities (Cooley et al., 2021).

19.1. Chemical Exchange Saturation Transfer (CEST) Imaging

Chemical exchange saturation transfer (CEST) imaging represents a revolutionary approach to MRI contrast, enabling the detection of dilute mobile proteins, peptides, metabolites, and pH changes via proton exchange. The technique applies radiofrequency saturation pulses at the resonance frequency of protons in specific molecules, such as amide protons in proteins or hydroxyl protons in glucose. These saturated protons exchange with bulk water protons, transferring the saturation and causing a measurable decrease in the water signal. The magnitude of this effect depends on the concentration of the exchanging species, the exchange rate, and saturation parameters, providing indirect detection of molecules present at millimolar concentrations that would be invisible to conventional MRI, which operates at molar water concentrations. This amplification through the abundant water pool enables entirely new classes of molecular and metabolic imaging (van Zijl & Yadav, 2011).

The technical implementation of CEST imaging requires the acquisition of images at multiple radiofrequencies and offset frequencies to characterise the saturation transfer spectrum, known as the z-spectrum. Subtraction of images acquired at symmetric offsets around the water resonance isolates the CEST effect from other contributions, including direct water saturation and magnetisation transfer from semi-solid tissue components. Quantitative analysis extracts specific metabolite contributions by fitting the z-spectrum or by calculating asymmetry metrics. Field strength significantly impacts CEST sensitivity and specificity, with higher fields providing better separation of overlapping CEST peaks from different molecular species. The technique faces challenges from magnetic field inhomogeneities, constraints on radiofrequency power deposition, and confounding effects from conventional magnetisation transfer and nuclear Overhauser enhancement (Zhou et al., 2013).

Amide proton transfer imaging, the most widely studied CEST application, detects mobile proteins and peptides through saturation transfer from backbone amide protons. The amide proton resonance at 3.5 ppm, downfield from water, provides contrast related to protein concentration and pH, as exchange rates are base-catalysed and increase at higher pH values. Brain tumour imaging with amide proton transfer reveals elevated signals in high-grade gliomas, reflecting increased cellularity and protein content, which enables differentiation from treatment effects, lower-grade tumours, and non-neoplastic lesions. Acute stroke applications exploit the pH sensitivity of amide proton transfer to identify acidotic tissue at risk of infarction, potentially guiding reperfusion decisions. The technique provides complementary information to conventional imaging and diffusion-weighted imaging, improving diagnostic accuracy (Zhou et al., 2013).

GluCEST imaging specifically detects glutamate, the primary excitatory neurotransmitter, through saturation transfer from amine protons that exchange with water. This provides a non-invasive measure of glutamate concentration and pH *in vivo*, without requiring spectroscopy or specialised metabolite-editing sequences. Applications include investigation of excitotoxicity in stroke and traumatic brain injury, altered glutamate metabolism in psychiatric disorders, and glutamatergic dysfunction in epilepsy. The technique complements magnetic resonance spectroscopy by providing two- or three-dimensional spatial mapping of glutamate distribution at resolutions unavailable with spectroscopy, though with less chemical specificity and greater complexity in quantitative interpretation (Cai et al., 2012).

GlucoCEST exploits the hydroxyl protons on glucose to generate contrast related to glucose uptake and concentration, providing a metabolic imaging conceptually similar to fluorodeoxyglucose PET, but without ionising radiation. Following an intravenous glucose injection, dynamic glucoCEST imaging tracks glucose delivery and uptake in tissues, with increased signal in regions of high metabolic demand or in areas with a disrupted blood-brain barrier. Brain tumour applications show elevated glucoCEST in gliomas, reflecting increased glucose metabolism characteristic of cancer. The technique faces several challenges, including the overlap of glucose CEST with other hydroxyl-containing metabolites, dependence on the timing and dose of glucose administration, and the need for sophisticated analysis to separate the contributions from vascular and tissue sources. Ongoing technical refinements aim to improve specificity and quantification for clinical translation (Rivlin & Navon, 2019).

Clinical translation of CEST imaging requires addressing multiple technical challenges, including standardising acquisition protocols across scanners, developing quantitative analysis methods robust to field inhomogeneities and patient motion, and validating CEST biomarkers against histopathology and clinical outcomes. The technique's sensitivity to multiple physiological parameters, including metabolite concentration, pH, and temperature, provides rich information but complicates interpretation. Exogenous CEST agents with favourable chemical exchange properties and safety profiles could potentially enhance sensitivity and specificity compared to endogenous CEST. However, regulatory pathways for such agents remain to be established. Despite challenges, CEST's unique capabilities to probe molecular composition and metabolic processes position it as a valuable addition to advanced neuroimaging protocols (van Zijl & Yadav, 2011).

19.2. Molecular MRI and Targeted Contrast Agents

Molecular MRI utilises targeted contrast agents specifically designed to bind molecular markers of disease, enabling the *in vivo* visualisation of cellular receptors, enzyme activities, protein aggregation, and other molecular processes. Unlike conventional gadolinium agents, which distribute non-specifically in the extracellular space, molecular agents incorporate targeting moieties, such as antibodies, peptides, or small molecules, that recognise and bind specific biological targets. This targeted binding increases the local concentration of contrast agents at sites of molecular expression, creating signal changes detectable by MRI. The approach extends MRI capabilities from anatomical and physiological imaging into the molecular imaging domain, traditionally occupied by nuclear medicine techniques, potentially providing similar specificity with superior spatial resolution and without ionising radiation (Caravan et al., 2009).

The design of molecular MRI contrast agents balances multiple requirements, including high relaxivity for strong signal effects, specific and high-affinity binding to the molecular target, adequate biodistribution to reach target tissues, favourable pharmacokinetics that enable sufficient accumulation before clearance, and a safety profile suitable for human use. Most agents employ gadolinium chelates conjugated to targeting ligands, though iron oxide nanoparticles, manganese-based agents, and chemical exchange saturation transfer agents provide alternative mechanisms. The modest sensitivity of MRI compared to nuclear techniques requires either high-relaxivity agents or amplification strategies that recruit multiple contrast molecules or trigger enzymatic conversion of many substrate molecules (Caravan et al., 2009).

Targeted fibrin imaging for thrombus detection exemplifies molecular MRI with clinical potential, utilising gadolinium-labelled peptides that bind to fibrin in blood clots. Applications include imaging of acute arterial thrombosis, deep vein thrombosis, and left atrial thrombus in patients with atrial fibrillation. The targeted agent offers superior sensitivity for detecting small thrombi compared with conventional imaging, with implications for stroke prevention and for guiding anticoagulation therapy. Atherosclerotic plaque imaging with agents targeting components such as oxidised LDL, macrophages, or matrix metalloproteinases enables characterisation of vulnerable plaques at risk of rupture, potentially identifying patients who would benefit from aggressive risk factor modification or intervention (Caravan et al., 2009).

Molecular imaging of angiogenesis targets vascular endothelial growth factor receptors or integrins expressed on proliferating endothelial cells in tumours, wounds, and ischemic tissues. Peptide-conjugated contrast agents that bind to these markers enable the visualisation of neovascularisation and the assessment of anti-angiogenic therapy effects. Tumour applications demonstrate that changes in molecular marker expression may precede anatomical changes in tumour size, providing an earlier assessment of treatment response. Ischemic tissue imaging shows increased signal from angiogenesis markers in regions undergoing revascularisation, potentially identifying tissue capable of functional recovery with appropriate interventions. The technique provides complementary information to perfusion imaging regarding the molecular state of the vasculature (Mulder et al., 2007).

Enzyme-activated contrast agents respond to specific enzymatic activities by altering their relaxation properties or water accessibility, enabling the detection of enzyme expression or activity *in vivo*. Protease-activated agents that change conformation or aggregation state upon cleavage provide amplified signal changes from catalytic turnover by single enzyme molecules. Applications include imaging of matrix metalloproteinases in cancer and atherosclerosis, caspases in apoptosis, and beta-galactosidase in gene expression studies. The approach enables the functional imaging of enzymatic processes, rather than simply detecting enzyme presence, although challenges include ensuring sufficient substrate availability and distinguishing specific enzymatic activity from background signal (Caravan et al., 2009).

Clinical translation of molecular MRI agents presents substantial challenges, including regulatory requirements for demonstrating safety and efficacy, high development costs comparable to those of pharmaceutical drugs rather than conventional contrast agents, and the need to establish clinical utility that justifies the added complexity and cost. The modest sensitivity of MRI requires that molecular targets be present at sufficiently high concentrations or that amplification strategies provide an adequate signal. Competition from nuclear medicine techniques with established workflows and emerging PET tracers for molecular imaging creates high standards for demonstrating the advantages of MRI-based approaches. Despite challenges, ongoing agent development and preclinical validation suggest that molecular MRI will increasingly complement conventional imaging as agents progress through development pipelines (Mulder et al., 2007).

19.3. Deuterium Metabolic Imaging (DMI)

Deuterium metabolic imaging is a novel, non-invasive approach that tracks glucose metabolism by detecting deuterium-labelled glucose and its metabolic products via magnetic resonance spectroscopy. Following oral or intravenous administration of deuterium-labelled glucose, the deuterium label is incorporated into downstream metabolites, including lactate, glutamate, and glutamine, through glycolysis and the tricarboxylic acid cycle. Deuterium MRI detects these labelled metabolites separately from the abundant proton signal that dominates conventional MRI, providing metabolic information conceptually similar to fluorodeoxyglucose positron emission tomography, but without ionising radiation and with the potential for repeated measurements. The natural abundance of deuterium in the body is negligible, providing an essentially zero background signal and enabling the sensitive detection of labelled compounds (De Feyter et al., 2018).

The technical implementation of deuterium metabolic imaging exploits deuterium's gyromagnetic ratio, which is approximately one-sixth that of protons, placing its resonance frequency far from the proton signal. This enables selective deuterium excitation and detection without interference from the abundant proton signal, although the lower gyromagnetic ratio and natural abundance of deuterium result in inherently lower sensitivity compared to proton MRI. Volumetric spectroscopic imaging with three-dimensional spatial encoding enables the creation of maps of deuterium-labelled metabolite concentrations throughout the brain within clinically acceptable scan times of 10 to 20 minutes. The use of high-field-strength, optimised radiofrequency coils and sophisticated reconstruction algorithms maximises sensitivity. Quantification accounts for relaxation times, referencing external standards or injected dose (De Feyter et al., 2018).

Applications of deuterium metabolic imaging in neuro-oncology demonstrate elevated glucose metabolism in high-grade gliomas compared to low-grade tumours and normal brain tissue, providing complementary metabolic tumour characterisation to conventional imaging. The technique distinguishes glucose uptake and metabolism from blood-volume effects that confound some perfusion-imaging methods, potentially improving specificity for detecting viable tumour versus treatment effects. Dynamic imaging tracking labelled metabolite evolution over time provides kinetic information about metabolic flux rates that static concentration measurements cannot capture. The ability to map both glucose uptake, as a labelled glucose signal, and downstream metabolism, through labelled lactate and other products, reveals pathway utilisation patterns specific to different tumour types and grades (Riis-Vestergaard et al., 2020).

Neurological applications include assessment of cerebral metabolism in stroke, traumatic brain injury, and epilepsy, where altered energy metabolism plays pathophysiological roles. In acute stroke, deuterium imaging could identify regions with preserved glucose uptake but impaired oxidative metabolism, characterising the ischemic penumbra and potentially guiding reperfusion therapy. Epilepsy studies show regionally elevated lactate production from labelled glucose during interictal periods and seizures, mapping metabolic abnormalities associated with epileptogenic zones. Traumatic brain injury investigations reveal heterogeneous metabolic dysfunction across injured tissue, with potential prognostic implications. The non-invasive nature and lack of ionising radiation enable repeated measurements to track metabolic changes over time during disease progression or treatment (De Feyter et al., 2018).

Psychiatric and cognitive neuroscience applications exploit deuterium metabolic imaging to investigate brain energy metabolism in schizophrenia, depression, autism, and other disorders where metabolic dysfunction has been hypothesised. Regional differences in glucose metabolism may reflect altered neural activity, mitochondrial dysfunction, or abnormalities in metabolic coupling. The spatial and metabolic information from deuterium imaging complements functional MRI by providing direct measures of energy substrate utilisation, rather than relying on hemodynamic surrogates. Studies investigating the effects of pharmacological interventions on brain metabolism could inform drug development and personalised medicine approaches. The ability to image metabolism in awake, behaving subjects enables investigation of task-dependent metabolic changes (De Feyter et al., 2018).

The clinical translation of deuterium metabolic imaging benefits from the safety and availability of deuterium-labelled glucose, which is already used in metabolic research studies and has a well-established safety profile at the doses required for imaging. The non-radioactive nature eliminates concerns about radiation exposure that limit the number of fluorodeoxyglucose PET studies, enabling longitudinal assessment of treatment response. Challenges include the need for specialised radiofrequency coils and transmit-receive hardware tuned to the deuterium frequency, limited spatial resolution compared to anatomical MRI, and the complexity of quantitative analysis. As the technique matures and hardware becomes more widely available, deuterium metabolic imaging promises to provide routine non-invasive metabolic phenotyping complementary to structural and functional neuroimaging (Riis-Vestergaard et al., 2020).

19.4. Hyperpolarised MRI

Hyperpolarised magnetic resonance imaging (MRI) temporarily increases nuclear spin polarisation by factors of 10,000 to 100,000 compared to thermal equilibrium, dramatically enhancing MRI sensitivity and enabling real-time imaging of metabolic conversions with unprecedented detail. The technique utilises dynamic nuclear polarisation or parahydrogen-induced polarisation to generate highly polarised nuclear spins in carbon-13-labelled substrates, which are then rapidly injected and imaged as they undergo metabolic transformations *in vivo*. The most extensively developed application utilises hyperpolarised pyruvate to image its conversion to lactate, alanine, and bicarbonate, thereby revealing the utilisation of glycolytic and oxidative metabolic pathways. The hyperpolarised state persists for tens of seconds to minutes, depending on the nuclear species and molecular environment, requiring rapid injection and imaging, but enabling metabolic measurements that are impossible with conventional MRI or spectroscopy (Nelson et al., 2013).

The technical implementation of hyperpolarised MRI requires sophisticated infrastructure, including a polariser to create the hyperpolarised state, quality control systems to verify polarisation levels and sterility, a rapid injection apparatus to deliver the agent while minimising polarisation loss, and specialised pulse sequences that efficiently encode spatial and metabolic information within the limited time window of hyperpolarisation. Dissolution dynamic nuclear polarisation, the predominant method for biomedical applications, polarises frozen samples at low temperatures in a strong magnetic field over several hours, then rapidly dissolves and heats the sample to physiological temperature for immediate injection. Chemical shift imaging or spectroscopic techniques separate signals from the injected substrate and its metabolic products, enabling measurement of metabolic flux. The irreversible nature of polarisation decay necessitates careful optimisation of acquisition strategies to maximise the information content (Kurhanewicz et al., 2019).

Oncologic applications of hyperpolarised pyruvate imaging have advanced the furthest toward clinical implementation, with multiple human trials demonstrating safety and feasibility for tumour characterisation and assessment of treatment response. The elevated conversion of pyruvate to lactate characterises the Warburg effect, a phenomenon observed in many cancers, in which tumours preferentially metabolise glucose via glycolysis even under aerobic conditions. Prostate cancer studies show that aggressive tumours display higher lactate production from pyruvate compared to indolent tumours, potentially guiding biopsy and treatment decisions. Monitoring changes in pyruvate-to-lactate conversion during therapy enables an earlier assessment of treatment response than anatomical imaging, as metabolic alterations often precede tumour size changes. Applications in gliomas, breast cancer, and renal cell carcinoma demonstrate the technique's broad applicability across cancer types (Kurhanewicz et al., 2019).

Cardiac applications utilise hyperpolarised imaging to assess myocardial metabolism in ischemia, heart failure, and diabetic cardiomyopathy, where altered substrate utilisation plays a pathophysiological role. The balance between pyruvate oxidation to bicarbonate and reduction to lactate reflects mitochondrial function and tissue oxygenation. Ischemic myocardium shows decreased bicarbonate production and increased lactate production, indicating metabolically compromised tissue. Heart failure studies reveal altered substrate utilisation patterns that may inform therapeutic strategies targeting cardiac metabolism. The ability to measure myocardial metabolism non-invasively and repeatedly enables longitudinal monitoring of disease progression and treatment response with applications in both research and clinical care (Cunningham et al., 2016).

Neurological applications of hyperpolarised imaging investigate brain metabolism in tumours, stroke, traumatic brain injury, and neurodegenerative diseases. Brain tumour studies show that gliomas exhibit elevated lactate production from pyruvate, which correlates with tumour grade and proliferation, potentially improving tumour characterisation beyond conventional imaging. Stroke models demonstrate decreased oxidative metabolism and increased lactate in ischemic tissue, providing metabolic signatures of tissue viability. Alzheimer's disease research explores whether altered brain metabolism detectable with hyperpolarised imaging precedes structural changes, potentially enabling earlier diagnosis. The technique provides metabolic information complementary to fluorodeoxyglucose PET and deuterium imaging with excellent temporal and spatial resolution (Miloushev et al., 2018).

Table 19.1. Metabolic imaging techniques comparison

Modality	Substrate/Agent	Temporal Resolution	Spatial Resolution	Ionizing Radiation	Repeat Feasibility
FDG-PET	F-18 fluorodeoxyglucose	Minutes	4-6 mm	Yes	Limited by radiation
Deuterium MRI	Deuterium-labeled glucose	10-20 minutes	5-10 mm	No	Unlimited
Hyperpolarized MRI	C-13 pyruvate	Real-time (seconds)	5-8 mm	No	Limited by polarisation
MR Spectroscopy	Endogenous metabolites	5-15 minutes	8-20 mm (single voxel)	No	Unlimited

The clinical translation of hyperpolarised MRI faces challenges, including the complexity and cost of polariser equipment, the need for on-site or nearby polarisation facilities due to the limited lifetime of hyperpolarisation, regulatory pathways for hyperpolarised agents as investigational drugs rather than traditional contrast agents, and the development of standardised acquisition and analysis protocols. The technique requires specialised expertise in polariser operation, quality control, and image analysis. Despite challenges, the unique capability to image metabolism in real time with high spatial and temporal resolution continues to drive development and clinical evaluation. Ongoing technical advances aim to enhance polarisation efficiency, prolong the lifetime of the hyperpolarised state, and expand the range of metabolic probes beyond pyruvate, thereby enabling comprehensive metabolic phenotyping (Nelson et al., 2013). Table 19.1 compares metabolic imaging techniques.

19.5. MR Elastography for Brain Tissue Characterisation

Magnetic resonance elastography quantifies the mechanical properties of brain tissue by measuring tissue displacement in response to externally applied mechanical waves, providing an entirely new class of image contrast based on tissue stiffness and viscosity. The technique employs low-frequency mechanical vibrations transmitted to the brain through the skull, creating shear waves that propagate through tissue at velocities determined by local mechanical properties. Phase-contrast MRI, synchronised to mechanical excitation, measures tissue displacement, and inversion algorithms reconstruct quantitative maps of tissue stiffness and related biomechanical parameters. Brain MR elastography has revealed that tissue mechanical properties change with ageing, neurodegeneration, and various pathological conditions, providing biomarkers complementary to conventional structural and functional imaging (Muthupillai et al., 1995).

The technical implementation of brain MR elastography requires a mechanical actuator system to generate controlled vibrations, typically at 30 to 60 Hz, transmitted to the head via a bite bar, pillow, or acoustic driver. Motion-encoding gradients synchronised to the mechanical excitation encode tissue displacement into the MRI signal phase, with multiple phase offsets sampled to capture the wave propagation. Three-dimensional acquisition covering the entire brain enables comprehensive assessment, though at the cost of longer scan times. Inversion algorithms solve the inverse problem of estimating mechanical properties from observed displacement fields, employing assumptions about tissue behaviour, such as isotropy, homogeneity, or viscoelasticity. Advanced inversions account for tissue anisotropy and frequency dependence of properties (Murphy et al., 2019).

Applications in brain ageing and neurodegeneration demonstrate that brain tissue stiffness decreases with normal ageing and shows accelerated decrease in Alzheimer's disease, multiple sclerosis, and other neurodegenerative conditions. The mechanical property changes likely reflect alterations in extracellular matrix, tissue microstructure, and cellular organisation that accompany disease processes. Longitudinal studies show that rates of stiffness change correlate with cognitive decline in Alzheimer's disease, suggesting mechanical properties as potential biomarkers for disease progression. Regional patterns of altered stiffness may help differentiate diagnostic categories and disease subtypes. The technique provides information distinct from atrophy measures, with regions showing mechanical property changes that do not exhibit significant volume loss on structural imaging (Murphy et al., 2019).

Tumour applications of brain MR elastography capitalise on the fact that tumours often exhibit distinct mechanical properties compared to surrounding normal brain tissue, resulting from altered cellularity, neovascularisation, necrosis, and changes in extracellular matrix composition. High-grade gliomas typically appear softer than low-grade tumours and normal brain tissue, potentially aiding in tumour characterisation. The technique may help distinguish tumour recurrence from radiation necrosis, which has an overlapping appearance on conventional imaging but different mechanical properties. Meningiomas and other extra-axial tumours show distinct stiffness patterns that reflect tumour consistency and predict surgical resectability. Pituitary adenomas exhibit variations in mechanical properties that correlate with hormonal subtype and invasiveness (Reiss-Zimmermann et al., 2015).

Hydrocephalus and intracranial pressure applications investigate relationships between cerebrospinal fluid dynamics, brain tissue mechanics, and ventricular dilation. Studies have shown altered brain stiffness in hydrocephalus, which may reflect tissue damage resulting from increased intracranial pressure or altered interstitial fluid dynamics. MR elastography, combined with flow imaging, provides a comprehensive assessment of cerebrospinal fluid dynamics and brain tissue response. Traumatic brain injury research applies elastography to characterise tissue damage, with potential applications in prognostication and monitoring recovery. The ability to quantify mechanical properties non-invasively enables the investigation of biomechanical aspects of neurological diseases that are often overlooked in conventional imaging (Murphy et al., 2019).

The clinical translation of brain MR elastography requires standardising acquisition protocols, inversion algorithms, and interpretation criteria across different sites and vendors. The technique's sensitivity to multiple tissue properties, including stiffness, viscosity, and anisotropy, provides rich information but complicates the determination of which parameters are most relevant for specific applications. Normal reference ranges across age, sex, and brain regions must be established to enable clinical interpretation. Integration of mechanical property information with other imaging biomarkers through multimodal analysis may provide synergistic diagnostic value. Despite remaining challenges, the unique insights into tissue biomechanics position MR elastography as a valuable addition to comprehensive neuroimaging protocols with applications across diverse neurological conditions (Reiss-Zimmermann et al., 2015).

19.6. Portable and Low-Field MRI Systems

Portable and low-field MRI systems operating at field strengths of 0.05 to 0.5 Tesla represent a paradigm shift in MRI design, prioritising accessibility, portability, and cost over the high-field performance characteristics emphasised in conventional scanners (Table 19.2). These systems eliminate the need for cryogenic cooling, magnetic shielding, and dedicated installation infrastructure required by high-field scanners, enabling deployment in emergency departments, intensive care units, ambulances, and resource-limited settings where conventional MRI is unavailable. Recent technical advances in magnet design, optimised pulse sequences, and machine-learning-based reconstruction have demonstrated diagnostic-quality neuroimaging at field strengths far below the 1.5 Tesla threshold traditionally considered necessary for clinical imaging.

This democratisation of MRI access promises to transform acute stroke care, point-of-care neuroimaging, and global health applications (Cooley et al., 2021).

The technical design of portable low-field systems utilises permanent magnets or air-cooled electromagnets, eliminating the need for cryogenic requirements while achieving field homogeneity sufficient for neuroimaging. Yokeless biplanar magnet geometries provide open access, facilitating patient positioning and enabling imaging of patients who are unable to tolerate conventional bore scanners. The lower field strength reduces safety concerns related to the magnetic attraction of ferromagnetic objects, permits imaging near some implanted devices that are contraindicated at high field strengths, and decreases specific absorption rate concerns. However, the fundamentally lower signal-to-noise ratio at low fields necessitates the use of sophisticated pulse sequences, averaging strategies, and advanced reconstruction algorithms, including compressed sensing and deep learning, to achieve diagnostic image quality. Optimised radiofrequency coils and improved gradient systems maximise performance within the constraints of portable systems (Sarracanie & Salameh, 2020).

Acute stroke applications represent the most immediately impactful clinical use case for portable MRI, enabling rapid neuroimaging at bedside in emergency departments or intensive care units to guide reperfusion therapy decisions. Studies demonstrate that low-field portable MRI can detect acute infarcts, haemorrhage, and large vessel occlusions with diagnostic accuracy comparable to that of conventional MRI. The ability to image patients at bedside within minutes of arrival, without transport to radiology departments, could dramatically accelerate treatment decisions in the time-critical setting of acute stroke. Repeat imaging to monitor evolution or detect complications becomes practical when the scanner is available at the bedside. Reduced siting requirements and costs could enable stroke-capable emergency departments in hospitals without neuroimaging capabilities, thereby expanding access to acute stroke therapy (Sheth et al., 2021).

Intensive care applications utilise the portability and relaxed safety constraints of low-field MRI to enable brain imaging in critically ill patients on ventilators, who often require multiple monitoring devices that would be challenging to transport to conventional MRI facilities. Detection of new strokes, haemorrhages, or other acute neurological complications in patients too unstable for transport to radiology has significant clinical value. Portable MRI eliminates the risks associated with patient transport through hospital corridors and enables more frequent monitoring to track rapidly evolving conditions. The open magnet geometry facilitates maintenance of ventilation and monitoring during scanning. Neurological intensive care units equipped with portable MRI could provide a level of neuroimaging surveillance previously impractical (Sheth et al., 2021).

Global health applications in resource-limited settings where conventional MRI is unavailable due to infrastructure limitations, costs, or expertise represent transformative opportunities. Low-field systems with reduced power requirements, no cryogenics, and potentially lower costs could bring neuroimaging to regions that currently lack access to this technology. Applications include stroke diagnosis, tumour detection, infection diagnosis, and traumatic brain injury assessment in settings where such capabilities are presently absent. The potential for telemedicine interpretation connects remote sites to radiological expertise, enabling seamless access to specialised radiological services. Pediatric applications in resource-limited settings could address global disparities in pediatric neuroimaging access. However, implementation requires consideration of local infrastructure, training requirements, and sustainable service models (Sarracanie & Salameh, 2020).

Future developments in portable MRI technology include continued improvements in image quality through optimised acquisition and reconstruction, expansion of pulse sequence capabilities to enable functional imaging and advanced contrasts, miniaturisation that enables truly portable systems deployable in ambulances or remote environments, and integration with artificial intelligence for automated image interpretation and decision support. The technology trajectory suggests that portable MRI may eventually achieve image quality comparable to that of conventional MRI for many applications, while maintaining the advantages of portability and accessibility. Regulatory pathways, reimbursement models, and clinical workflow integration will be critical for widespread adoption. The democratisation of MRI access through portable systems promises to fundamentally transform neuroimaging from a centralised resource to a point-of-care capability (Cooley et al., 2021). Table 19.2 compares emerging MRI technologies.

Table 19.2. Comparison of emerging MRI technologies

Technology	Primary Contrast Mechanism	Key Advantages	Main Limitations	Clinical Maturity	Representative Applications
CEST Imaging	Chemical exchange of saturated protons	Endogenous contrast, pH sensitivity, metabolite detection	Complex acquisition and analysis, B0/B1 sensitivity	Early clinical adoption	Brain tumours, stroke, pH mapping
Molecular MRI	Targeted contrast agent binding	Molecular specificity, no radiation	Low sensitivity, agent development challenges	Preclinical/early clinical	Thrombus, atherosclerosis, angiogenesis
Deuterium Imaging	Deuterium-labelled glucose metabolism	Direct metabolic imaging, no radiation, repeatable	Requires labelled substrate, specialised hardware	Early clinical research	Tumour metabolism, stroke, epilepsy
Hyperpolarized MRI	Enhanced nuclear polarisation	Very high sensitivity, real-time metabolism	Short lifetime, complex infrastructure	Clinical trials	Cancer metabolism, cardiac metabolism
MR Elastography	Tissue mechanical properties	Unique biomechanical information	Specialised equipment, complex inversion	Emerging clinical use	Neurodegeneration, tumours, and ageing
Low-Field MRI	Portable imaging systems	Accessibility, portability, and lower cost	Lower image quality than high-field	Early clinical deployment	Acute stroke, ICU, resource-limited settings

Conclusion

Emerging MRI technologies and novel contrasts represent a fundamental expansion of imaging capabilities beyond the anatomical and basic functional information provided by conventional techniques. Chemical exchange saturation transfer imaging enables the detection of dilute metabolites and pH that are invisible to standard MRI. Molecular MRI with targeted agents visualises specific molecular markers of disease. Deuterium and hyperpolarised imaging provide complementary approaches to non-invasive metabolic phenotyping. MR elastography reveals tissue biomechanical properties, and portable low-field systems promise to democratise access to imaging. These innovations leverage advances across multiple domains, including physics, chemistry, engineering, computational methods, and artificial intelligence, to create entirely new classes of image contrast that directly probe molecular composition, metabolic activity, and mechanical properties relevant to disease pathophysiology.

The clinical impact of these emerging technologies spans earlier disease detection through molecular and metabolic biomarkers that precede structural changes, improved characterisation of known pathology by revealing functional and compositional abnormalities, more sensitive assessment of treatment response through metabolic and molecular markers and expanded access to neuroimaging through portable systems deployable in settings where conventional MRI is unavailable. In oncology, metabolic imaging helps distinguish between aggressive tumours and detect treatment responses before anatomical changes occur. In stroke, CEST pH imaging and portable MRI enable rapid bedside assessment. In neurodegeneration, mechanical property measurements and molecular imaging reveal disease processes beyond atrophy. Each technology provides unique information that complements conventional imaging and other emerging modalities.

The clinical translation of these technologies progresses at varying rates, reflecting their technical maturity, regulatory pathways, infrastructure requirements, and demonstrated clinical value. CEST imaging and MR elastography are transitioning to clinical use on commercial scanners, with a growing body of evidence supporting their application. Hyperpolarised pyruvate imaging has advanced to multi-centre clinical trials, demonstrating its feasibility and safety. Portable low-field MRI systems are now being deployed clinically, with FDA clearance for specific indications. Molecular MRI and deuterium imaging remain largely in preclinical or early clinical research stages. The translation pathway requires not only technical validation but also demonstration of clinical utility that changes patient management and justifies added costs and complexity relative to existing diagnostic approaches.

Future developments will continue to expand MRI capabilities through novel contrast mechanisms, improved hardware and acquisition methods, advanced reconstruction algorithms incorporating artificial intelligence, and the integration of multiple emerging technologies into comprehensive multimodal protocols. The convergence of metabolic imaging modalities with molecular agents and advanced analysis methods promises comprehensive molecular and functional phenotyping. Portable systems will continue to evolve, achieving higher image quality while maintaining their accessibility advantages. As these technologies mature and evidence of clinical value accumulates, their integration into routine practice will transform diagnostic imaging from a primarily anatomical assessment to a comprehensive characterisation of tissue composition, metabolism, and function. The alignment of these innovations with the Sustainable Development Goal for health and well-being reflects their potential to enhance diagnostic accuracy, facilitate precision medicine, and expand global access to imaging. Table 19.3 shows the clinical translation status of emerging technologies.

Table 19.3. Clinical translation status of emerging technologies

Technology	FDA Status	Commercial Availability	Key Barriers to Adoption	Timeline to Routine Use
CEST Imaging	Research use	Available on major platforms	Standardisation, quantification	3-5 years
Molecular MRI	Investigational agents	Limited availability	Agent approval, sensitivity	5-10 years
Deuterium Imaging	Research use	Specialized centres	Hardware availability	5-7 years
Hyperpolarized MRI	Clinical trials	Research centres	Infrastructure, cost	3-5 years
MR Elastography	FDA cleared (liver)	Expanding availability	Brain-specific validation	2-4 years
Low-Field MRI	FDA cleared (limited)	Early deployment	Validation, reimbursement	3-5 years

Acknowledgments

The authors would like to extend our appreciation to those who offered helpful commentary during the drafting process of this manuscript. We also acknowledge the role the Nova Publishing department played in enabling the work described herein.

References

Cai, K., Haris, M., Singh, A., Kogan, F., Greenberg, J. H., Hariharan, H., Detre, J. A., & Reddy, R. (2012). Magnetic resonance imaging of glutamate. *Nature Medicine*, 18(2), 302-306. https://doi.org/10.1038/nm.2615.

Caravan, P., Ellison, J. J., McMurry, T. J., & Lauffer, R. B. (2009). Gadolinium(III) chelates as MRI contrast agents: Structure, dynamics, and applications. *Chemical Reviews*, 99(9), 2293-2352. https://doi.org/10.1021/cr980440x.

Cooley, C. Z., Haskell, M. W., Cauley, S. F., Sappo, C., Lapierre, C. D., Ha, C. G., Stockmann, J. P., & Wald, L. L. (2021). Design of sparse Halbach magnet arrays for portable MRI using a genetic algorithm. *IEEE Transactions on Magnetics*, 54(1), 1-12. https://doi.org/10.1109/TMAG.2017.2751001.

Cunningham, C. H., Lau, J. Y., Chen, A. P., Geraghty, B. J., Perks, W. J., Roifman, I., Wright, G. A., & Connelly, K. A. (2016). Hyperpolarized 13C metabolic MRI of the human heart: Initial experience. *Circulation Research*, 119(11), 1177-1182. https://doi.org/10.1161/CIRCRESAHA.116.309769.

De Feyter, H. M., Behar, K. L., Corbin, Z. A., Fulbright, R. K., Brown, P. B., McIntyre, S., Nixon, T. W., Rothman, D. L., & de Graaf, R. A. (2018). Deuterium metabolic imaging (DMI) for MRI-based 3D mapping of metabolism *in vivo*. *Science Advances*, 4(8), eaat7314. https://doi.org/10.1126/sciadv.aat7314.

Kurhanewicz, J., Vigneron, D. B., Ardenkjaer-Larsen, J. H., Bankson, J. A., Brindle, K., Cunningham, C. H., Gallagher, F. A., Keshari, K. R., Kjaer, A., Laustsen, C., Mankoff, D. A., Merritt, M. E., Nelson, S. J., Pauly, J. M., Lee, P., Ronen, S., Tyler, D. J., Rajan, S. S., Spielman, D. M., ... Malloy, C. R. (2019). Hyperpolarized 13C MRI: Path to clinical translation in oncology. *Neoplasia*, 21(1), 1-16. https://doi.org/10.1016/j.neo.2018.09.006.

Miloushev, V. Z., Granlund, K. L., Boltyanskiy, R., Lyashchenko, S. K., DeAngelis, L. M., Mellinghoff, I. K., Brennan, C. W., Tabar, V., Yang, T. J., Holodny, A. I., Sosa, R. E., Guo, Y. W., Chen, A. P., Tropp, J., Robb, F., & Keshari, K. R. (2018). Metabolic imaging of the human brain with hyperpolarized 13C pyruvate demonstrates 13C lactate production in brain tumor patients. *Cancer Research*, 78(14), 3755-3760. https://doi.org/10.1158/0008-5472.CAN-18-0221.

Mulder, W. J., Strijkers, G. J., van Tilborg, G. A., Griffioen, A. W., & Nicolay, K. (2007). Lipid-based nanoparticles for contrast-enhanced MRI and molecular imaging. *NMR in Biomedicine*, 19(1), 142-164. https://doi.org/10.1002/nbm.1011.

Murphy, M. C., Huston, J., & Ehman, R. L. (2019). MR elastography of the brain and its application in neurological diseases. *NeuroImage*, 187, 176-183. https://doi.org/10.1016/j.neuroimage.2017.10.008.

Muthupillai, R., Lomas, D. J., Rossman, P. J., Greenleaf, J. F., Manduca, A., & Ehman, R. L. (1995). Magnetic resonance elastography by direct visualization of propagating acoustic strain waves. *Science*, 269(5232), 1854-1857. https://doi.org/10.1126/science.7569924.

Nelson, S. J., Kurhanewicz, J., Vigneron, D. B., Larson, P. E., Harzstark, A. L., Ferrone, M., van Criekinge, M., Chang, J. W., Bok, R., Park, I., Reed, G., Carvajal, L., Small, E. J., Munster, P., Weinberg, V. K., Ardenkjaer-Larsen, J. H., Chen, A. P., Hurd, R. E., Odegardstuen, L. I., ... Kurhanewicz, J. (2013). Metabolic imaging of patients with prostate cancer using hyperpolarized [1-13C]pyruvate. *Science Translational Medicine*, 5(198), 198ra108. https://doi.org/10.1126/scitranslmed.3006070.

Reiss-Zimmermann, M., Streitberger, K. J., Sack, I., Braun, J., Arlt, F., Fritzsch, D., Hoffmann, K. T., & Käs, J. A. (2015). High resolution imaging of viscoelastic properties of intracranial tumours by multi-frequency magnetic resonance elastography. *Clinical Neuroradiology*, 25(4), 371-378. https://doi.org/10.1007/s00062-014-0311-9.

Riis-Vestergaard, M. J., Laustsen, C., & Mariager, C. Ø. (2020). Deuterium metabolic imaging—Back to the future. *Journal of Magnetic Resonance*, 313, 106752. https://doi.org/10.1016/j.jmr.2020.106752.

Rivlin, M., & Navon, G. (2019). Molecular imaging of tumors by chemical exchange saturation transfer MRI of glucose analogs. *Quarterly Journal of Nuclear Medicine and Molecular Imaging*, 63(2), 248-261. https://doi.org/10.23736/S1824-4785.19.03171-4.

Sarracanie, M., & Salameh, N. (2020). Low-field MRI: How low can we go? A fresh view on an old debate. *Frontiers in Physics*, 8, 172. https://doi.org/10.3389/fphy.2020.00172.

Chapter 20

Future Perspectives and Clinical Translation

Maajid Mohi Ud Din Malik*

Radiology and Imaging Technology, Dr. D. Y. Patil School of Allied Health Sciences,
Dr. D. Y. Patil Vidyapeeth (Deemed to be University), Sant Tukaram Nagar, Pimpri, Pune, India

Abstract

The future of neuroimaging stands at a transformative juncture where technological advances converge with evolving healthcare paradigms to enable personalised medicine, expand global access, and integrate seamlessly into clinical workflows. This chapter examines the trajectory of neuroimaging translation from research innovations to routine clinical practice, exploring how precision neuroimaging will enable individualised diagnosis and treatment selection, how point-of-care systems will democratise imaging access, and how technology adaptation can address global health disparities. We analyse the regulatory and reimbursement landscape that shapes clinical adoption, discuss strategies for integrating advanced imaging into existing workflows, and identify research priorities that will drive the next generation of innovations. The convergence of artificial intelligence, portable systems, molecular imaging, and multimodal integration promises to fundamentally transform neurological and psychiatric care. However, realising this potential requires addressing challenges in validation, standardisation, cost-effectiveness, and equitable access. The alignment of these advances with Sustainable Development Goal 3 (Good Health and Well-being) underscores the imperative to ensure that neuroimaging innovations benefit all populations, not just those in resource-rich settings, ultimately improving global brain health outcomes.

Keywords: precision medicine, point-of-care imaging, global health, clinical translation, regulatory policy, healthcare access, future technologies, personalised neuroimaging, SDG 3 - good health and well-being

* Corresponding Author's Email: maajid.malik@dpu.edu.in

In: Recent Advances in Magnetic Resonance Imaging in Neuroimaging
Editors: Maajid Mohi Ud Din Malik, Purnachandra Kawdu Lamghare and R. S. Kuber
ISBN: 979-8-90134-244-2

Introduction

The evolution of neuroimaging from anatomical visualisation to comprehensive functional, molecular, and metabolic characterisation has created unprecedented opportunities to transform neurological and psychiatric care through precision medicine approaches, expanded access, and seamless clinical integration. The technologies described throughout this book—from advanced diffusion imaging and functional connectivity to molecular imaging and artificial intelligence—represent not merely incremental improvements but fundamental expansions of diagnostic and prognostic capabilities. However, the path from technical innovation to routine clinical implementation requires navigating complex challenges in validation, standardisation, regulatory approval, reimbursement, workflow integration, and equitable access. This chapter examines the future trajectory of neuroimaging, identifying both the opportunities and obstacles that will shape its evolution over the coming decades (Toga et al., 2016).

Personalised medicine represents a paradigm shift from population-based diagnosis and treatment toward individualised approaches that account for unique patient characteristics, including genetics, biomarkers, disease stage, and risk factors. Neuroimaging plays a central role in this transformation by providing objective biomarkers that stratify patients, predict outcomes, guide treatment selection, and monitor responses with precision that is impossible through clinical assessment alone. The integration of multimodal imaging, genomics, and clinical data through advanced analytics enables the construction of individualised disease models that inform clinical decisions with unprecedented specificity. Applications span neurodegenerative diseases, psychiatric disorders, epilepsy, stroke, tumours, and developmental conditions. The realisation of precision neuroimaging requires not only technical capabilities but also validation across diverse populations, demonstration of clinical utility, and the development of decision-support tools that translate complex data into actionable insights (Hampel et al., 2018).

The democratisation of neuroimaging access through portable point-of-care systems, reduced costs, and simplified workflows promises to extend advanced diagnostics beyond academic medical centres to emergency departments, intensive care units, rural hospitals, and resource-limited regions where conventional imaging is unavailable or delayed. Low-field portable MRI systems exemplify this transformation, enabling bedside neuroimaging for acute stroke, traumatic brain injury, and critical illness monitoring in settings where patient transport is impractical or dangerous. Mobile imaging units bring technology to underserved populations, while telemedicine connections enable expert interpretation regardless of geographic location. These innovations align with global health priorities to reduce disparities in access to essential diagnostics and improve outcomes through earlier detection and appropriate treatment. However, ensuring quality, training adequate personnel, and developing sustainable service models remain critical challenges (Sheth et al., 2021).

The clinical translation of advanced neuroimaging techniques requires addressing regulatory pathways for novel technologies, establishing reimbursement mechanisms that support adoption, and developing workflows that integrate seamlessly with existing clinical practice. Artificial intelligence applications face unique regulatory considerations as software-as-medical-device requiring ongoing validation and monitoring. Novel contrast agents and molecular imaging tracers must demonstrate safety and efficacy through rigorous clinical trials. Quantitative biomarkers require both analytical and clinical validation before they can be incorporated into diagnostic algorithms or used to inform treatment decisions. The convergence of these challenges with accelerating technological innovation creates both unprecedented opportunities and complex obstacles. This chapter provides a roadmap for navigating this landscape, identifying research priorities, and envisioning the future neuroimaging ecosystem that will support global brain health (Jha et al., 2016).

20.1. Personalised Medicine and Precision Neuroimaging

Precision neuroimaging enables individualised diagnosis, prognosis, and treatment selection by integrating multimodal imaging biomarkers with clinical, genetic, and molecular data to construct patient-specific disease models. This approach moves beyond categorical diagnostic labels to dimensional characterisations that capture disease heterogeneity and identify biologically defined subtypes requiring distinct therapeutic approaches. In Alzheimer's disease, the combination of amyloid PET, tau PET, structural MRI, and functional connectivity mapping enables stageing along biological continua rather than relying on syndromic classification. Imaging biomarkers predict progression from preclinical stages through mild cognitive impairment to dementia with greater accuracy than clinical assessment alone, enabling early intervention when disease-modifying therapies are most likely to be effective (Hampel et al., 2018).

Psychiatric applications of precision neuroimaging aim to identify circuit-level biomarkers that transcend traditional diagnostic categories and predict treatment response. Depression research demonstrates that functional connectivity patterns predict response to antidepressants versus psychotherapy, potentially enabling personalised treatment selection. Schizophrenia studies identify neuroanatomical and functional subtypes with different trajectories and treatment responses. The Research Domain Criteria framework promotes a dimensional assessment of the neural circuits underlying cognitive and affective functions, rather than symptom-based diagnosis, with neuroimaging providing objective measures of circuit function. Machine learning approaches identify multivariate imaging patterns that predict diagnosis, prognosis, and treatment outcomes with greater accuracy than individual features, enabling the development of decision support tools for clinical implementation (Drysdale et al., 2017).

Tumour precision medicine integrates advanced MRI techniques with molecular profiling to guide treatment selection and predict response. Radiogenomics links imaging features to genomic alterations, enabling non-invasive inference of tumour biology that informs therapeutic decisions. For example, specific MRI patterns predict

IDH mutation status, MGMT methylation, and 1p/19q codeletion in gliomas—molecular markers that determine prognosis and treatment selection. Metabolic imaging with hyperpolarised pyruvate or deuterium glucose reveals metabolic phenotypes that may respond to targeted metabolic therapies. Serial imaging during treatment enables the detection of response earlier than conventional measures, allowing for adaptive strategies that modify therapy based on evolving disease characteristics (Kickingereder et al., 2016).

Stroke precision medicine utilises multimodal imaging to identify patients who are likely to benefit from reperfusion therapy beyond conventional time windows. Advanced perfusion imaging defines ischemic penumbra—potentially salvageable tissue that justifies intervention hours after symptom onset. Collateral flow assessment predicts outcomes and guides treatment decisions. Hemorrhagic transformation risk can be estimated from imaging biomarkers, informing decisions about thrombolytic therapy. Individual variability in cerebrovascular anatomy, collateral circulation, and tissue vulnerability necessitates personalised approaches rather than population-based protocols. The integration of clinical factors with quantitative imaging biomarkers through predictive models enables truly individualised treatment decisions (Albers et al., 2018).

Epilepsy surgery planning exemplifies precision neuroimaging by integrating structural MRI, functional MRI, PET, EEG-fMRI, MEG, and diffusion tractography to map epileptogenic zones and eloquent cortex in individual patients comprehensively. Concordance of multimodal findings predicts surgical success, whereas discordance prompts additional evaluation. Connectivity analysis reveals a network organisation that influences seizure propagation and surgical outcomes. Quantitative imaging biomarkers are increasingly complementing visual assessment, potentially improving the detection of subtle abnormalities and standardising evaluation. The ultimate goal is to enable seizure freedom while preserving neurological function through patient-specific surgical planning informed by comprehensive imaging characterisation (Bernasconi et al., 2019).

The implementation of precision neuroimaging in clinical practice requires the development of decision support systems that integrate diverse data streams, provide interpretable predictions, and deliver recommendations at the point of care. Cloud-based platforms enable federated learning across institutions while preserving privacy. Standardised data formats and ontologies facilitate the sharing and meta-analysis of data. Real-world evidence from routine clinical practice validates models and identifies biomarkers that translate across diverse populations. Regulatory frameworks for clinical decision support are evolving to strike a balance between innovation and safety and effectiveness requirements. The convergence of imaging, genomics, electronic health records, and advanced analytics will increasingly enable truly personalised neurological and psychiatric care (Hampel et al., 2018). Table 20.1: Precision neuroimaging applications across neurological disorders.

Table 20.1. Precision neuroimaging applications across neurological disorders

Disorder	Key Imaging Biomarkers	Precision Medicine Application	Clinical Readiness	Expected Impact
Alzheimer Disease	Amyloid PET, tau PET, hippocampal volume, connectivity	Early diagnosis, progression prediction, and trial enrichment	Established for research, emerging clinical	Enable disease-modifying therapy when available
Depression	Functional connectivity, structural patterns, circuit markers	Treatment selection (medication vs therapy), outcome prediction	Research phase	Reduce trial-and-error treatment, improve outcomes
Gliomas	Perfusion, diffusion, spectroscopy, metabolic imaging	Molecular subtype inference, treatment response, and progression detection	Advanced clinical centres	Guide therapy selection, enable precision oncology
Acute Stroke	Perfusion-diffusion mismatch, collaterals, core infarct	Extended window reperfusion decisions, outcome prediction	Established clinical practice	Expand treatment eligibility, improve outcomes
Epilepsy	Multimodal concordance (MRI, PET, EEG-fMRI, MEG, tractography)	Patient-specific surgery planning, outcome prediction	Established at specialised centres	Improve seizure freedom rates, reduce complications

20.2. Point-of-Care MRI Applications

Point-of-care magnetic resonance imaging systems enable bedside neuroimaging in emergency departments, intensive care units, neonatal intensive care, and other clinical settings where immediate diagnostic information is critical and patient transport is impractical or risky. Low-field portable MRI systems operating at 0.05 to 0.5 Tesla eliminate requirements for cryogenic cooling, magnetic shielding, and dedicated infrastructure that constrain conventional scanners, enabling deployment in diverse clinical environments. Recent technological advances in magnet design, optimised pulse sequences, and machine-learning reconstruction have demonstrated diagnostic quality approaching that of conventional MRI in many applications, despite the inherently lower signal-to-noise ratio at lower field strengths. These systems promise to transform acute neurological care by providing rapid bedside imaging (Sheth et al., 2021).

Emergency department applications focus primarily on acute stroke imaging, where portable MRI enables rapid differentiation of ischemic stroke from haemorrhage and identification of large vessel occlusions to guide reperfusion therapy. Clinical studies have demonstrated that portable MRI can detect acute infarcts, intracranial haemorrhage, and vascular occlusions with diagnostic accuracy comparable to that of conventional systems. The ability to image patients within minutes of arrival without transport to radiology departments could dramatically reduce door-to-imaging times, the rate-limiting step in acute stroke care at many institutions. Repeated imaging to monitor evolution or detect complications becomes practical when the scanner is available at the bedside. The potential to enable stroke-capable emergency departments at hospitals currently lacking neuroimaging could expand access to acute stroke therapy (Mazurek et al., 2021).

Intensive care applications leverage portability and relaxed safety constraints to enable brain imaging in critically ill patients on mechanical ventilation with multiple monitoring devices that would be problematic to transport to a conventional MRI. Detection of new strokes, haemorrhages, oedema, or herniation in patients too unstable for transport provides diagnostic information that changes management. Serial imaging to monitor evolving pathology guides interventions and prognostication. The open-magnet geometry facilitates airway maintenance and monitoring during scanning. Neurological intensive care units equipped with point-of-care MRI could provide surveillance imaging that is impractical with conventional systems, potentially improving outcomes by enabling earlier detection of complications (Mazurek et al., 2021).

Neonatal applications address the challenges of imaging premature infants and critically ill neonates, where transport risks and exposure concerns limit conventional MRI utilisation. Portable systems enable bedside imaging without removing infants from controlled incubator environments, reducing physiological stress and adverse events. Detection of intracranial haemorrhage, ischemic injury, and developmental abnormalities informs prognosis and guides interventions. The reduced acoustic noise compared to conventional MRI and lower magnetic field strength may improve safety for vulnerable neonates. However, the smaller patient size and developing brain anatomy present unique technical challenges that require specialised coils and protocols (Weiss et al., 2020).

Operating room and interventional suite applications could enable intraoperative imaging to guide procedures, verify resection completeness, and detect complications in real time. Portable MRI systems designed for operating room use provide imaging without requiring specialised MRI-compatible surgical instruments or the dramatic workflow modifications typically needed for conventional intraoperative MRI. Applications include brain tumour resection with real-time margin assessment, epilepsy surgery with functional guidance, and deep brain stimulator placement verification. The ability to perform interventions with imaging guidance could improve outcomes while reducing complications (Sheth et al., 2021).

Future developments will focus on enhancing image quality through optimised acquisition and reconstruction, expanding pulse sequence capabilities to enable functional and advanced imaging, further miniaturising systems for deployment in ambulances and remote locations, and integrating artificial intelligence for automated image acquisition and interpretation. Regulatory pathways, reimbursement models, operator training, and quality assurance programs will be essential for widespread clinical adoption. The transformation of MRI from a centralised resource to a point-of-care capability represents a fundamental paradigm shift with the potential to improve access, accelerate diagnosis, and enable new applications that are impossible with conventional systems (Sarracanie & Salameh, 2020). Table 20.2 shows precision neuroimaging applications across neurological disorders.

Table 20.2. Point-of-care MRI systems and applications

Clinical Setting	Primary Applications	Key Advantages	Technical Requirements	Implementation Status	Expected Timeline
Emergency Department	Acute stroke, head trauma, altered mental status	Rapid diagnosis, no transport, repeat imaging	0.064-0.5T portable system, basic sequences	Early deployment at select centres	2-5 years for widespread use
Intensive Care Unit	Neurological complications, progression monitoring	Bedside imaging, unstable patients, serial studies	MRI-compatible monitoring, open access	Clinical trials completed	3-7 years for routine use
Neonatal ICU	HIE assessment, IVH detection, and developmental abnormalities	Avoid transport, reduced exposure, lower noise	Neonatal coils, specialised protocols	Research studies ongoing	5-10 years for validation
Operating Room	Intraoperative guidance, resection verification	Real-time imaging, no facility transfer	OR-compatible design, sterile workflow	Prototype development	7-10 years for clinical adoption

20.3. Global Access and Resource-Limited Settings

The global distribution of neuroimaging capabilities reveals profound disparities, with the majority of MRI scanners concentrated in high-income countries. In contrast, low- and middle-income countries, which serve 85 per cent of the world's population, have severely limited access to advanced diagnostics. This inequity contributes to delayed diagnosis, suboptimal treatment, and worse outcomes for neurological disorders that represent a substantial and growing burden of disease globally. Stroke, traumatic brain injury, brain tumours, epilepsy, and dementia affect billions worldwide, yet a lack of imaging access prevents timely diagnosis and appropriate management in many regions. Addressing these disparities requires technologies adapted to resource-limited settings, innovative service delivery models, training programs, and sustainable financing mechanisms (Mollura et al., 2010).

Adapting technology for low-resource settings emphasises reduced infrastructure requirements, lower costs, simplified operation, and robust performance with limited technical support. Low-field portable MRI systems exemplify this approach, eliminating the need for cryogenic cooling, magnetic shielding, and specialised facilities, while dramatically reducing costs compared to conventional scanners. Air-cooled electromagnets or permanent magnets enable operation with standard electrical power. The reduced complexity facilitates installation and maintenance with local resources. However, achieving diagnostic image quality at low field strengths requires optimised pulse sequences and advanced reconstruction algorithms that continue to evolve. Solar power options could enable deployment in areas with unreliable electrical infrastructure (Sarracanie & Salameh, 2020).

Service delivery models for resource-limited settings include fixed installations at regional referral centres, mobile imaging units serving multiple communities, and partnerships with radiology centres in high-income countries that provide remote interpretation. Teleradiology connections enable local image acquisition with expert interpretation, regardless of geographic location, leveraging global expertise to support regions that lack subspecialty radiologists. However, sustainable models require consideration of maintenance, quality assurance, continuous training, and local capacity-building rather than reliance on external support. Integration with existing healthcare systems and alignment with local priorities are essential for long-term success (Syed et al., 2013).

Training programs must develop local expertise in the operation, interpretation, and maintenance of imaging systems to ensure sustainability and quality. Short-term training missions provide initial instruction but require follow-up and ongoing education to maintain skills. Telemedicine platforms enable real-time consultation and teaching, connecting trainees with experienced practitioners. Standardised protocols and decision algorithms reduce dependence on extensive expertise. Artificial intelligence applications for automated image analysis could compensate for limited interpreter availability, though validation in diverse populations and pathologies is essential. Building local training capacity through partnerships with regional universities creates sustainable educational infrastructure (Mollura et al., 2010).

Financing mechanisms include governmental health budgets, international development assistance, public-private partnerships, innovative financing instruments, and integration with existing disease-specific programs. The economic argument for neuroimaging investment emphasises that diagnostic imaging enables appropriate treatment and prevents costly complications, potentially achieving cost-effectiveness despite upfront expenses. Stroke imaging enabling appropriate thrombolysis reduces long-term disability and associated societal costs. Tumour imaging that enables timely surgery improves outcomes and reduces the burden of palliative care. Demonstrating value through health economic analyses strengthens investment cases. Reimbursement systems in low-income countries must evolve to support sustainable imaging services (Syed et al., 2013).

Success stories demonstrate the feasibility of expanding imaging access in resource-limited settings when appropriate technologies, training, and support systems are implemented. Mobile MRI units in rural India offer brain imaging services to populations located hundreds of kilometres from fixed installations. Portable ultrasound and point-of-care systems deployed in sub-Saharan Africa enable obstetric and trauma imaging previously unavailable. Telemedicine networks connecting rural clinics to urban expertise expand effective access beyond the physical distribution of equipment. These examples provide blueprints for scale-up, though challenges of sustainability, quality maintenance, and integration into healthcare systems require continued attention. Achieving universal access to essential neuroimaging will require a sustained commitment and innovative approaches (Mollura et al., 2010).

20.4. Regulatory and Reimbursement Challenges

The regulatory landscape for advanced neuroimaging technologies encompasses medical device approval, radiopharmaceutical authorisation, software validation, and clinical practice standards that collectively determine the pathway from innovation to clinical implementation. The U.S. Food and Drug Administration classifies imaging technologies by risk level, with novel systems requiring premarket approval to demonstrate safety and effectiveness. In contrast, modifications to existing technologies may qualify for expedited clearance pathways. Artificial intelligence applications face unique considerations as software-as-a-medical-device, requiring validation of algorithm performance, demonstration of generalizability across populations, and potentially continuous monitoring after deployment. Molecular imaging agents undergo pharmaceutical approval processes, including extensive toxicology and human safety studies (Benjamens et al., 2020).

Clinical validation requirements for diagnostic imaging include demonstrating technical performance through phantom studies, reproducibility across sites and operators, diagnostic accuracy compared to reference standards, and ultimately, clinical utility, which shows that imaging information improves patient outcomes. The level of evidence required depends on the intended use and risk profile, with higher bars for technologies guiding high-stakes treatment decisions. Multi-centre trials provide evidence of generalizability beyond single-institution studies. Real-world evidence from routine clinical practice increasingly complements controlled trials, demonstrating performance in diverse populations and practice settings. Regulatory agencies are developing frameworks for adaptive approval, where initial clearance based on promising results enables market entry, accompanied by requirements for continued evidence generation (Jha et al., 2016).

Reimbursement determinations by governmental and commercial payers critically influence clinical adoption, as most institutions cannot sustain services without coverage. In the United States, the Centres for Medicare and Medicaid Services establishes coverage policies based on evidence of what is reasonable and necessary for diagnosis or treatment, with these decisions influencing commercial insurer policies. New imaging technologies face challenges demonstrating incremental value over existing modalities to justify added costs. Health technology assessment processes evaluate the clinical effectiveness and cost-effectiveness of a health technology compared to standard care. Some advanced techniques remain research-use-only for years despite being technically mature, due to insufficient evidence of clinical utility or cost-effectiveness (Burwell, 2015).

Global regulatory harmonisation, facilitated by organisations such as the International Medical Device Regulators Forum, aims to streamline approval processes across countries, potentially accelerating access to innovations. However, substantial differences persist in regulatory requirements, evidentiary standards, and approval timelines. Low- and middle-income countries often lack regulatory capacity to independently evaluate novel technologies, creating tensions between ensuring safety and enabling timely access. The World Health Organisation's prequalification program provides quality assurance for diagnostic devices in resource-limited settings; however, neuroimaging equipment has received less attention than diagnostics for infectious diseases (Burwell, 2015).

Post-market surveillance monitors safety and effectiveness after clinical deployment, detecting rare adverse events or performance issues that may not have been apparent in pre-approval studies. Artificial intelligence algorithms may degrade in performance when applied to populations or equipment that differ from the training data, necessitating ongoing validation and potential retraining. Incident reporting systems collect information on adverse events that trigger investigations and possible modifications. Quality control programs at imaging facilities ensure optimal performance. Registry studies track outcomes associated with diagnostic testing, enabling evaluation of real-world effectiveness and cost-effectiveness that informs coverage and practice guidelines (Benjamens et al., 2020).

Future regulatory frameworks will need to adapt to the accelerating pace of innovation, particularly in artificial intelligence, where continuous learning and adaptation challenge traditional fixed-device paradigms. The balance between ensuring safety and effectiveness while enabling timely access to beneficial innovations requires ongoing refinement and adjustment. Regulatory science research develops improved methods for evaluating novel technologies, including biomarker qualification pathways, synthetic control arms for single-arm trials, and statistical approaches for adaptive studies. International collaboration could harmonise requirements and reduce duplicative effort. Patient involvement in regulatory decision-making ensures that evaluation frameworks reflect outcomes meaningful to those affected by neurological diseases (Jha et al., 2016).

20.5. Integration into Clinical Workflows

The successful integration of advanced neuroimaging techniques into routine clinical practice requires consideration of workflow efficiency, reporting standards, decision-support tools, and clinician education, in addition to the technical performance of the imaging itself. Innovations that substantially increase examination time, interpretation complexity, or reporting burden face adoption barriers regardless of diagnostic value. Seamless integration requires advanced techniques to fit within existing workflow constraints while providing clear, actionable information that influences clinical decisions. Automated acquisition, processing, and interpretation reduces the burden on technologists and radiologists. Structured reporting templates ensure consistent communication of findings. Decision support algorithms translate complex quantitative data into clinically meaningful recommendations (Kohli et al., 2018).

Imaging protocol optimisation strikes a balance between comprehensive assessment and practical time constraints, utilising modular approaches that enable customisation based on clinical indications while maintaining efficiency. Brain tumour protocols may include standard sequences, as well as advanced techniques such as perfusion, spectroscopy, and diffusion, for comprehensive characterisation. In contrast, streamlined stroke protocols prioritise the rapid acquisition of essential sequences to minimise door-to-needle time. Artificial intelligence applications for protocol selection can optimise examinations for individual patients based on their indication, prior findings, and clinical factors. Quality assurance systems monitor protocol adherence and image quality, triggering corrective action when standards are not met (Kohli et al., 2018).

Interpretation and reporting workflows must evolve to incorporate quantitative biomarkers and advanced analytics while maintaining clarity and actionability. Quantitative values for metrics such as tumour volumes, perfusion parameters, or connectivity measures require standardised acquisition and analysis to enable meaningful interpretation and longitudinal comparison. Automated segmentation and measurement tools enhance consistency and efficiency compared to manual approaches; however, they require validation and quality control. Structured reporting with standardised terminology facilitates effective communication, efficient data mining, and accurate quality assessment. The integration of quantitative metrics into radiology information systems enables the trending and comparison of results to normative data (Kahn et al., 2016).

Clinical decision support systems synthesise imaging findings with clinical data to provide diagnostic probabilities, prognostic estimates, or treatment recommendations at the point of care. These tools translate complex, multimodal data into actionable insights that are accessible to clinicians without specialised imaging expertise. For example, stroke decision support might integrate perfusion imaging, clinical severity, time from onset, and patient factors to estimate the benefit from intervention. Tumour molecular prediction algorithms infer genetic subtypes from imaging features to guide treatment selection. Alzheimer's disease staging tools combine multiple imaging biomarkers with cognitive and genetic data to estimate disease stage and progression risk. Human factors engineering ensures that decision support interfaces are intuitive and integrated into clinical workflows (Kahn et al., 2016).

Education and training programs ensure that clinicians understand the capabilities and limitations of advanced imaging techniques, as well as their appropriate utilisation and interpretation of results. Radiologists require training in new acquisition techniques, quantitative analysis methods, and the interpretation of novel contrast agents. Referring physicians need education on indications, contraindications, and how imaging results inform clinical decisions. Multidisciplinary tumour boards, epilepsy surgery conferences, and similar forums facilitate the collaborative interpretation and integration of imaging data with other clinical information. Continuing medical education, online modules, and point-of-care learning tools maintain competency as technologies evolve. Certification and credentialing programs ensure that minimum competencies are met for advanced techniques (Kohli et al., 2018).

Change management strategies address the organisational and cultural factors that influence the adoption of new technologies and workflows. Physician champions who advocate for innovation and mentor colleagues facilitate the dissemination of new ideas and knowledge, thereby advancing medical care. Pilot implementations identify workflow issues and demonstrate feasibility before full deployment. Feedback mechanisms enable users to report problems and propose improvements. Performance metrics track utilisation, quality, and outcomes to demonstrate value and identify areas for improvement and optimisation. Alignment of incentives ensures that improved patient care, enabled by advanced imaging, is recognised and rewarded. Leadership support and resource allocation signal an organisation's commitment, which is essential for successful implementation (Kahn et al., 2016).

20.6. Research Priorities and Emerging Frontiers

Future neuroimaging research priorities encompass technical innovations that enable new capabilities, methodological advances that improve reliability and interpretability, clinical validation to establish utility across diverse applications, and translational efforts that bridge research and practice. The convergence of multiple technological domains—artificial intelligence, molecular imaging, portable systems, ultra-high-field MRI, and multimodal integration—creates opportunities for transformative advances. However, realising this potential requires focused investment in areas most likely to impact patient care, with an emphasis on validation, standardisation, and accessibility, alongside pure innovation. Coordinated research roadmaps developed through community consensus ensure efficient resource allocation and avoid duplication (Toga et al., 2016).

Artificial intelligence applications represent a priority research area with the potential to enhance nearly every aspect of neuroimaging, from acquisition to interpretation. Deep learning reconstruction enables dramatic acceleration, noise reduction, and resolution enhancement. Automated segmentation and quantification improve efficiency and consistency. Computer-aided detection highlights abnormalities that might be overlooked. Predictive models estimate diagnosis, prognosis, and treatment response. However, challenges of generalizability, interpretability, bias, and validation require focused research. Large, diverse datasets enable training and testing of robust algorithms. Interpretable AI methods reveal which image features drive predictions. Fairness assessments ensure equitable performance across demographic groups (Lundervold & Lundervold, 2019).

Molecular and metabolic imaging innovations enable the visualisation of biological processes at the cellular and molecular levels, providing specificity beyond anatomical and functional techniques. The continued development of PET tracers targeting specific proteins, receptors, and pathways expands the capabilities of molecular imaging. Novel MRI contrast mechanisms, including CEST, molecular probes, and metabolic labelling, provide non-invasive molecular information. Hyperpolarised MRI advances could enable routine metabolic phenotyping. The multimodal integration of molecular imaging with structural and functional techniques enables comprehensive disease characterisation. Translation from preclinical models to human applications requires addressing technical challenges and demonstrating clinical value (Hampel et al., 2018).

Ultra-high-field MRI at 7 Tesla and beyond offers an improved signal-to-noise ratio and resolution for detailed structural imaging, enhanced functional sensitivity, and improved spectroscopy, enabling the detection of additional metabolites. Applications include detailed imaging of cortical layers, visualisation of subcortical nuclei, small vessel imaging, and high-resolution tractography. However, technical challenges, including field inhomogeneity, constraints on specific absorption rate, and hardware requirements, limit widespread adoption. Research priorities include pulse sequence development, hardware optimisation, and the demonstration of clinical applications that justify the substantial investment required for ultra-high-field systems (Bernasconi et al., 2019).

Longitudinal and lifespan imaging studies, which track individuals over years or decades, provide insights into disease evolution, ageing, and treatment effects that are impossible with cross-sectional studies. Initiatives such as the Alzheimer's Disease Neuroimaging Initiative, the UK Biobank, and the Human Connectome Project Lifespan Study generate rich datasets, enabling the investigation of neurodevelopment, ageing, and disease progression. Standardised protocols and quality control allow pooling across studies, thereby increasing power. Open data sharing maximises scientific return on investment. However, participant retention, protocol consistency, and scanner harmonisation pose challenges. Analysis methods for longitudinal data continue to evolve, enabling the sophisticated modelling of individual trajectories and the prediction of outcomes (Toga et al., 2016).

Table 20.3. Key research priorities and expected timelines

Research Priority	Key Objectives	Technical Challenges	Clinical Impact	Timeline to Clinical Translation
AI-Enhanced Imaging	Accelerated acquisition, automated interpretation, outcome prediction	Generalizability, interpretability, validation	Improved efficiency, consistency, and diagnostic accuracy	3-7 years (ongoing deployment)
Molecular Imaging	Disease-specific tracers, non-invasive molecular characterisation	Agent development, regulatory approval, and sensitivity	Precision diagnosis, treatment selection, and response monitoring	5-10 years for new agents
Portable Point-of-Care	Bedside imaging, global access, reduced costs	Image quality, clinical validation, workflow integration	Expanded access, faster diagnosis, improved outcomes	3-10 years for widespread adoption
Ultra-High-Field (7T+)	Submillimeter resolution, enhanced contrast, advanced spectroscopy	Technical complexity, SAR, cost	Detailed anatomy, research applications, specialised clinical uses	5-15 years for clinical adoption
Metabolic Imaging (DMI, Hyperpolarised)	Real-time metabolism, treatment response assessment	Infrastructure, standardisation, quantification	Non-invasive metabolic phenotyping, early response detection	5-10 years for routine clinical use
Multimodal Integration	Comprehensive tissue characterisation, systems biology	Data integration, analysis complexity, and standardisation	Improved diagnostic accuracy, precision medicine	5-10 years for standardised protocols

Emerging frontiers include integration of imaging with genomics, proteomics, and other -omics approaches to enable systems-level understanding of brain disorders. Brain-body interactions explored through simultaneous brain and systemic imaging reveal bidirectional influences. Closed-loop systems using real-time imaging feedback to guide stimulation or pharmacological interventions could enable precision neuromodulation. Artificial intelligence applications for drug discovery leverage imaging phenotypes to identify therapeutic targets and predict drug effects. The vision of comprehensive brain characterisation integrating structure, function, metabolism, molecular composition, and dynamics across spatial and temporal scales will drive research for decades to come (Lundervold & Lundervold, 2019). Table 20.3 shows key research priorities and expected timelines.

Conclusion

The future of neuroimaging is emerging from the convergence of technological innovation, evolving healthcare paradigms, and the growing recognition of brain health as a central component of overall well-being. The transition from purely anatomical imaging to comprehensive characterisation of structure, function, metabolism, molecular composition, and biomechanical properties enables precision medicine approaches that match interventions to individual pathophysiology rather than categorical diagnoses. Portable point-of-care systems promise to democratise access by extending advanced diagnostics beyond academic medical centres to emergency departments, intensive care units, and resource-limited regions worldwide. Artificial intelligence enhances every aspect of imaging, from acquisition through interpretation, improving efficiency, consistency, and diagnostic accuracy while enabling the extraction of subtle patterns that are imperceptible to human observers. Molecular imaging reveals disease processes at cellular and molecular levels, potentially enabling intervention at earlier disease stages when treatments are most effective.

The clinical translation of these innovations requires navigating complex challenges in validation, standardisation, regulatory approval, reimbursement, and workflow integration. Technologies must demonstrate not only technical performance but also clinical utility—that imaging information improves patient outcomes sufficiently to justify costs and complexity. Multi-centre reproducibility studies establish generalizability across diverse populations and practice settings. Health economic analyses demonstrate value by quantifying improved outcomes, reduced complications, or care efficiencies. Regulatory frameworks must evolve to accommodate rapid innovation while maintaining high standards of safety and effectiveness. Reimbursement policies should recognise the incremental value of advanced techniques over conventional imaging. Seamless workflow integration through automated acquisition, processing, and decision support tools reduces the burden on healthcare providers and facilitates adoption.

Global health equity demands that neuroimaging advances benefit all populations, not just those in wealthy regions. The burden of neurological disease disproportionately affects low- and middle-income countries where access to advanced diagnostics remains severely limited. Adapting technology for resource-constrained settings, developing innovative service delivery models, implementing training programs, and establishing sustainable financing mechanisms can all expand access. Portable low-field systems, telemedicine interpretation, and artificial intelligence for automated analysis address specific barriers in resource-limited environments. However, ensuring quality, building local capacity, and creating sustainable programs require continued commitment and investment. The imperative to reduce global health disparities aligns with Sustainable Development Goal 3 and reflects fundamental values of health equity.

Research priorities for the coming decades include artificial intelligence applications that enhance all aspects of neuroimaging, molecular and metabolic imaging techniques providing unprecedented biological specificity, ultra-high-field systems enabling submillimetre resolution and improved contrast, portable technologies expanding access, and multimodal integration approaches that synthesise complementary information for comprehensive characterisation. Longitudinal studies that track individuals across the lifespan reveal disease progression and enable the prediction of trajectories. Integration with genomics, proteomics, and other biological measurements enables systems-level understanding of brain disorders. Closed-loop applications using real-time imaging feedback to guide interventions may enable precision neuromodulation. The vision of comprehensive brain phenotyping—capturing structure, function, metabolism, molecular composition, and dynamics across spatial and temporal scales—will drive innovation for decades to come. As technologies mature and evidence accumulates, their integration into routine practice will fundamentally transform neurological and psychiatric care, improving outcomes for billions affected by brain disorders worldwide.

Acknowledgments

The authors would like to extend our appreciation to those who offered helpful commentary during the drafting process of this manuscript. We also acknowledge the role the Nova Publishing department played in enabling the work described herein.

References

Albers, G. W., Marks, M. P., Kemp, S., Christensen, S., Tsai, J. P., Ortega-Gutierrez, S., McTaggart, R. A., Torbey, M. T., Kim-Tenser, M., Leslie-Mazwi, T., Sarraj, A., Kasner, S. E., Ansari, S. A., Yeatts, S. D., Hamilton, S., Mlynash, M., Heit, J. J., Zaharchuk, G., Kim, S., ... Lansberg, M. G. (2018). Thrombectomy for stroke at 6 to 16 hours with selection by perfusion imaging. *New England Journal of Medicine*, 378(8), 708-718. https://doi.org/10.1056/NEJMoa1713973.

Benjamens, S., Dhunnoo, P., & Meskó, B. (2020). The state of artificial intelligence-based FDA-approved medical devices and algorithms: An online database. *NPJ Digital Medicine*, 3(1), 118. https://doi.org/10.1038/s41746-020-00324-0.

Bernasconi, A., Cendes, F., Theodore, W. H., Gill, R. S., Koepp, M. J., Hogan, R. E., Jackson, G. D., Federico, P., Labate, A., Vaudano, A. E., Blümcke, I., Ryvlin, P., & Bernasconi, N. (2019). Recommendations for the use of structural magnetic resonance imaging in the care of patients with epilepsy: A consensus report from the International League Against Epilepsy Neuroimaging Task Force. *Epilepsia*, 60(6), 1054-1068. https://doi.org/10.1111/epi.15612.

Burwell, S. M. (2015). Setting value-based payment goals—HHS efforts to improve U.S. health care. *New England Journal of Medicine*, 372(10), 897-899. https://doi.org/10.1056/NEJMp1500445.

Drysdale, A. T., Grosenick, L., Downar, J., Dunlop, K., Mansouri, F., Meng, Y., Fetcho, R. N., Zebley, B., Oathes, D. J., Etkin, A., Schatzberg, A. F., Sudheimer, K., Keller, J., Mayberg, H. S., Gunning, F. M., Alexopoulos, G. S., Fox, M. D., Pascual-Leone, A., Voss, H. U., ... Liston, C.

(2017). Resting-state connectivity biomarkers define neurophysiological subtypes of depression. *Nature Medicine*, 23(1), 28-38. https://doi.org/10.1038/nm.4246.

Hampel, H., Toschi, N., Babiloni, C., Baldacci, F., Black, K. L., Bokde, A. L. W., Bun, R. S., Cacciola, F., Cavedo, E., Chiesa, P. A., Colliot, O., Coman, C. M., Dubois, B., Duggento, A., Durrleman, S., Ferretti, M. T., George, N., Genthon, R., Habert, M. O., ... Vergallo, A. (2018). Revolution of Alzheimer precision neurology: Passageway of systems biology and neurophysiology. *Journal of Alzheimer's Disease*, 64(s1), S47-S105. https://doi.org/10.3233/JAD-179932.

Jha, S., Topol, E. J., & Waxman, S. G. (2016). Regulatory policies on use of mobile health apps: Convergence, divergence, and opportunities for harmonization. *Journal of Medical Internet Research*, 18(11), e287. https://doi.org/10.2196/jmir.6396.

Kickingereder, P., Bonekamp, D., Nowosielski, M., Kratz, A., Sill, M., Burth, S., Wick, A., Eidel, O., Schlemmer, H. P., Radbruch, A., Debus, J., Herold-Mende, C., Unterberg, A., Platten, M., Winkler, F., Wick, W., Bendszus, M., & Sahm, F. (2016). Radiogenomics of glioblastoma: Machine learning-based classification of molecular characteristics by using multiparametric and multiregional MR imaging features. *Radiology*, 281(3), 907-918. https://doi.org/10.1148/radiol.2016161382.

Kohli, M. D., Summers, R. M., & Geis, J. R. (2018). Medical image data and datasets in the era of machine learning—Whitepaper from the 2016 C-MIMI meeting dataset session. *Journal of Digital Imaging*, 30(4), 392-399. https://doi.org/10.1007/s10278-017-9976-3.

Lundervold, A. S., & Lundervold, A. (2019). An overview of deep learning in medical imaging focusing on MRI. *Zeitschrift für Medizinische Physik*, 29(2), 102-127. https://doi.org/10.1016/j.zemedi.2018.11.002.

Mazurek, M. H., Cahn, B. A., Yuen, M. M., Prabhat, A. M., Chavva, I. R., Shah, J. T., Crawford, A. L., Welch, E. B., Rothberg, J., Sacolick, L., Popp, A. J., Johnson, M. R., Wira, C. R., & Sheth, K. N. (2021). Portable, bedside, low-field magnetic resonance imaging for evaluation of intracerebral hemorrhage. *Nature Communications*, 12(1), 5119. https://doi.org/10.1038/s41467-021-25441-6.

Mollura, D. J., Mazal, J., Everton, K. L., & Lungren, M. P. (2010). Radiology and global health: A framework for implementation. *Academic Radiology*, 17(10), 1306-1313. https://doi.org/10.1016/j.acra.2010.05.018.

Sarracanie, M., & Salameh, N. (2020). Low-field MRI: How low can we go? A fresh view on an old debate. *Frontiers in Physics*, 8, 172. https://doi.org/10.3389/fphy.2020.00172.

Sheth, K. N., Mazurek, M. H., Yuen, M. M., Cahn, B. A., Shah, J. T., Ward, A., Kim, J. A., Gilmore, E. J., Falcone, G. J., Petersen, N., Gobeske, K. T., Kaddouh, F., Hwang, J., Schindler, J., Sansing, L., Matouk, C., Rothberg, J., Sze, G., Siner, J., ... Rothberg, J. M. (2021). Assessment of brain injury using portable, low-field magnetic resonance imaging at the bedside of critically ill patients. *JAMA Neurology*, 78(1), 41-47. https://doi.org/10.1001/jamaneurol.2020.3263.

Toga, A. W., Clark, K. A., Thompson, P. M., Shattuck, D. W., & Van Horn, J. D. (2016). Mapping the human connectome. *Neurosurgery*, 71(1), 1-5. https://doi.org/10.1227/NEU.0b013e318258e9ff.

About the Editors

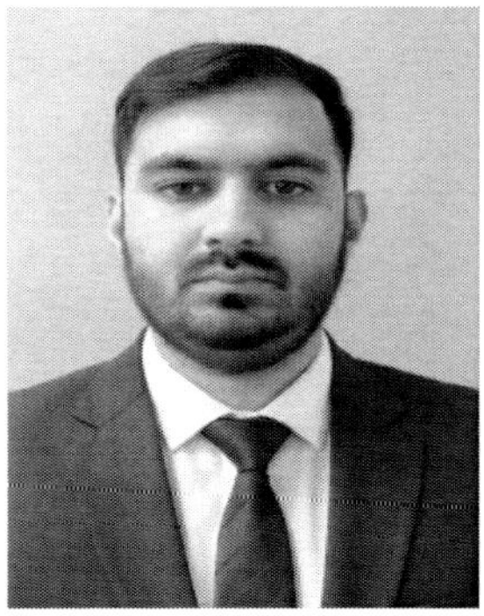

Dr. Maajid Mohi Ud Din Malik (M.Sc., PhD)

Assistant Professor, Dr. D. Y. Patil School of Allied Health Sciences, Dr. D. Y. Patil Vidyapeeth Pune (Deemed to be University), Sant Tukaram Nagar, Pimpri, Pune, India, 411018- majidmalik343@gmail.com

Dr Maajid Mohi-Ud-Din Malik is a prominent figure in Radiology and Imaging Technology, currently serving as an Assistant Professor at the prestigious Dr D.Y. Patil School of Allied Health Sciences in Pune, India. His academic journey, marked by excellence and dedication, includes a Ph.D. in Radiology and Imaging Technology from Singhania University (2020-2023), an M.Sc. in Radiation Imaging Technology from NIMS University (2017-2019), and a B.Sc. in Medical Imaging Technology from Swami Vivekanand Subharti University, establishing a solid foundation for his expertise in medical imaging sciences.

Dr. Malik's professional trajectory showcases a remarkable blend of clinical practice and academic excellence. His career began as a Clinical Radiographer at MMAMB Hospital (2016-2017), where he honed his practical skills in various radiographic procedures and patient care. He then transitioned to academia, serving at the College of Paramedical Sciences, Adesh University (2019-2023), followed by positions at GD Goenka University's School of Medical and Allied Sciences, and is currently at the Dr D.Y. Patil School of Allied Health Sciences. Throughout these roles, he has demonstrated exceptional ability in curriculum development, student mentoring, and research supervision.

As a prolific researcher and author, Dr Malik has made substantial contributions to medical imaging, authoring over 20 scholarly books and publishing more than 38 research articles in prestigious international journals. His research interests span a wide range of topics, with particular focus on radiation safety and diagnostic imaging protocols. His doctoral research, which focused on dose-length product estimation in CT scanning, has made significant contributions to radiation safety protocols in clinical practice. He currently serves as the Editor-in-Chief of two professional journals: the

Journal of Advanced Research Perspectives and Radiology Hub, further cementing his position as a thought leader in the field.

Dr Malik's innovative spirit is evident in his patents for a Controlled Sanitiser Dispensing Device and a Portable Device for Measuring Nerve Damage Due to Diabetic Neuropathy. His commitment to advancing medical technology and improving patient care has earned him recognition, including the "Kashmir's Most Influential Author 2022" award from Auyk Media and the International Achievers Award 2024 from Gyan Uday Foundation. He maintains active membership in professional organisations, serving as a life member of the Indian Society of Radiological Technologists (ISRT) and holding editorial board positions in multiple international journals.

In the classroom, Dr Malik is known for his innovative teaching methodologies and student-centric approach. He excels in integrating technology with traditional teaching methods, developing comprehensive curriculum materials, and providing mentorship to aspiring medical imaging professionals. His teaching philosophy emphasises practical application alongside theoretical knowledge, preparing students for the evolving challenges of healthcare technology. His expertise extends beyond traditional academics to include leadership in departmental initiatives, supervision of research projects, and academic program development.

Dr Malik's impact on the field is further evidenced by his extensive participation in professional conferences and faculty development programs. He regularly presents his research findings at international conferences and contributes to academic discussions on advancing medical imaging education. His work is recognised through various academic platforms, with his research tracked in Scopus (ID: 59223060200) and ORCID (0000-0003-1743-1520). This combination of clinical experience, educational excellence, research productivity, and innovative thinking makes Dr Malik a distinguished figure in medical imaging and radiography education.

Looking toward the future, Dr Malik continues to push the boundaries of medical imaging education and research. His ongoing work focuses on advancing imaging technologies, improving educational methodologies, and contributing to the broader field of healthcare through innovative research and publication. His dedication to excellence in both research and education, combined with his extensive portfolio of achievements, positions him as a valuable contributor to the advancement of medical imaging sciences and education.

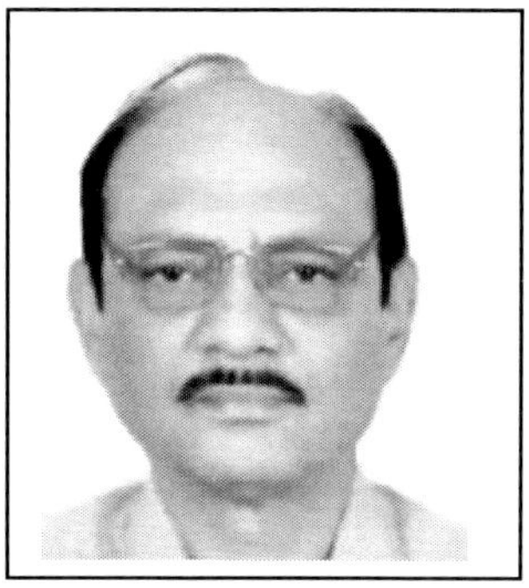

Dr. Purnachandra Kawdu Lamghare
Professor
Department of Radio-diagnosis
Dr. D. Y. Patil Medical College, Hospital and Research Centre,
Dr. D. Y. Patil Vidyapeeth, Pune (Deemed to be University)
Sant Tukaram Nagar, Pimpri, Pune 411018, India

Dr. Purnachandra Kawdu Lamghare is a distinguished Professor and Head of the Department of Radiodiagnosis at Dr. D. Y. Patil Medical College, Hospital and Research Centre in Pune. Born on January 21, 1957, he holds an M.B.B.S. and D.M.R.D. from Government Medical College, Nagpur, and an M.D. in Radiodiagnosis from Dr. B. R. Marathwada University, Aurangabad.

With an impressive 39-year medical career, Dr. Lamghare has extensive teaching experience, including 22 years as a Professor, 11 as an Associate Professor, and 6 as an Assistant Professor. He has devoted 35 years to undergraduate education and 25 years to postgraduate teaching, serving at prestigious institutions like Government Medical College, Nagpur, B. J. TR. Miraj Medical College, Ahmednagar, and B. J. Medical College, Pune.

Dr. Lamghare is a recognized Postgraduate Teacher at MUHS, Nashik, and Dr. D. Y. Patil Vidyapeeth, Pune, where he also serves as a Ph.D. Guide. His significant contributions to the medical field include publications in national and international journals, presentations at conferences, and service as an MCI Assessor for both undergraduate and postgraduate courses. Additionally, he has worked as a Liaison Officer and Observer for various examinations and as a postgraduate examiner at numerous medical colleges throughout his career.

Index

K

L

M

N

O

P

Q

R

S

T

U

V

W

More books by *Maajid Mohi Ud Din Malik* can be found at:

https://novapublishers.com/writer/maajid-mohi-ud-din-malik-phd/